Manual of Botulinum Toxin Therapy

Manual of Botulinum Toxin Therapy

Edited by

Daniel Truong

The Parkinson's and Movement Disorder Institute, Orange Coast Memorial Medical Center, USA

Dirk Dressler

Hanover Medical School, Hanover, Germany

Mark Hallett

NINDS, National Institutes of Health, USA

Medical illustrator
Mayank Pathak

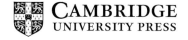
CAMBRIDGE
UNIVERSITY PRESS

CAMBRIDGE UNIVERSITY PRESS
Cambridge, New York, Melbourne, Madrid, Cape Town, Singapore,
São Paulo, Delhi, Dubai, Tokyo

Cambridge University Press
The Edinburgh Building, Cambridge CB2 8RU, UK

Published in the United States of America by
Cambridge University Press, New York

www.cambridge.org
Information on this title: www.cambridge.org/9780521694421

First published 2009
Reprinted 2010

Printed in the United Kingdom at the University Press, Cambridge

A catalog record for this publication is available from the British Library

Library of Congress Cataloging-in-Publication Data

Manual of botulinum toxin therapy / edited by Daniel Truong, Dirk Dressler, Mark Hallett.
    p. ; cm.
  Includes bibliographical references and index.
  ISBN 978-0-521-69442-1 (hardback)
1. Botulinum toxin – Therapeutic use – Handbooks, manuals, etc.   I. Truong, Daniel, M.D.
II. Dressler, Dirk.   III. Hallett, Mark, 1943–
  [DNLM: 1. Botulinum Toxins – pharmacology.   2. Botulinum Toxins – therapeutic use.
3. Movement Disorders – drug therapy.   4. Neuromuscular Diseases – drug therapy.   QV 140 M144 2009]
  RL120.B66M36 2009
  615′.778–dc22

                                 2008038897

ISBN 978-0-521-69442-1 hardback

Dedication

To my parents, Te Truong and Cam Tran,
who sacrificed for my opportunity; to my wife,
Diane Truong, who lovingly endured the
unrelenting commitments of my career; to
my teachers, Stanley Fahn and Edward Hogan, who
opened my door to neurology; to Victor Tsao and
Suzanne Mellor, for whose support and wisdom
I am grateful; finally, to all my patients from whom
I've learned so much.

DT

I am most grateful to my colleagues for their
discussions, my patients for their encouragement
and most of all to my wife Dr Fereshte Adib Saberi
for her professional and emotional support.

DD

I am grateful to the contributors to our book and to
my wife for her continuous support, and dedicate it
to the patients who participate in research studies,
helping others as well as themselves.

MH

Contents

Contributors

Vito Annese
Department of Medical Sciences, Unit of GI Endoscopy, IRCCS Hospital "Casa Sollievo della Sofferenza", San Giovanni Rotondo, Italy

Mary S. Babcock
Department of Orthopedics and Rehabilitation, Walter Reed Army Medical Center, Washington, DC, USA

Reiner Benecke
Department of Neurology, University of Rostock, Rostock, Germany

Alfredo Berardelli
Department of Neurological Sciences and Neuromed Institute (IRCSS), Sapienza, University of Rome, Rome, Italy

Roongroj Bhidayasiri
Division of Neurology, Chulalongkorn University Hospital, Bangkok, Thailand; The Parkinson's and Movement Disorder Institute, Fountain Valley, CA, USA; Department of Neurology, UCLA Medical Center, David Geffen School of Medicine at UCLA, Los Angeles, CA, USA

Hans Bigalke
Institute of Toxicology, Medizinische Hochschule, Hannover, Germany

Allison Brashear
Department of Neurology, Wake Forest University Baptist Medical Center, Winston-Salem, NC, USA

Francisco Cardoso
Departamento de Clínica Médica, Setor de Neurologia, Universidade Federal de Minas Gerais Belo Horizonte, Minas Gerais, Brazil

Carlo Colosimo
Department of Neurological Sciences and Neuromed Institute (IRCSS), Sapienza, University of Rome, Rome, Italy

Cynthia L. Comella
Department of Neurological Sciences, Rush University Medical Center, Chicago, IL, USA

Chandi Prasad Das
Department of Neurology, Postgraduate Institute of Medical Education and Research, Chandigarh, India

Dirk Dressler
Department of Neurology, Hanover Medical School, Hanover, Germany

Dennis D. Dykstra
Department of Physical Medicine and Rehabilitation, University of Minnesota, Minneapolis, MN, USA

Frank J. Erbguth
Department of Neurology, Nuremberg Municipal Academic Hospital, Nuremberg, Germany

Karen Frei
The Parkinson's and Movement Disorder Institute, Orange Coast Memorial Medical Center, Fountain Valley, CA, USA

Jürgen Frevert
Institute of Toxicology, Medizinische Hochschule, Hannover, Germany

Dee Anna Glaser
Department of Dermatology, Saint Louis University School of Medicine, St. Louis, MO, USA

H. Kerr Graham
University of Melbourne, Royal Children's Hospital, Parkville, Victoria, Australia

Daniele Gui
Department of Surgery, Università Cattolica del Sacro Cuore, Policlinico "A. Gemelli", Rome, Italy

Mark Hallett
Human Motor Control Section, NINDS, National Institutes of Health, Bethesda, MD, USA

Henning Hamm
Department of Dermatology, University of Würzburg, Würzburg, Germany

Bahman Jabbari
Department of Neurology, Yale University School of Medicine, New Haven, CT, USA

Joseph Jankovic
Parkinson's Disease Center and Movement Disorder Clinic, Department of Neurology, Baylor College of Medicine, Houston, TX, USA

Amy M. Lang
Department of Rehabilitation Medicine, Emory University School of Medicine, Atlanta, GA, USA

Rainer Laskawi
Department of Otolaryngology, Head and Neck Surgery, University of Göttingen, Göttingen, Germany

Markus K. Naumann
Department of Neurology, Klinikum Augsburg, Augsburg, Germany

Arno Olthoff
Department of Phoniatrics and Pediatric Audiology, University of Göttingen, Göttingen, Germany

Mayank S. Pathak
The Parkinson's and Movement Disorder Institute, Orange Coast Memorial Medical Center, Fountain Valley, CA, USA

Diana Richardson
Department of Neurology, Yale University School of Medicine, New Haven, CT, USA

Peter Roggenkaemper
Department of Ophthalmology, University of Bonn, Bonn, Germany

Brigitte Schurch
Neurourology, Spinal Cord Injury Centre, University Hospital Balgrist, Zurich, Switzerland

Alan B. Scott
Smith-Kettlewell Eye Research Institute, San Francisco, CA, USA

James K. Sheffield
Parkinson's Disease Center and Movement Disorder Clinic, Department of Neurology, Baylor College of Medicine, Houston, TX, USA

Stephen D. Silberstein
Jefferson Headache Center, Thomas Jefferson University Philadelphia, PA, USA

Ann Tilton
Louisiana State University Health Sciences Center, New Orleans, LA, USA

Dorina Tiple
Department of Neurological Sciences and Neuromed Institute (IRCSS), Sapienza, University of Rome, Rome, Italy

Daniel Truong
The Parkinson's and Movement Disorder Institute, Orange Coast Memorial Medical Center, Fountain Valley, CA, USA

Foreword

Thirty years after treatment of the first human with botulinum toxin, application of the drug has expanded to an extraordinary variety of conditions. I did not initially anticipate use in the gastrointestinal tract, the bladder wall, pathological sweating, reduction of saliva and tears, and surely not widespread cosmetic use. Yet, a look back at Kerner's descriptions of botulism shows us that each of those areas, even the flat and featureless face, was impacted by the toxin. Use in migraine and pain disorders is entirely new and unpredicted; surely further valuable uses of botulinum toxin and of new drugs based on the toxin molecule will continue to emerge.

The expert authors of this volume, several of them originators of the applications described in their particular chapters, carry to us and to our patients masterly teaching of the techniques for botulinum toxin's safe and effective use.

Alan B. Scott, San Francisco

Preface

Botulinum toxin is an exciting therapy that is applicable to a wide variety of disorders in many fields of medicine. Because botulinum toxins must be injected locally, physicians must possess the appropriate expertise in order to deliver the therapy effectively. Occasionally, unique approaches to muscles are required, which may differ from those used by electromyographers. Additionally, many physicians are not accustomed to giving injection therapy. A simple anatomical atlas or even an atlas for electromyography will not be helpful in all circumstances – hence the need for this book. We have assembled a team of international experts in the use of botulinum toxin to give guidance on exactly how to administer the injections. The emphasis in this book is on technique, and it is profusely illustrated for maximal advantage. The book can be read as a teaching aid, but may also be useful at the bedside for immediate guidance. We are grateful to the contributors of this book and trust that physicians who employ this therapy in their practices will find it valuable.

Our special thanks to the Parkinson's and Movement Disorders Foundation, which provided a grant for the graphics in this book, Anne Kenton and Laura Wood from Cambridge University Press for their tireless assistance during the preparation, and Mary Ann Chapman for her many suggestions and encouragement. We are also blessed by having a talented and patient neurologist and artist, Dr Mayank Pathak, who drew all the original anatomical illustrations. Even with all this help, the three-year preparation of this book seemed like an eternity.

We also express our appreciation to our family and friends for their support and understanding during the preparation of this book.

Daniel Truong, M.D., Dirk Dressler, M.D. and
Mark Hallett, M.D.

The pretherapeutic history of botulinum toxin

Frank J. Erbguth

Unintended intoxication with botulinum toxin (botulism) occurs only rarely, but its high fatality rate makes it a great concern for those in the general public and in the medical community. In the United States an average of 110 cases of botulism are reported each year. Of these, approximately 25% are food borne, 72% are infant botulism, and the rest are wound botulism. Outbreaks of food-borne botulism involving two or more persons occur most years and are usually caused by eating contaminated home-canned foods.

Botulism in ancient times

Botulinum toxin poisoning probably has afflicted humankind through the mists of time. As long as humans have preserved and stored food, some of the chosen conditions were optimal for the presence and growth of the toxin-producing pathogen *Clostridium botulinum*: for example, the storage of ham in barrels of brine, poorly dried and stored herring, trout packed to ferment in willow baskets, sturgeon roe not yet salted and piled in heaps on old horsehides, lightly smoked fish or ham in poorly heated smoking chambers, and insufficiently boiled blood sausages.

However, in ancient times there was no general knowledge about the causal relationship between the consumption of spoiled food and a subsequent fatal paralytic disease, nowadays recognized as botulism. Only some historical sources reflect a potential understanding of the life-threatening consumption of food intoxicated with botulinum toxin. Louis Smith, for example, reported in his textbook on botulism a dietary edict announced in the tenth century by Emperor Leo VI of Byzantium (886–911), in which manufacturing of blood sausages was forbidden (Smith, 1977). This edict may have its origin in the recognition of some circumstances connected with cases of food poisoning. Also, some ancient formulas suggested by shamans to Indian maharajas for the killing of personal enemies give hint to an intended lethal application of botulinum toxin: a tasteless powder extracted from blood sausages dried under anaerobic conditions should be added to the enemies' food at an invited banquet. Because the consumer's death occurred after he or she had left the murderer's place with a latency of some days, the host was probably not suspected (Erbguth, 2007).

Botulism outbreaks in Germany in the eighteenth and nineteenth centuries

Accurate descriptions of botulism emerge in the German literature from two centuries ago when the consumption of improperly preserved or stored meat and blood sausages gave rise to many deaths throughout the kingdom of Württemberg in Southwestern Germany. This area near the city of Stuttgart developed as the regional focus of botulinum toxin investigations in the eighteenth and nineteenth centuries. In 1793, 13 people of whom 6 died were involved in the first well-recorded outbreak of botulism in the small southwest German village of Wildbad. Based on the observed mydriasis in all affected victims, the first official medical speculation was that the outbreak was caused by an atropine (*Atropa belladonna*) intoxication. However, in the controversial scientific discussion, the term "sausage poison" was introduced by the exponents of the opinion that the fatal disease in Wildbad was caused by the consumption of "Blunzen," a popular local food from cooked pork stomach filled with blood and spices.

The number of cases with suspected sausage poisoning in Southwestern Germany increased rapidly at the end of the eighteenth century. Poverty ensuing from the devastating Napoleonic Wars (1795–1813) had led to the neglect of sanitary measures in rural food production (Grüsser, 1986). In July 1802, the Royal Government of Württemberg in Stuttgart issued a public warning about the "harmful consumption of smoked blood-sausages." In August 1811, the medical section of the Department of Internal Affairs of the Kingdom of Württemberg on Stuttgart again addressed the problem of "sausage poisoning," considering it to be caused by hydrocyanic acid, known at that time as "prussic acid." However, the members of the near Medical Faculty of the University of Tübingen disputed that prussic acid could be the toxic agent in sausages, suspecting a biological poison. One of the important medical professors of the University of Tübingen, Johann Heinrich Ferdinand Autenrieth (1772–1835), asked the Government to collect the reports of general practitioners and health officers on cases of food poisoning for systematic scientific analyses. After Autenrieth had studied these reports, he issued a list of symptoms of the so-called "sausage poisoning" and added a comment, in which he blamed the housewives for the poisoning, because they did not dunk the sausages long enough in

boiling water, thus trying to prevent the sausages from bursting (Grüsser, 1998). The list of symptoms was distributed by a public announcement and contained characteristic features of food-borne botulism such as gastrointestinal problems, double vision, mydriasis, and muscle paralysis.

In 1815, a health officer in the village of Herrenberg, J. G. Steinbuch (1770–1818), sent the case reports of seven intoxicated patients who had eaten liver sausage and peas to Professor Autenrieth. Three of the patients had died and the autopsies had been carried out by Steinbuch himself (Steinbuch, 1817).

Justinus Kerner's observations and publications on botulinum toxin 1817–1822

Contemporaneously with Steinbuch, the 29-year-old physician and Romantic poet Justinus Kerner (1786–1862) (Figure 1.1), then medical officer in a small village, also reported of a lethal food poisoning. Autenrieth considered the two reports from Steinbuch and Kerner as accurate and important observations and decided to publish them both in 1817 in the "*Tübinger Blätter für Naturwissenschaften und Arzneykunde*" ["*Tübinger Papers for Natural Sciences and Pharmacology*"] (Kerner, 1817; Steinbuch, 1817).

Kerner again disputed that an inorganic agent such as hydrocyanic acid could be the toxic agent in the sausages, suspecting a biological poison instead. After he had observed further cases, Kerner published a first monograph in 1820 on "sausage poisoning" in which he summarized the case histories of 76 patients and gave a complete clinical description of what we now recognize as botulism. The monograph was entitled "Neue Beobachtungen über die in Württemberg so häufig vorfallenden tödtlichen Vergiftungen durch den Genuß geräucherter Würste" ["New observations on the lethal poisoning that occurs so frequently in Württemberg owing to the consumption of smoked sausages"] (Kerner, 1820). Kerner compared the various recipes and ingredients of all sausages which had produced intoxication and found out that among

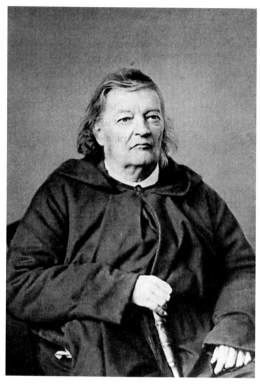

Figure 1.1 Justinus Kerner; photograph of 1855.

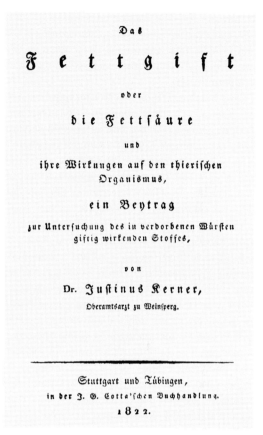

Figure 1.2 Title of Justinus Kerner's second monograph on sausage poisoning 1822.

the ingredients blood, liver, meat, brain, fat, salt, pepper, coriander, pimento, ginger, and bread the only common ones were fat and salt. Because salt was probably known to be "innocent," Kerner concluded that the toxic change in the sausage must take place in the fat and therefore called the suspected substance "sausage poison," "fat poison" or "fatty acid." Later Kerner speculated about the similarity of the "fat poison" to other known poisons, such as atropine, scopolamine, nicotine, and snake venom, which led him to the conclusion that the fat poison was probably a biological poison (Erbguth, 2004).

In 1822, Kerner published 155 case reports including postmortem studies of patients with botulism and developed hypotheses on the "sausage poison" in a second monograph "Das Fettgift oder die Fettsäure und ihre Wirkungen auf den thierischen Organismus, ein Beytrag zur Untersuchung

des in verdorbenen Würsten giftig wirkenden Stoffes" ["The fat poison or the fatty acid and its effects on the animal body system, a contribution to the examination of the substance responsible for the toxicity of bad sausages"] (Kerner, 1822) (Figure 1.2). The monograph contained an accurate description of all muscle symptoms and clinical details of the entire range of autonomic disturbances occurring in botulism, such as mydriasis, decrease of lacrimation and secretion from the salivary glands, and gastrointestinal and bladder paralysis. Kerner also experimented on various animals (birds, cats, rabbits, frogs, flies, locusts, snails) by feeding them with extracts from bad sausages and finally carried out high-risk experiments on himself. After he had tasted some drops of a sausage extract he reported: ". . . some drops of the acid brought onto the tongue cause great drying out of the palate and the pharynx" (Erbguth & Naumann, 1999).

Kerner deduced from the clinical symptoms and his experimental observations that the toxin acts by interrupting the motor and autonomic nervous signal transmission (Erbguth, 1996). He concluded: "The nerve conduction is brought by the toxin into a condition in which its influence on the chemical process of life is interrupted. The capacity of nerve conduction is interrupted by the toxin in the same way as in an electrical conductor by rust" (Kerner, 1820). Finally, Kerner tried in vain to produce an artificial "sausage poison." In summary, Kerner's hypotheses concerning "sausage poison" were (1) that the toxin develops in bad sausages under anaerobic conditions, (2) that the toxin acts on the motor nerves and the autonomic nervous system, and (3) that the toxin is strong and lethal even in small doses (Erbguth & Naumann, 1999).

In the eighth chapter of the 1822 monograph, Kerner speculated about using the "toxic fatty acid" botulinum toxin for therapeutic purposes. He concluded that small doses would be beneficial in conditions with pathological hyperexcitability of the nervous system (Erbguth, 2004). Kerner wrote: "The fatty acid or zoonic acid administered in such doses, that its action could be restricted to the sphere of the sympathetic nervous system only, could be of benefit in the many diseases which originate from hyperexcitation of this system" and "by analogy it can be expected that in outbreaks of sweat, perhaps also in mucous hypersecretion, the fatty acid will be of therapeutic value." The term "sympathetic nervous system" as used during the Romantic period, encompassed nervous functions in general. "Sympathetic overactivity" then was thought to be the cause of many internal, neurological, and psychiatric diseases. Kerner favored the "Veitstanz" (St. Vitus dance – probably identical with Chorea minor) with its "overexcited nervous ganglia" to be a promising indication for the therapeutic use of the toxic fatty acid. Likewise, he considered other diseases with assumed nervous overactivity to be potential candidates for the toxin treatment: hypersecretion of body fluids, sweat or mucus; ulcers from malignant diseases; skin alterations after burning; delusions; rabies; plague; consumption from lung tuberculosis; and yellow-fever. However, Kerner conceded self-critically that all the possible indications mentioned were only hypothetical and wrote: "What is said here about the fatty acid as a therapeutic drug belongs to the realm of hypothesis and may be confirmed or disproved by observations in the future" (Erbguth, 1998).

Justinus Kerner also advanced the idea of a gastric tube suggested by the Scottish physician Alexander Monro in 1811 and adapted it for the nutrition of patients with botulism; he wrote: "if dysphagia occurs, softly prepared food and fluids should be brought into the stomach by a flexible tube made from resin." He considered all characteristics of modern nasogastric tube application: the use of a guide wire with a cork at the tip and the lubrication of the tube with oil.

Botulism research after Kerner

After his publications on food-borne botulism, Kerner was well known to the German public and amongst his contemporaries as an expert on sausage poisoning, as well as for his melancholic poetry. Many of his poems were set to music by the great German Romantic composer Robert Schumann (1810–56) who had to quit his piano career due to the development of a pianist's focal finger dystonia. Kerner's poem "The Wanderer in the Sawmill" was the favourite poem of the twentieth-century poet Franz Kafka (Appendix 1.1). The nickname "Sausage Kerner" was commonly used and "sausage poisoning" was known as "Kerner's disease." Further publications in the nineteenth century by various authors, for example Müller (Müller, 1869), increased the number of reported cases of "sausage poisoning," describing the fact that the food poisoning had occurred after the consumption not only of meat but also of fish. However, these reports

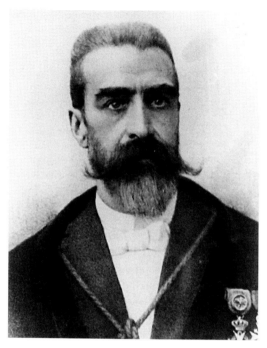

Figure 1.3 Emile Pierre Marie van Ermengem 1851–1922.

added nothing substantial to Kerner's early observations. The term "botulism" (from the Latin word *botulus* meaning sausage) appeared at first in Müller's reports and was subsequently used. Therefore, "botulism" refers to the poisoning due to sausages and not to the sausage-like shape of the causative bacillus discovered later (Torrens, 1998). The next and most important scientific step was the identification of *Clostridium botulinum* in 1895–6 by the Belgian microbiologist Emile Pierre Marie van Ermengem of the University of Ghent (Figure 1.3).

The discovery of *"Bacillus botulinus"* in Belgium

On December 14, 1895 an extraordinary outbreak of botulism occurred amongst the 4000 inhabitants of the small Belgian village of Ellezelles. The musicians of the local brass band "Fanfare Les Amis Réunis" played at the funeral of the 87-year-old

Antoine Creteur and as it was the custom gathered to eat in the inn "Le Rustic" (Devriese, 1999). Thirty-four people were together and ate pickled and smoked ham. After the meal the musicians noticed symptoms such as mydriasis, diplopia, dysphagia, and dysarthria followed by increasing muscle paralysis. Three of them died and ten nearly died. A detailed examination of the ham and an autopsy were ordered and conducted by van Ermengem who had been appointed Professor of Microbiology at the University of Ghent in 1888 after he had worked in the laboratory of Robert Koch in Berlin in 1883. van Ermengem isolated the bacterium in the ham and in the corpses of the victims (Figure 1.4), grew it, used it for animal experiments, characterized its culture requirements, described its toxin, called it *"Bacillus botulinus,"* and published his observations in the German microbiological journal *"Zeitschrift für Hygiene und Infektionskrankheiten"* [*"Journal of Hygiene and Infectious Diseases"*] in 1897 (an English translation was published in 1979) (van Ermengem, 1897). The pathogen was later renamed *"Clostridium botulinum."* van Ermengem was the first to correlate "sausage poisoning" with the newly discovered anaerobic microorganism and concluded that "it is highly probable that the poison in the ham was produced by an anaerobic growth of specific microorganisms during the salting process." van Ermengem's milestone investigation yielded all clinical facts about botulism and botulinum toxin: (1) botulism is an intoxication, not an infection, (2) the toxin is produced in food by a bacterium, (3) the toxin is not produced if the salt concentration in the food is high, (4) after ingestion, the toxin is not inactivated by the normal digestive process, (5) the toxin is susceptible to inactivation by heat, and (6) not all species of animals are equally susceptible.

Botulinum toxin research in the early twentieth century

In 1904, when an outbreak of botulism in the city of Darmstadt, Germany was caused by canned white beans, the opinion that the only botulinogenic

(a) 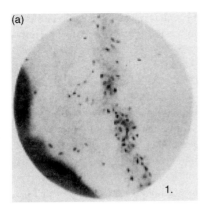 1.

(b) 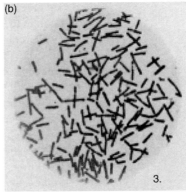 3.

Figure 1.4 Microscopy of the histological section of the suspect ham at the Ellezelles botulism outbreak. (a) Numerous spores among the muscle fibers (Ziehl × 1000). (b) Culture (gelatine and glucose) of mature rod-shaped forms of "Bacillus botulinus" from the ham; eighth day (× 1000) (from van Ermengem, 1897).

foods were meat or fish had to be revised. The bacteria isolated from the beans by Landmann (Landmann, 1904) and from the Ellezelles ham were compared by Leuchs (Leuchs, 1910) at the Royal Institute of Infectious Diseases in Berlin. He found that the strains differed and the toxins were serologically distinct. The two types of Bacillus botulinus did not receive their present letter designations of serological subtypes until Georgina Burke, who worked at Stanford University, designated them as types A and B (Burke, 1919). Over the next decades, increases in food canning and food-borne botulism went hand in hand (Cherington, 2004). The first documented outbreak of food-borne botulism in the United States was caused by commercially conserved pork and beans, and dates from 1906 (Drachmann, 1971; Smith, 1977). Techniques for killing the spores during the canning process were subsequently developed. The correct pH (< 4.0), the osmolarity needed to prevent clostridial growth and toxin production, and the requirements for toxin inactivation by heating were defined.

In 1922, type C was identified in the United States by Bengston and in Australia by Seddon, type D and type E were characterized some years later (type D: USA 1928 by Meyer and Gunnison; type E: Ukraine 1936 by Bier) (Kriek & Odendaal, 1994; Geiges, 2002). Type-F and type-G toxins were identified in 1960 in Scandinavia by Moller and Scheibel and in 1970 in Argentina by Gimenex and Ciccarelli (Gunn, 1979; Geiges, 2002). In 1949, Burgen and

his colleagues (Burgen *et al.*, 1949) in London discovered that botulinum toxin blocked the release of acetylcholine at neuromuscular junctions. The essential insights into the molecular actions of botulinum toxin were gained by various scientists after 1970 (Dolly *et al.*, 1990; Schiavo *et al.*, 1992, 1993; Dong *et al.*, 2006; Mahrhold *et al.*, 2006), when its use as a therapeutic agent was pioneered by Edward J. Schantz and Alan B. Scott.

Until the last century, botulism was thought to be caused exclusively by food that was contaminated with preformed toxin. This view has changed during the last 50 years, due to spores of *C. botulinum* being discovered in the intestines of babies first in 1976 (infant botulism) and in contaminated wounds (wound botulism) in the 1950s (Merson & Dowell, 1973; Picket *et al.*, 1976; Arnon *et al.*, 1977). The number of cases of food-borne and infant botulism has changed little in recent years, but wound botulism has increased because of the use of black-tar heroin, especially in California.

Swords to ploughshares

Before the therapeutic potential of botulinum toxin was discovered around 1970, its potential use as a weapon was recognized during World War I (Lamb, 2001). The basis for its use as a toxin was investigations by Hermann Sommer and colleagues working at the Hooper Foundation, University of

California, San Francisco in the 1920s: the researchers were the first to isolate pure botulinum toxin type A as a stable acid precipitate (Snipe & Sommer, 1928; Schantz, 1994). With the outbreak of World War II, the United States government began intensive research into biological weapons, including botulinum toxin, especially in the laboratory at Camp Detrick (later named Fort Detrick) in Maryland. Development of concentration and crystallization techniques at Fort Detrick was pioneered by Carl Lamanna and James Duff in 1946. The methodology was subsequently used by Edward J. Schantz to produce the first batch of toxin which was the basis for the later clinical product (Lamanna *et al.*, 1946). The entrance of botulinum toxin into the medical therapeutic armament in Europe also led from military laboratories to hospitals: in the United Kingdom, botulinum toxin research was conducted in the Porton Down laboratories of the military section of the "Centre for Applied Microbiology and Research" (CAMR), which later provided British clinicians with a therapeutic formulation of the toxin (Hambleton *et al.*, 1981).

APPENDIX 1.1

The Wanderer in the Sawmill (*by Justinus Kerner 1826*)

Down yonder in the sawmill
I sat in good repose
and saw the wheels go spinning
and watched the water too.

I saw the shiny saw blade,
as if I had a dream,
which carved a lengthy furrow
into a fir tree trunk.

The fir tree as if living,
in saddest melody,
through all its trembling fibers
sang out these words for me:

At just the proper hour,
o wanderer! you come,
it's you for whom this wounding
invades my heart inside.

It's you, for whom soon will be,
when wanderings cut short,
these boards in earth's deep bosom,
a box for lengthy rest.

Four boards I then saw falling,
my heart was turned to stone,
one word I would have stammered,
the blade went 'round no more.

REFERENCES

Arnon, S. S., Midura, T. F., Clay, S. A., Wood, R. M. & Chin, J. (1977). Infant botulism: epidemiological, clinical and laboratory aspects. *JAMA*, **237**, 1946–51.

Burgen, A., Dickens, F. & Zatman, L. (1949). The action of botulinum toxin on the neuromuscular junction. *J Physiol*, **109**, 10–24.

Burke, G. S. (1919). The occurrence of Bacillus botulinus in nature. *J Bacteriol*, **4**, 541–53.

Cherington, M. (2004). Botulism: update and review. *Semin Neurol*, **24**, 155–63.

Devriese, P. P. (1999). On the discovery of Clostridium botulinum. *J Hist Neurosci*, **8**, 43–50.

Dolly, J. O., Ashton, A. C., McInnes, C., *et al.* (1990). Clues to the multi-phasic inhibitory action of botulinum neurotoxins on release of transmitters. *J Physiol*, **84**, 237–46.

Dong, M., Yeh, F., Tepp, W. H., *et al.* (2006). SV2 is the protein receptor for botulinum neurotoxin A. *Science*, **312**, 592–6.

Drachmann, D. B. (1971). Botulinum toxin as a tool for research on the nervous system. In L. L. Simpson, ed., *Neuropoisons: Their Pathophysiology Actions*, Vol. 1. New York: Plenum Press, pp. 325–47.

Erbguth, F. (1996). Historical note on the therapeutic use of botulinum toxin in neurological disorders. *J Neurol Neurosurg Psychiatry*, **60**, 151.

Erbguth, F. (1998). Botulinum toxin, a historical note. *Lancet*, **351**, 1280.

Erbguth, F. J. (2004). Historical notes on botulism, Clostridium botulinum, botulinum toxin, and the idea of the therapeutic use of the toxin. *Mov Disord*, **19**(Suppl 8), S2–6.

Erbguth, F. J. (2008). From poison to remedy: the chequered history of botulinum toxin. *J Neural Transm*, **115**(4), 559–65.

Erbguth, F. & Naumann, M. (1999). Historical aspects of botulinum toxin: Justinus Kerner (1786–1862) and the "sausage poison". *Neurology*, **53**, 1850–3.

Geiges, M. L. (2002). The history of botulism. In O. P. Kreyden, R. Böne & G. Burg, eds., *Hyperhidrosis and Botulinum Toxin in Dermatology. Curr Probl Dermatol*, Vol. 30. Basel: Karger, pp. 77–93.

Grüsser, O. J. (1986). Die ersten systematischen Beschreibungen und tierexperimentellen Untersuchungen des Botulismus. Zum 200. Geburtstag von Justinus Kerner am 18. September 1986. *Sudhoffs Arch*, **10**, 167–87.

Grüsser, O. J. (1998). Der "Wurstkerner". Justinus Kerners Beitrag zur Erforschung des Botulismus. In H. Schott, ed., *Justinus Kerner als Azt und Seelenforscher*, 2nd edn. Weinsberg: Justinus Kerner Verein, pp. 232–56.

Gunn, R. A. (1979). Botulism: from van Ermengem to the present. A comment. *Rev Infect Dis*, **1**, 720–1.

Hambleton, P., Capel, B., Bailey, N., Tse, C. K. & Dolly, O. (1981). Production, purification and toxoiding of clostridium botulinum A toxin. In G. Lewis, ed., *Biomedical Aspects of Botulism*. New York: Academic Press, pp. 247–60.

Kerner, J. (1817). Vergiftung durch verdorbene Würste. *Tübinger Blätter für Naturwissenschaften und Arzneykunde*, **3**, 1–25.

Kerner, J. (1820). Neue Beobachtungen über die in Württemberg so häufig vorfallenden tödlichen Vergiftungen durch den Genuss geräucherter Würste. Tübingen: Osiander.

Kerner, J. (1822). Das Fettgift oder die Fettsäure und ihre Wirkungen auf den thierischen Organismus, ein Beytrag zur Untersuchung des in verdorbenen Würsten giftig wirkenden Stoffes. Stuttgart, Tübingen: Cotta.

Kriek, N. P. J. & Odendaal, M. W. (1994). Botulism. In J. A. W. Coetzer, G. R. Thomson & R. C. Tustin, eds., *Infectious Diseases of Livestock*. Cape Town: Oxford University Press, pp. 1354–71.

Lamanna, C., Eklund, H. W. & McElroy, O. E. (1946). Botulinum Toxin (Type A); Including a Study of Shaking with Chloroform as a Step in the Isolation Procedure. *J Bacteriol*, **52**, 1–13.

Lamb, A. (2001). Biological weapons: the Facts not the Fiction. *Clin Med*, **1**, 502–4.

Landmann, G. (1904). Über die Ursache der Darmstädter Bohnenvergiftung. *Hyg Rundschau*, **10**, 449–52.

Leuchs, J. (1910). Beiträge zur Kenntnis des Toxins und Antitoxins des Bacillus botulinus. *Ztschr Hyg u Infekt*, **65**, 55–84.

Mahrhold, S., Rummel, A., Bigalke, H., Davletov, B. & Binz, T. (2006). The synaptic vesicle protein 2C mediates the uptake of botulinum neurotoxin A into phrenic nerves. *FEBS Lett*, **580**, 2011–14.

Merson, M. H. & Dowell, J. (1973). Epidemiologic, clinical and laboratory aspects of wound botulism. *N Engl J Med*, **289**, 1105–10.

Müller, H. (1869). Das Wurstgift. Deutsche Klinik, pulserial publication: **35**, 321–3, **37**, 341–3, **39**, 357–9, **40**, 365–7, 381–3, **49**, 453–5.

Pickett, J., Berg, B., Chaplin, E. & Brunstetter-Shafer, M. A. (1976). Syndrome of botulism in infancy: clinical and electrophysiologic study. *N Engl J Med*, **295**, 770–2.

Schantz, E. J. (1994). Historical perspective. In J. Jankovic & M. Hallett, eds., *Therapy with Botulinum Toxin*. New York: Marcel Dekker, pp. xxiii–vi.

Schiavo, G., Benfenati, F., Poulain, B., *et al.* (1992). Tetanus and botulinum-B toxins block transmitter release by proteolytic cleavage of synaptobrevin. *Nature*, **359**, 832–5.

Schiavo, G., Cantucci, A., Das Gupta, B. R., *et al.* (1993). Botulinum neurotoxin serotypes A and E cleave SNAP-25 at distinct COOH-terminal peptide bonds. *FEBS Lett*, **335**, 99–103.

Smith, L. D. (1977). *Botulism. The Organism, its Toxins, the Disease*. Springfield USA: Charles C Thomas Publishers.

Snipe, P. T. & Sommer, H. (1928). Studies on botulinus toxin. 3. Acid preparation of botulinus toxin. *J Infect Dis*, **43**, 152–60.

Steinbuch, J. G. (1817). Vergiftung durch verdorbene Würste. *Tübinger Blätter für Naturwissenschaften und Arzneykunde*, **3**, 26–52.

Torrens, J. K. (1998). Clostridium botulinum was named because of association with "sausage poisoning". *BMJ*, **316**, 151.

van Ermengem, E. P. (1897). Über einen neuen anaeroben Bacillus und seine Beziehung zum Botulismus. *Z Hyg Infektionskrankh*, **26**, 1–56 (English version: Van Ermengem, E. P. (1979). A new anaerobic bacillus and its relation to botulism. *Rev Infect Dis*, **1**, 701–19).

2

Botulinum toxin: history of clinical development

Daniel Truong, Dirk Dressler and Mark Hallett

The clinical development of botulinum toxin began in the late 1960s with the search for an alternative to surgical realignment of strabismus. At that time, surgery of the extraocular muscles was the sole treatment. However, it was unsatisfactory due to variable results, consequent high reoperation rates, and its invasive nature. In an attempt to find an alternative, Alan B. Scott, an ophthalmologist from the Smith-Kettlewell Eye Research Institute in San Francisco, CA, USA, had been investigating the effects of different compounds injected into the extraocular muscles to chemically weaken them. The drugs tested initially proved unreliable, short acting or necrotizing (Scott *et al.*, 1973). About this time, Scott became aware of Daniel Drachman, a renowned neuroscientist at Johns Hopkins University, and his work, in which he had been injecting minute amounts of botulinum toxin directly into the hind limbs of chicken to achieve local denervation (Drachman, 1972). Drachman introduced Scott to Edward Schantz (1908–2005) who was producing purified botulinum toxins for experimental use and generously making them available to the academic community. Schantz himself credits Vernon Brooks with the idea that botulinum toxin might be used for weakening muscle (Schantz, 1994). Brooks worked on the mechanism of action of botulinum toxin for his Ph.D. under the mentorship of Arnold Burgen, who suggested the project to him (Brooks, 2001). Schantz had left the US Army Chemical Corps

at Fort Detrick, Maryland in 1972 to work at the Department of Microbiology and Toxicology, University of Wisconsin, Madison, WI, USA. Using acid precipitation purification techniques worked out at Fort Detrick by Lamanna and Duff, Schantz was able to make the purified botulinum toxins. In extensive animal experiments botulinum toxin produced the desired long-lasting, localized, dose-dependent muscle weakening without any systemic toxicity and without any necrotizing side effects (Scott *et al.*, 1973). Based on these results the US Food and Drug Administration (FDA) permitted Scott in 1977 to test botulinum toxin in humans under an Investigative New Drug (IND) license for the treatment of strabismus. These tests proved successful and the results of 67 injections were published in 1980 (Scott, 1980). With this publication botulinum toxin was established as a novel therapeutic agent. Before botulinum toxin could be registered as a drug the US FDA required numerous tests including tests for safety, potency, stability, sterility, and water retention in the freeze-dried product. In addition to establishing a laboratory for the tests, a sterile facility for filling and freeze-drying was set up by Scott, Schantz, and Eric Johnson, who joined the team in 1985.

By the early 1980s, Scott and colleagues had injected botulinum toxin for the treatment of strabismus, blepharospasm, hemifacial spasm, cervical dystonia, and thigh adductor spasm (Scott, 1994).

During the 1980s, the use of botulinum toxin for therapeutic purposes increased substantially as Scott supplied investigators with various interests. In 1985, Tsui and colleagues reported the successful use of botulinum toxin for the treatment of cervical dystonia in 12 patients based on the earlier dosage data from Scott's injections (Tsui *et al.*, 1985). This was followed by a double-blind, crossover study in which botulinum toxin was found to be significantly superior to placebo at reducing the symptoms of cervical dystonia, including pain (Tsui *et al.*, 1986). Soon, botulinum toxin became the treatment of choice for cervical dystonia. The therapeutic use of botulinum toxin for the treatment of blepharospasm and hemifacial spasm proceeded along similar lines, with several groups reporting success in these indications by the mid 1980s and documenting the benefits of repeated injections after the effects waned (Frueh *et al.*, 1984; Mauriello, 1985; Scott *et al.*, 1985). Reports of the successful use of botulinum toxin in many conditions of focal muscle overactivity followed, including spasmodic dysphonia (Blitzer *et al.*, 1986), oromandibular dystonia (Jankovic & Orman, 1987), dystonias of the hand (Cohen *et al.*, 1989), and limb spasticity (Das & Park, 1989).

In December 1989, the FDA licensed the manufacturing facilities and a batch of botulinum toxin type A manufactured by Scott and Schantz in November 1979, the so-called batch 11/79. The therapeutic preparation contained 100 mouse units of toxin per vial. The FDA identified this product named Oculinum® (**ocul** and **lin**ing-up) as an orphan drug for the treatment of strabismus, hemifacial spasm, and blepharospasm. For about 2 years, Scott's Oculinum Inc. was the licensed manufacturer with Allergan Inc., Irvine, CA, USA acting as the sole distributor. The manufacturing facilities and the license were turned over to Allergan in late 1991 and the product was later renamed Botox® (**bo**tulinum **tox**in). The name Botox was perhaps first used by Stanley Fahn, but he did not think of it as a possible trade name. A different batch of Botox was prepared in 1988 and served as the basis for European licensing. This and subsequent batches of Botox contain less neurotoxin complex protein per mouse unit, which may make them less liable to elicit antibodies than batch 11/79.

In 2000 NeuroBloc®/Myobloc® was registered with the US FDA by Elan Pharmaceuticals, South San Francisco, CA, USA with the indication of cervical dystonia. Myobloc is the trade name in the USA and NeuroBloc is the trade name used elsewhere. It was eventually sold to Solstice Neurosciences Inc., Malvern, PA, USA. Botox was also approved for cervical dystonia in 2000.

In Europe botulinum toxin was first produced for therapeutic purposes at the Defence Science and Technology Laboratory in Porton Down, Salisbury Plain, Wilts., UK. When the product was commercialized the manufacturing operations were renamed several times to Centre of Applied Microbiology and Research (CAMR), Porton Products, Public Health Laboratory Service (PHLS), and Speywood Pharmaceuticals. In 1994 Speywood Pharmaceuticals was acquired by Ipsen, Paris, France. The UK botulinum toxin product was first registered in 1991 as Dysport® (**Dys**tonia **Port**on Products). It is now distributed worldwide by Ipsen Ltd., Slough, Berks., UK. A US registration for cervical dystonia as well as a cosmetic registration under the name Reloxin is in preparation. The UK product was first used in the UK to treat strabismus and blepharospasm not long after Scott's initial reports (Elston, 1985; Elston *et al.*, 1985). C. David Marsden's movement disorders group at the National Hospital of Neurology and Neurosurgery, Queen Square, London, UK, pioneered its use in neurology (Stell *et al.*, 1988). Soon afterwards, Dirk Dressler, a student of Marsden, introduced this product to continental European neurology (Dressler *et al.*, 1989). More details about the continental European spread of the botulinum toxin therapy are described elsewhere (Homann *et al.*, 2002).

Recently, another botulinum toxin drug named Xeomin® has been marketed by Merz Pharmaceuticals from Frankfurt/M, Germany. It is a botulinum toxin type A preparation with high specific biological activity, and, as a consequence, a reduced protein load (Dressler & Benecke, 2006). Structurally, it is free of the complexing botulinum toxin proteins. It is currently approved in many countries in Europe and in trials in other countries.

An additional source of therapeutic botulinum toxin type A is the Lanzhou Institute of Biological Products, Lanzhou, Gansu Province, China, where the manufacturing expertise comes from Wang Yinchun, a former collaborator of Schantz. Its product was registered as Hengli® in China in 1993. In some other Asian and South American markets it is distributed as CBTX-A, Redux or Prosigne®. The international marketing is provided by Hugh Source International Ltd., Kowloon, Hong Kong. A registration of this product in the USA and in Europe seems unlikely. Publications about this product are scarce.

In South Korea and some other Asian countries Neuronox®, a botulinum toxin type A drug manufactured by Medy-Tox, Ochang, South Korea, is distributed. Other botulinum toxin drugs are under development at Tokushima University, Tokushima City, Japan, and at the Mentor Corporation, Santa Barbara, CA, USA.

In the 1990s the clinical applications for botulinum toxin continued to expand. Botox was approved by the FDA for glabellar rhytides in 2002 and for primary axillary hyperhidrosis in 2004. Off-label use is widespread and includes tremor, spasticity, overactive bladder, anal fissure, achalasia, various conditions of pain such as headache, and others (Dressler, 2000; Moore & Naumann, 2003; Truong & Jost, 2006). Outside of the USA, there are 20 indications in 75 countries. Numerous formal therapeutic trials for registration are in progress. The use of Botox for wrinkles has been very popular and is perhaps the best known indication in the public.

These expanded uses were paralleled by an increased understanding of the mechanism of action of botulinum neurotoxins from basic research (Lalli et al., 2003). The multistep mechanism of action postulated by Simpson (1979) was verified, and research on botulinum toxin has itself contributed much to the understanding of vesicular neurotransmitter release. We have also learned that botulinum toxin, which was once believed to exert its activity solely on cholinergic neurons, can, under certain conditions, inhibit the evoked release of several other neurotransmitters (Welch et al., 2000; Durham et al., 2004). These discoveries continue to intrigue basic scientists and clinicians alike, as the therapeutic uses and applications of botulinum toxin appear destined to increase still further in the years to come.

REFERENCES

Blitzer, A., Brin, M. F., Fahn, S., Lange, D. & Lovelace, R. E. (1986). Botulinum toxin (BOTOX) for the treatment of "spastic dysphonia" as part of a trial of toxin injections for the treatment of other cranial dystonias. *Laryngoscope*, **96**, 1300–1.

Brooks, V. (2001). In L. R. Squire, ed., *The History of Neuroscience in Autobiography*. Vol. 3. New York: Academic Press, pp. 76–116.

Cohen, L. G., Hallett, M., Geller, B. D. & Hochberg, F. (1989). Treatment of focal dystonias of the hand with botulinum toxin injections. *J Neurol Neurosurg Psychiatry*, **52**, 355–63.

Das, T. K. & Park, D. M. (1989). Effect of treatment with botulinum toxin on spasticity. *Postgrad Med J*, **65**, 208–10.

Drachman, D. B. (1972). Neurotrophic regulation of muscle cholinesterase: effects of botulinum toxin and denervation. *J Physiol*, **226**, 619–27.

Dressler, D. (2000). *Botulinum Toxin Therapy*. Stuttgart, New York: Thieme-Verlag.

Dressler, D. & Benecke, R. (2006). Xeomin® eine neue therapeutische Botulinum Toxin Typ A-Präparation. *Akt Neurol*, **33**, 138–41.

Dressler, D., Benecke, R. & Conrad, B. (1989). Botulinum Toxin in der Therapie kraniozervikaler Dystonien. *Nervenarzt*, **60**, 386–93.

Durham, P. L., Cady, R. & Cady, R. (2004). Regulation of calcitonin gene-related peptide secretion from trigeminal nerve cells by botulinum toxin type A: implications for migraine therapy. *Headache*, **44**, 35–42.

Elston, J. S. (1985). The use of botulinum toxin A in the treatment of strabismus. *Trans Ophthalmol Soc UK*, **104**(Pt 2), 208–10.

Elston, J. S., Lee, J. P., Powell, C. M., Hogg, C. & Clark, P. (1985). Treatment of strabismus in adults with botulinum toxin A. *Br J Ophthalmol*, **69**, 718–24.

Frueh, B. R., Felt, D. P., Wojno, T. H. & Musch, D. C. (1984). Treatment of blepharospasm with botulinum toxin. A preliminary report. *Arch Ophthalmol*, **102**, 1464–8.

Homann, C. N., Wenzel, K., Kriechbaum, N., *et al.* (2002). Botulinum Toxin – Die Dosis macht das Gift. Ein historischer Abriß. *Nervenheilkunde*, **73**, 519–24.

Jankovic, J. & Orman, J. (1987). Botulinum A toxin for cranial-cervical dystonia: a double-blind, placebo-controlled study. *Neurology*, **37**, 616–23.

Lalli, G., Bohnert, S., Deinhardt, K., Verastegui, C. & Schiavo, G. (2003). The journey of tetanus and botulinum neurotoxins in neurons. *Trends Microbiol*, **11**, 431–7.

Mauriello, J. A. Jr. (1985). Blepharospasm, Meige syndrome, and hemifacial spasm: treatment with botulinum toxin. *Neurology*, **35**, 1499–500.

Moore, P. & Naumann, M. *Handbook of Botulinum Toxin Treatment*, 2nd edn. Maulden, Mass: Blackwell Science.

Schantz, E. J. (1994). Historical perspective. In J. Jankovic & M. Hallett, eds., *Therapy with Botulinum Toxin*. New York: Marcel Dekker, Inc., pp. xxiii–vi.

Scott, A. B. (1980). Botulinum toxin injection into extraocular muscles as an alternative to strabismus surgery. *Ophthalmology*, **87**, 1044–9.

Scott, A. B. (1994). Foreword. In J. Jankovic & M. Hallett, eds., *Therapy with Botulinum Toxin*. New York: Marcel Dekker, Inc., pp. vii–ix.

Scott, A. B., Rosenbaum, A. & Collins, C. C. (1973). Pharmacologic weakening of extraocular muscles. *Invest Ophthalmol*, **12**(12), 924–7.

Scott, A. B., Kennedy, R. A. & Stubbs, H. A. (1985). Botulinum A toxin injection as a treatment for blepharospasm. *Arch Ophthalmol*, **103**, 347–50.

Simpson, L. L. (1979). The action of botulinal toxin. *Rev Infect Dis*, **1**, 656–62.

Stell, R., Thompson, P. D. & Marsden, C. D. (1988). Botulinum toxin in spasmodic torticollis. *J Neurol Neurosurg Psychiatry*, **51**, 920–3.

Truong, D. D. & Jost, W. H. (2006). Botulinum toxin: clinical use. *Parkinsonism Relat Disord*, **12**, 331–55.

Tsui, J. K., Eisen, A., Mak, E., *et al.* (1985). A pilot study on the use of botulinum toxin in spasmodic torticollis. *Can J Neurol Sci*, **12**, 314–16.

Tsui, J. K., Eisen, A., Stoessl, A. J., Calne, S. & Calne, D. B. (1986). Double-blind study of botulinum toxin in spasmodic torticollis. *Lancet*, **2**(8501), 245–7.

Welch, M. J., Purkiss, J. R. & Foster, K. A. Sensitivity of embryonic rat dorsal root ganglia neurons to Clostridium botulinum neurotoxins. *Toxicon*, **38**, 245–58.

3

Pharmacology of botulinum toxin drugs

Dirk Dressler and Hans Bigalke

Introduction

Botulinum toxin (BT) drugs consist of a complex mixture of substances. All of those components can differ between BT drugs. Therapeutically the most important difference refers to the botulinum neurotoxin (BNT) serotype used. So far, only types A and B are commercially available, whereas types C and F have been tried in humans on an experimental basis only. Types A and B have a substantially different affinity to the motor and to the autonomic nervous system (Dressler & Benecke, 2003). Other ingredients can also vary. The pH 5.4 buffer system of NeuroBloc®/Myobloc® increases the injection site pain as compared to all other BT drugs using pH 7.4 buffer systems. Hengli® is the only BT drug applying gelatine stabilization, which may cause allergic reactions. Other differences in protein content may affect tissue perfusion and antigenicity. Clearly, the commercially available BT drugs are not identical. Some of their differences matter therapeutically, others, however, seem not to matter. Contrary to a commercially biased belief BT drugs can be compared and should be compared. "Uniqueness" does not exist amongst BT drugs, whereas differentiation does.

Structure

As shown in Figure 3.1, BT drugs consist of the BT component and excipients. Excipients include lactose, sucrose, and serum albumin for stabilization purposes and buffer systems for pH calibration. The BT component is formed by BNT and by non-toxic proteins also known as complexing proteins. The BT component should be abbreviated as BT, botulinum neurotoxin as BNT. Different BT types, such as type A, type B, type C, type D, type E, type F, and type G can be abbreviated as BT-A, BT-B, BT-C, BT-D, BT-E, BT-F and BT-G. Occasionally the abbreviations BoNT, Botx, BoTX, BoTx and Botox are used without a definition of the BT components they are referring to. Botox®, additionally, is the brand name for the BT drug manufactured by Allergan Inc. The abbreviation BTX is also used for the dart frog toxin batrachotoxin.

Botulinum neurotoxin consists of a heavy amino acid chain with a molecular weight of 100 kDa and a light amino acid chain with a molecular weight of 50 kDa. Both chains are formed from a single stranded circular progenitor toxin by proteolysis. They are interconnected by a single disulfide-bridge. The integrity of this disulfide bridge is essential for BT's biological activity making BT a compound highly fragile to various environmental influences. As shown in Figure 3.2 BNT and complexing proteins form BT with a molecular weight of 450 kDa. Two BT molecules associate to a dimer with a molecular weight of 900 kDa. In Xeomin® the complexing proteins could be removed during the manufacturing process so that Xeomin contains isolated

Note: This chapter uses a different abbreviation for botulinum toxin to the rest of the book.
Manual of Botulinum Toxin Therapy, ed. Daniel Truong, Dirk Dressler and Mark Hallett. Published by Cambridge University Press.

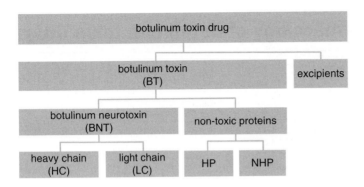

Figure 3.1 Contents of botulinum toxin drugs. HP, hemagglutinating protein; NHP, non-hemagglutinating protein.

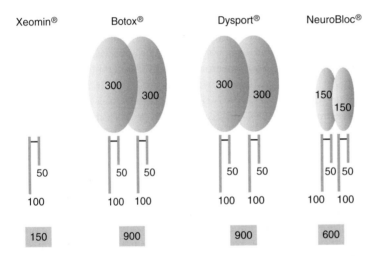

Figure 3.2 Configuration of the botulinum toxin component of botulinum toxin drugs. The botulinum toxin component of Xeomin® consists of a botulinum neurotoxin monomer, whereas all other botulinum toxin drugs contain dimer-forming non-toxic proteins each with molecular weights of 150 kDa or 300 kDa. From: Dressler D. & Benecke, R. (2006). Xeomin®: Eine neue therapeutische Botulinum Toxin Typ A-Präparation. *Akt Neurol*, **33**, 138–41.

monomeric BNT only. Other BT types contain different complexing protein aggregates so that their total molecular weight is different from that of BT-A.

Mode of action

When BT is injected into a target tissue it is bound with astounding selectivity to glycoprotein structures located on the cholinergic nerve terminal. Subsequently BNT's light chain is internalized and cleaves different proteins of the acetylcholine transport protein cascade (**s**oluble **N**-ethylmaleimide-sensitive factor **a**ttachment protein **re**ceptor, SNARE proteins) transporting the acetylcholine vesicle from the intracellular space into the synaptic cleft (Pellizzari *et al.*, 1999). Different BT types target different SNARE proteins. Whereas BT-A, BT-C, and BT-E target SNAP 25 (Schiavo *et al.*, 1993; Binz *et al.*, 1994; Foran *et al.*, 1996), BT-B, BT-D, and BT-F target VAMP (**v**esicle-**a**ssociated **m**embrane **p**rotein = Synaptobrevin) (Schiavo *et al.*, 1992; Yamasaki *et al.*, 1994).

When BT blocks the cholinergic synapse the neuron forms new synapses replacing its original ones. This process is known as sprouting (Duchen, 1971a, b). Whereas it was originally thought that sprouting is responsible for the termination of BT's action, it recently became clear that sprouting

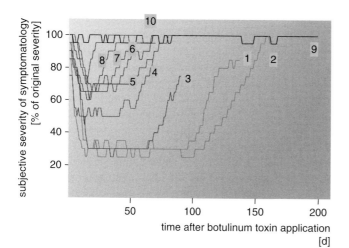

Figure 3.3 Therapeutic effect of botulinum toxin in a patient with cervical dystonia documented with a treatment calendar. Injection series 1 and 2 (light gray) show normal treatment results. Injection series 10 represents a complete secondary therapy failure (black). All other injection series show normal treatment results. From: Dressler D. (2000). *Botulinum Toxin Therapy*. Stuttgart, New York: Thieme Verlag with permission.

is a temporary recovery process only and that the original synapses are eventually regenerated while the sprouts are being removed (de Paiva *et al.*, 1999). Botulinum toxin, therefore, is interrupting the synaptic transmission only temporarily. Structural neuronal changes or functional neuronal impairment other than the synaptic blockade itself cannot be detected. Recently, we therefore suggested classifying BT not as a neurotoxin, but as a temporary neuromodulator (Brin *et al.*, 2004). Depending on the target tissue, BT can block the cholinergic neuromuscular transmission, but also the cholinergic autonomic innervation of the sweat glands, the tear glands, the salivary glands, and the smooth muscles. As shown in Figure 3.3 first BT effects can be detected after intramuscular injection within 2 to 3 days depending on the detection methods used. Botulinum toxin reaches its maximal effect after about 2 weeks, stays at this and then gradually starts to decline after 2.5 months. Botulinum toxin injections into glandular tissue can exert prolonged effects of up to 6 or 9 months.

Botulinum toxin's action features a dose–effect correlation (Dressler & Rothwell, 2000). It can be used for patient-based antibody testing (Dressler *et al.*, 2000). Additionally a dose–duration correlation can be described. Both correlations are valid only within certain limits. They can be used for

comparison of different BT drugs and for modeling of optimal BT dosing. When the dose–duration correlation is not considered together with the dose–effect correlation comparison of BT drugs becomes inaccurate. For comprehensive drug comparison adverse effect profiles also need to be considered.

Apart from a direct action upon the striate muscle BT can act upon the muscle spindle organ reducing its centripetal information traffic (Dressler *et al.*, 1993; Filippi *et al.*, 1993; Rosales *et al.*, 1996). Whether this muscle afferent blockade is relevant to BT's therapeutic action remains unclear (Kaji *et al.*, 1995a, b). Although BT can produce numerous indirect central nervous system effects, direct ones beyond the alpha motoneuron have not been described after intramuscular injection (Wiegand *et al.*, 1976). Although BT is transported centripetally by retrograde axonal transport, this transport is so slow that BT is inactivated by the time it reaches the central nervous system. Affection of the central nervous system via transport through the blood–brain barrier is excluded due to BT's molecular size. Despite its almost complete binding to the cholinergic nerve terminal (Takamizawa *et al.*, 1986) minute amounts of BT can be distributed with the blood circulation. This systemic spread can be detected by an increased neuromuscular jitter in muscles distant from the injection site (Sanders *et al.*, 1986; Lange *et al.*, 1987; Olney *et al.*, 1988; Girlanda *et al.*, 1992).

Systemic spread of BT-A is minute, so that it can be detected clinically only when extremely high BT-A doses are used. Systemic spread of BT-B is substantially higher and autonomic adverse effects occur frequently even when low or intermediate BT-B doses are used (Dressler & Benecke, 2003).

In addition to the blockade of acetylcholine secretion, animal experiments indicate BT induced blockade of transmitters involved in pain perception, pain transmission, and pain processing. Apart from substance P (Ishikawa *et al.*, 2000; Purkiss *et al.*, 2000; Welch *et al.*, 2000), glutamate (McMahon *et al.*, 1992; Cui *et al.*, 2002), calcitonin gene-related peptide (CGRP) (Morris *et al.*, 2001), and noradrenaline (Shone & Melling, 1992) could be blocked by BT. Whether these data derived from animal experiments translate into a genuine clinical nociceptive effect, remains open at this point of time.

Botulinum toxin drugs

Currently available BT drugs are Botox (Allergan Inc., Irvine, CA, USA), Dysport® (Ipsen Ltd., Slough, Berks., UK), NeuroBloc/Myobloc (Solstice Neurosciences Inc., Malvern, PA, USA) and Xeomin (Merz Pharmaceuticals, Frankfurt/M, Germany). From 1989 to 1992 Botox's trade name was Oculinum®. In the USA and in some other countries NeuroBloc is distributed as Myobloc.

Additional BT drugs include Hengli (Lanzhou Institute of Biological Products, Lanzhou, Gansu Province, China), which is based upon BT type A and which is distributed in some other Asian and South American markets as CBTX-A or Prosigne®, and Neuronox® (Medy-Tox, Ochang, South Korea), which is sold in South Korea and in some other Asian countries. New BT drugs are under development at Tokushima University, Tokushima City, Japan and at the Mentor Corporation, Santa Barbara, CA, USA.

Botox was the first BT drug to be registered in 1989, whilst Dysport was registered in 1991, Hengli in 1993, NeuroBloc/Myobloc in 2000, and Xeomin in 2005.

Most of the currently available BT drugs are shown in Figure 3.4. Their properties are summarized in Table 3.1. All BT-A drugs are powders which need to be reconstituted with 0.9%NaCl/H$_2$O prior to application. Only NeuroBloc/Myobloc is a ready-to-use solution. For all BT drugs special storage temperatures are required. Xeomin is the only drug which can be stored at room temperature. The shelf lives of all BT drugs are similar. The long shelf life of Xeomin is remarkable, since it was originally believed that the lack of complexing proteins would destabilize its BNT. Since NeuroBloc/Myobloc is stabilized by a reduced pH value, about half of the patients receiving NeuroBloc/Myobloc report intensified application pain (Dressler *et al.*, 2002).

All BT drugs are manufactured biologically. For this, *Clostridium botulinum* selected from a special strain is bred in special high-security converters. After about 72 hours the BT concentration is maximal and the culture is inactivated by acidification. After centrifugation the raw BT is purified in a special process applying several precipitation steps and ion exchange chromatography. At the end of the purification process half of the initial amount of BT is retrieved as sterile and highly purified BT. Some of this material is inactivated by conformational changes as a result of the purification process. Depending on the biological activity measured the stem solution is diluted by addition of lactose, sucrose or NaCl solutions until the required biological activity is obtained. Production variability of the biological activity for the main four BT drugs is in the order of approximately ±15%.

The biological activity of therapeutic BT preparations is given in mouse units (MU) although doses are sometimes shortened to units (U). One mouse unit describes the amount of BT which would kill 50% of a BT-intoxicated mouse population. Mouse units therefore describe a biological activity and – according to the amount of inactivated BT contained – correspond to different mass units. Although mouse units are defined by international convention, the activity assays used by the manufacturers are performed differently so that the activity labeling of the different BT drugs cannot be

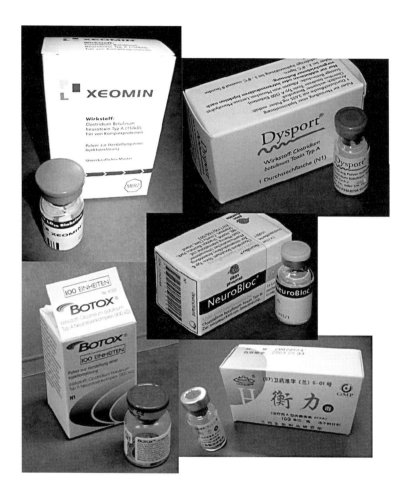

Figure 3.4 Some of the commercially available botulinum toxin drugs.

compared directly. One mouse unit of Botox is equivalent to approximately 3 MU of Dysport, whereas the activity labeling of Botox and Xeomin seems to be identical (Benecke *et al.*, 2005, Dressler & Adib Saberi, 2006). The potency labeling of different BT types can also not be compared directly. The motor effects of Botox and NeuroBloc/Myobloc seem to be comparable on a 1:40 ratio. For treatment of autonomic disorders this conversion ratio could be different (Dressler *et al.*, 2002). Overall, BT-B has relatively stronger autonomic and relatively weaker motor effects as compared to BT-A (Dressler & Benecke, 2003).

Immunological quality

One of the risk factors for antibody-induced therapy failure (ABTF) is the single dose, i.e. the amount of BT applied at each injection series (Dressler & Dirnberger, 2000). The single dose is determined by the amount of biological activity required to produce the necessary therapeutic effect. Only recently it became clear that the single dose as a risk factor implicitly includes the immunological quality of the BT drug applied. The risk of ABTF is not associated with the biological activity as such, but with the amount of antigen presented to the immune

Table 3.1. Properties of different botulinum toxin drugs

	Botox	Dysport	Xeomin	NeuroBloc/Myobloc
Manufacturer	Allergan Inc. Irvine, CA, USA	Ipsen Ltd. Slough, Berks., UK	Merz Pharmaceuticals Frankfurt/M, Germany	Solstice Neurosciences Inc. Malvern, PA, USA
Pharmaceutical preparation	powder	powder	powder	ready-to-use solution 5000 MU-E/cc
Storage conditions	below 8 °C	below 8 °C	below 25 °C	below 8 °C
Shelf life	36 months	24 months	36 months	24 months
Botulinum toxin type	A	A	A	B
Clostridium botulinum strain	Hall A	Ipsen strain	Hall A	Bean B
SNARE target	SNAP25	SNAP25	SNAP25	VAMP
Purification process	precipitation and chromatography	precipitation and chromatography	precipitation and chromatography	precipitation and chromatography
pH-value of the reconstituted preparation	7.4	7.4	7.4	5.6
Stabilization	vacuum drying	freeze-drying (lyophilizate)	vacuum drying	pH-reduction
Excipients	human serum albumin 500 μg/vial NaCl 900 μg/vial buffer system	human serum albumin 125 μg/vial lactose 2500 μg/vial buffer system	human serum albumin 1 mg/vial sucrose 4.7 mg/vial buffer system	human serum albumin 0.5 mg/cc disodium succinate 0.01 M NaCl 0.1 M H$_2$O hydrochloric acid
Biological activity	100 MU-A/vial	500 MU-I/vial	100 MU-M/vial	1.0/2.5/10.0 kMU-E/vial
Biological activity in relation to Botox	1	1/3	1	1/40
Specific biological activity	60 MU-EV/ngBNT	100 MU-EV/ngBNT	167 MU-EV/ngBNT	5 MU-EV/ngBNT

Notes:
BNT: botulinum neurotoxin
MU-A: mouse unit in the Allergan mouse lethality assay
MU-E: mouse unit in the Solstice mouse lethality assay
MU-I: mouse unit in the Ipsen mouse lethality assay
MU-M: mouse unit in the Merz mouse lethality assay
MU-EV: equivalence mouse unit (approximate, for motor effects), 1 MU-EV = 1 MU-A = 1 MU-M = 3 MU-I = 40 MU-E.

system. When BNT is manufactured and stored conformational changes can inactivate it. Although inactivated BNT has lost its biological activity, it can still act as an antigen for BT antibody (BT-AB) formation. The amount of inactivated BT contained, therefore, determines the immunological quality of a BT drug. When the immunological quality is high, the amount of inactivated BT contained is low, i.e. the drug has a high biological activity per mass unit of BT antigen resulting in a low antigenicity. When the immunological quality is low, the drug has a low biological activity per mass unit of BT antigen resulting in a high antigenicity. The relationship between biological potency and the amount of BNT is called the specific biological activity and serves as a parameter for the immunological quality of a BT drug. Its dimension is MU/ng BNT. The inversed ratio is called the protein load and is given in ng BNT/MU. As shown in Table 3.1 the specific biological activity varies substantially between different therapeutic preparations with Xeomin having the highest and Neuro-Bloc/Myobloc the lowest values (Setler, 2000; Jankovic *et al.*, 2003; Pickett *et al.*, 2003; Dressler & Benecke, 2006).

Safety aspects and adverse effects

Based upon a broad therapeutic window and strictly local effects avoiding contact with excretion organs, BT excels with a remarkably advantageous adverse effects profile. Adverse effects can be classified as obligate, local or systemic. Obligate adverse effects are inborn effects caused by the therapeutic principle itself. Local adverse effects are caused by diffusion of BT from the target tissue into adjacent tissues. Systemic adverse effects are adverse effects in tissues distant from the injection site and based upon BT transport within the blood circulation. Botulinum toxin adverse effects occur in a typical time window after BT application, usually starting after one week and lasting for one to two weeks. Severity and duration of adverse effects depend on the BT dose applied. Central

nervous system adverse effects have not been reported so far. As described above, there is no centripetal transport of active BT after intramuscular BT application and no transsynaptic BT transport beyond the alpha motoneuron. Systemic spread of BT becomes clinically relevant only when BT doses applied are very high. Transport of BT through the blood–brain barrier is not possible due to BT's molecular size. The use of BT during pregnancy is contraindicated as a precautionary measure until further experience is gained. Few accidental BT applications during pregnancies did not induce any developmental abnormalities. Extremely rarely, BT applications can trigger acute autoimmune brachial plexopathies (Probst *et al.*, 2002). If they occur, continuation of BT therapy seems to be safe, since reoccurrence is rare.

Caution is required when using BT in patients with pre-existing pareses, as in amyotrophic lateral sclerosis, myopathies, and motor polyneuropathies, or in patients with impaired neuromuscular transmission, such as myasthenia gravis and Lambert-Eaton syndrome (Erbguth *et al.*, 1993). Increased paresis seen in patients with botulism receiving aminoglycoside antibiotics has led to warnings about using BT therapy and aminoglycosides at the same time. Whether these interactions are relevant in a therapeutic situation remains open.

When patients with chronic disorders are treated with a symptomatic therapy, issues of long-term safety become relevant. Since BT therapy was introduced in the late 1980s, large numbers of patients have been exposed to BT. Many of them have received BT in high doses over prolonged periods of time. However, none of these patients has experienced additional long-term adverse effects.

All BT-A drugs have similar adverse effect profiles. However, recent observations suggest an increased frequency of local adverse effects after Dysport as compared to Botox (Dressler, 2002). Reasons for this are unclear, but may include increased diffusion as demonstrated in animal experiments (Brin *et al.*, 2004), or conversion factors incorrectly underestimating Dysport's biological activity. Based upon a conversion factor of 1:1 the adverse effect profiles of Xeomin and of Botox seem to be identical (Benecke *et al.*, 2005; Dressler & Adib Saberi, 2006).

The adverse effect profile of the BT-B drug NeuroBloc/Myobloc is substantially different from the adverse effect profiles of BT-A drugs. Whereas even low and intermediate BT-B doses are frequently producing autonomic adverse effects, including dryness of mouth, corneal irritation, accommodation difficulties, and irritation of the nasal or genital mucosa, the frequency of motor adverse effects is similar after BT-B and BT-A (Dressler & Benecke, 2003). Comparison of injection sites and localization of autonomic adverse effects suggests a systemic spread of BT-B. Whereas BT-A has a relatively strong effect on the motor system and a relatively weak effect on the autonomic nervous system this correlation is reversed in BT-B. Whether – compared to BT-A – BT-B has a particular strong effect on the autonomous system or whether it has a particular weak effect on the motor system remains unclear. High doses necessary to treat motor symptoms could point towards a genuinely weak motor effect (Dressler & Eleopra, 2006). Because of its systemic autonomic adverse effects BT-B should be used with caution in patients with pre-existing autonomic dysfunction or in connection with anticholinergics. Since identical therapeutic effects can be produced with BT-A, therapeutic use of BT-B is limited and may just include patients with ABTF after BT-A application. Whether BT-B drugs have advantages over BT-A drugs in the treatment of autonomic disorders remains open.

Therapeutic dosages for BT drugs vary more widely than with almost any other drug. Whereas minimum therapeutic BT doses used for spasmodic dysphonia are as low as 5 MU Botox, maximum reported BT doses used for generalized spasticity and generalized dystonia can reach 850 MU Botox or 850 MU Xeomin (Dressler & Adib Saberi, 2006). When Botox and Xeomin are used in high doses systemic motor and systemic autonomic adverse effects are very rare. When Dysport is used in doses of more than 1500 MU systemic motor adverse

effects can occur. Since this dose is considered to be equivalent to 500 MU of Botox or 500 MU of Xeomin, Dysport seems to produce more adverse effects in high dose applications than Botox and Xeomin. Whether this reflects different diffusion properties or an inappropriate potency labeling conversion factor is still unclear. For the use of NeuroBloc/Myobloc systemic autonomic adverse effects can occur with doses as low as 4000 MU, and with doses of 10 000 MU they are frequent. Despite excellent tolerability BT starting doses should be moderate when BT therapy is initiated and the patient's reagibility is unknown.

Outlook

Botulinum toxin drugs are a group of highly potent drugs with an intriguing mechanism of action. With the advent of new competitors comparative studies amongst different BT drugs will become more and more interesting.

REFERENCES

Benecke, R., Jost, W. H., Kanovsky, P., *et al.* (2005). A new botulinum toxin type A free of complexing proteins for treatment of cervical dystonia. *Neurology*, **64**, 1949–51.

Binz, T., Blasi, J., Yamasaki, S., *et al.* (1994). Proteolysis of SNAP-25 by types E and A botulinal neurotoxins. *J Biol Chem*, **269**, 1617–20.

Brin, M. F., Dressler, D. & Aoki, R. Pharmacology of botulinum toxin therapy. In J. Jankovic, C. Comella & M. F. Brin, eds., *Dystonia: Etiology, Clinical Features, and Treatment*. Philadelphia: Lippincott Williams & Wilkins, pp. 93–112.

Cui, M., Li, Z., You, S., Khanijou, S. & Aoki, R. (2002) Mechanisms of the antinociceptive effect of subcutaneous Botox: inhibition of peripheral and central nociceptive processing. *Arch Pharmacol*, **365**, R17.

de Paiva, A., Meunier, F. A., Molgo, J., Aoki, K. R. & Dolly, J. O. (1999). Functional repair of motor endplates after botulinum neurotoxin type A poisoning: biphasic switch of synaptic activity between nerve sprouts and their parent terminals. *Proc Natl Acad Sci USA*, **96**, 3200–5.

Dressler, D. (2000). *Botulinum Toxin Therapy*. Stuttgart, New York: Thieme Verlag.

Dressler, D. (2002). Dysport produces intrinsically more swallowing problems than Botox: unexpected results from a conversion factor study in cervical dystonia. *J Neurol Neurosurg Psychiatry*, **73**, 604.

Dressler, D. & Adib Saberi, F. (2006). Safety aspects of high dose Xeomin® therapy. *J Neurol*, **253**(Suppl 2), II/141.

Dressler, D. & Benecke, R. (2003). Autonomic side effects of botulinum toxin type B treatment of cervical dystonia and hyperhidrosis. *Eur Neurol*, **49**, 34–8.

Dressler, D. & Benecke, R. (2006). Xeomin® eine neue therapeutische Botulinum Toxin Typ A-Präparation. *Akt Neurol*, **33**, 138–41.

Dressler, D. & Dirnberger, G. (2000). Botulinum toxin therapy: risk factors for therapy failure. *Mov Disord*, **15**(Suppl 2), 51.

Dressler, D. & Eleopra, R. (2006). Clinical use of non-A botulinum toxins: botulinum toxin type B. *Neurotox Res*, **9**, 121–5.

Dressler, D. & Rothwell, J. C. (2000). Electromyographic quantification of the paralysing effect of botulinum toxin. *Eur Neurol*, **43**, 13–16.

Dressler, D., Eckert, J., Kukowski, B. & Meyer, B. U. (1993). Somatosensorisch Evozierte Potentiale bei Schreibkrampf: Normalisierung pathologischer Befunde unter Botulinum Toxin Therapie. *Z EEG EMG*, **24**, 191.

Dressler, D., Adib Saberi, F. & Benecke, R. (2002). Botulinum toxin type B for treatment of axillar hyperhidrosis. *J Neurol*, **249**, 1729–32.

Dressler, D., Rothwell, J. C. & Bigalke, H. (2000). The sternocleidomastoid test: an in-vivo assay to investigate botulinum toxin antibody formation in man. *J Neurol*, **247**, 630–2.

Duchen, L. W. (1971a). An electron microscopic study of the changes induced by botulinum toxin in the motor end-plates of slow and fast skeletal muscle fibres of the mouse. *J Neurol Sci*, **14**, 47–60.

Duchen, L. W. (1971b). Changes in the electron microscopic structure of slow and fast skeletal muscle fibres of the mouse after the local injection of botulinum toxin. *J Neurol Sci*, **14**, 61–74.

Erbguth, F., Claus, D., Engelhardt, A. & Dressler, D. (1993). Systemic effect of local botulinum toxin injections unmasks subclinical Lambert-Eaton myasthenic syndrome. *J Neurol Neurosurg Psychiatry*, **56**, 1235–6.

Filippi, G. M., Errico, P., Santarelli, R., Bagolini, B. & Manni, E. (1993). Botulinum A toxin effects on rat jaw muscle spindles. *Acta Otolaryngol*, **113**, 400–4.

Foran, P., Lawrence, G. W., Shone, C. C., Foster, K. A. & Dolly, J. O. (1996). Botulinum neurotoxin C1 cleaves both syntaxin and SNAP-25 in intact and permeabilized chromaffin cells: correlation with its blockade of catecholamine release. *Biochemistry*, **35**, 2630–6.

Girlanda, P., Vita, G., Nicolosi, C., Milone, S. & Messina, C. (1992). Botulinum toxin therapy: distant effects on neuromuscular transmission and autonomic nervous system. *J Neurol Neurosurg Psychiatry*, **55**, 844–5.

Ishikawa, H., Mitsui, Y., Yoshitomi, T., *et al.* (2000). Presynaptic effects of botulinum toxin type A on the neuronally evoked response of albino and pigmented rabbit iris sphincter and dilator muscles. *Jpn J Ophthalmol*, **44**, 106–9.

Jankovic, J., Vuong, K. D. & Ahsan, J. (2003). Comparison of efficacy and immunogenicity of original versus current botulinum toxin in cervical dystonia. *Neurology*, **60**, 1186–8.

Kaji, R., Kohara, N., Katayama, M., *et al.* (1995a). Muscle afferent block by intramuscular injection of lidocaine for the treatment of writer's cramp. *Muscle Nerve*, **18**, 234–5.

Kaji, R., Rothwell, J. C., Katayama, M., *et al.* (1995b). Tonic vibration reflex and muscle afferent block in writer's cramp. *Ann Neurol*, **138**, 155–62.

Lange, D. J., Brin, M. F., Warner, C. L., Fahn, S. & Lovelace, R. E. (1987). Distant effects of local injection of botulinum toxin. *Muscle Nerve*, **10**, 552–5.

McMahon, H., Foran, P. & Dolly, J. (1992). Tetanus toxin and botulinum toxins type A and B inhibit glutamate, gamma-aminobutyric acid, aspartate, and met-enkephalin release from synaptosomes: clues to the locus of action. *J Biol Chem*, **267**, 21338–43.

Morris, J., Jobling, P. & Gibbins, I. (2001). Differential inhibition by botulinum neurotoxin A of cotransmitters released from autonomic vasodilator neurons. *Am J Physiol Heart Circ Physiol*, **281**, 2124–32.

Olney, R. K., Aminoff, M. J., Gelb, D. J. & Lowenstein, D. H. (1988). Neuromuscular effects distant from the site of botulinum neurotoxin injection. *Neurology*, **38**, 1780–3.

Pellizzari, R., Rossetto, O., Schiavo, G. & Montecucco, C. (1999). Tetanus and botulinum neurotoxins: mechanism of action and therapeutic uses. *Philos Trans R Soc Lond B Biol Sci*, **354**, 259–68.

Pickett, A., Panjwani, N., O'Keeffe, R. S. (2003). Potency of type A botulinum toxin preparations in clinical use. 40th Annual Meeting of the Interagency Botulism Research Coordinating Committee (IBRCC), Nov. 2003, Atlanta, USA.

Probst, T. E., Heise, H., Heise, P., Benecke, R. & Dressler, D. (2002). Rare immunologic side effects of botulinum toxin therapy: brachial plexus neuropathy and dermatomyositis. *Mov Disord*, **17**(Suppl 5), S49.

Purkiss, J., Welch, M., Doward, S. & Foster, K. (2000). Capsaicin-stimulated release of substance P from cultured dorsal root ganglion neurons: involvement of two distinct mechanisms. *Biochem Pharmacol*, **59**, 1403–6.

Rosales, R. L., Arimura, K., Takenaga, S. & Osame, M. (1996). Extrafusal and intrafusal muscle effects in experimental botulinum toxin-A injection. *Muscle Nerve*, **19**, 488–96.

Sanders, D. B., Massey, E. W. & Buckley, E. G. (1986). Botulinum toxin for blepharospasm: single-fibre EMG studies. *Neurology*, **36**, 545–7.

Schiavo, G., Benfenati, F., Poulain, B., *et al.* (1992). Tetanus and botulinum-B neurotoxins block neurotransmitter release by proteolytic cleavage of synaptobrevin. *Nature*, **359**, 832–5.

Schiavo, G., Santucci, A., Dasgupta, B. R., *et al.* (1993). Botulinum neurotoxins serotypes A and E cleave SNAP-25 at distinct COOH-terminal peptide bonds. *FEBS Lett*, **335**, 99–103.

Setler, P. (2000). The biochemistry of botulinum toxin type B. *Neurology*, **55**(Suppl 5), S22–8.

Shone, C. C. & Melling, J. (1992). Inhibition of calcium-dependent release of noradrenaline from PC12 cells by botulinum type-A neurotoxin. Long-term effects of the neurotoxin on intact cells. *Eur J Biochem*, **207**, 1009–16.

Takamizawa, K., Iwamori, M., Kozaki, S., *et al.* (1986). TLC immunostaining characterization of Clostridium botulinum type A neurotoxin binding to gangliosides and free fatty acids. *FEBS Lett*, **201**, 229–32.

Welch, M. J., Purkiss, J. R. & Foster, K. A. (2000). Sensitivity of embryonic rat dorsal root ganglia neurons to Clostridium botulinum neurotoxins. *Toxicon*, **38**, 245–58.

Wiegand, H., Erdmann, G. & Wellhoner, H. H. (1976). 125I-labelled botulinum A neurotoxin: pharmacokinetics in cats after intramuscular injection. *Naunyn Schmiedebergs Arch Pharmacol*, **292**, 161–5.

Yamasaki, S., Baumeister, A., Binz, T., *et al.* (1994). Cleavage of members of the synaptobrevin/VAMP family by types D and F botulinal neurotoxins and tetanus toxin. *J Biol Chem*, **269**, 12764–72.

4

Immunological properties of botulinum toxins

Hans Bigalke, Dirk Dressler and Jürgen Frevert

Introduction

Botulinum toxins are used to treat a large number of muscle hyperactivity disorders, including dystonia, spasticity, and tremor, autonomic disorders, such as hyperhidrosis and hypersalivation, as well as facial wrinkles. Commercially available products differ with respect to serotype, formulation, and purity. Not all products are approved in all countries. Serotype A-containing products are Botox®, Dysport®, Chinese BoNT-A (CBTX-A) and Xeomin®, whereas NeuroBloc®/Myobloc® contains serotype B. The active ingredient in all products is botulinum neurotoxin (BoNT), a di-chain protein with a molecular weight of 150 kDa. Botulinum toxin type A (BoNT-A) inhibits release of acetylcholine by cleaving the soluble N-ethylmaleimide-sensitive factor attachment protein receptor (SNARE) protein SNAP 25 while BoNT type B (BoNT-B) cleaves vesicle-associated membrane protein (VAMP) II. Since BoNTs are foreign proteins, the human immune system may respond to them with the production of specific anti-BoNT antibodies (BoNT-AB). The probability of developing BoNT-AB increases with the BoNT doses applied (Göschel et al., 1997). Whether other drug-related factors might contribute to immune responses is discussed below. Patient-related factors may also be involved in triggering BoNT-AB formation. Recently, a patient was reported who was treated with Dysport for several years with good results until he developed BoNT-AB-induced therapy failure after he received BoNT following a wasp sting (Paus et al., 2006). Since components of wasp poison are effective immunostimulants, a preactivation of lymphocytes may have triggered BoNT-A-AB formation. In the following a method is presented for the quantification of BoNT-AB in sera, the immune cell reactions to antigens are described, and drug-related immune responses are discussed.

Methods for the detection and quantification of neutralizing BoNT-AB

A method used for detection of BoNT-AB must test the function of each domain of the neurotoxin: binding, translocation, as well as the catalytic activity of the enzyme in one assay or in a set of assays, because antibodies can be directed against each domain. If a single assay is to be developed, this can only be achieved by using intact cellular systems. The easiest method is to inject the toxin into animals, e.g. mice, and determine their survival rate. This assay, the so-called mouse bioassay, is presently considered the gold standard because the median lethal dose (MLD) can be determined very accurately. The MLD increases when BoNT-AB are present. With the help of a calibration curve, based upon standard BoNT-AB concentration, titers in patients' sera can be calculated. The test has, however, many disadvantages. It is

Manual of Botulinum Toxin Therapy, ed. Daniel Truong, Dirk Dressler and Mark Hallett. Published by Cambridge University Press.
© Cambridge University Press 2009.

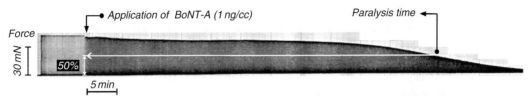

Figure 4.1 Development of paralysis. A mouse hemidiaphragm was continuously stimulated via the phrenic nerve at a frequency of 1 Hz. After equilibration the muscle was exposed to 1 ng/cc of BoNT-A. The arrows indicate when the toxin was applied and when the amplitude was reduced by 50% of its initial value, respectively. Paralysis time is defined as the time elapsed till the contraction amplitude has been halved.

costly, requires several days before it can be evaluated, and, most important, exposes the test animals to prolonged agony including respiratory failure. Since the end point of the test is the paralysis of the respiratory muscle, a truncated version of the test is represented by an isolated nerve-muscle, the phrenic-hemidiaphragm preparation (mouse diaphragm assay; MDA). When BoNT is applied to an organ bath in which a muscle has been placed, the contraction amplitude of the nerve-stimulated muscle continuously declines until it disappears completely (Figure 4.1). The contractions of the diaphragm can be recorded isometrically, using a commercially available force transducer, while commercially available software allows the analysis of the contraction amplitude over time. The time period between application of toxin to the organ bath and the point when the contraction amplitude is reduced to half of its original height (paralysis time or $t_{1/2}$) is used to characterize the efficacy and potency of the toxin. This paralysis time is closely correlated to the toxicity as measured in the MLD (Figure 4.2) (for details see Wohlfarth *et al.* [1997]). With the help of the MDA, it is possible to detect BoNT-AB quantitatively. Using a calibration curve with increasing concentrations of either standard BoNT-A-AB or BoNT-B-AB, antibody titers in sera can be measured (Figure 4.3) (Göschel *et al.*, 1997; Dressler *et al.*, 2005).

Reactions of the organism to botulinum toxin

A BoNT is a foreign protein that might be recognized by B-cells. B-cells bind BoNT with the help of

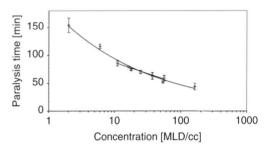

Figure 4.2 Concentration–response curves of a standard batch of BoNT-A. One curve was constructed using samples containing pure BoNT-A in a concentration range between 2 and 162 MLD/cc, the other from the same batch, however, in a range from 11 to 56 MLD/cc. The curve with the lower range was fitted by linear regression.

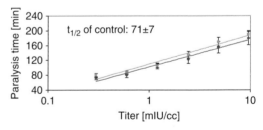

Figure 4.3 Calibration curves of anti-BoNT-A and -B. Antibody titers of anti-BoNT-A (upper) and anti-BoNT-B (lower) were plotted against the respective paralysis times in the *ex vivo* model ($n = 3 \pm$ SD). The standard antibody was taken from Botulism Antitoxin from Behring, Marburg, Germany (750 U/cc). Paralysis time in the antibody free control was 71 min. With increasing titers the paralysis time was prolonged. With the help of the paralysis time antibody titers in patients' sera can be calculated when these sera are supplemented with the same toxin concentration as used for the calibration curves.

specific, preformed antigen receptors. Subsequently, the BoNT is internalized and proteolysed to small peptides of 9–20 amino acids. These peptides are presented to the outside of the B-cells via the major histocompatability complex (MHC). T-helper cells bind to the antigen-presenting B-cells in addition to co-stimulatory molecules. As a result the T-cells release cytokines which, together with the MHC-bound peptides, stimulate the B-cells to differentiate into plasma cells. Plasma cells then produce and release specific BoNT-binding immunoglobulins, the BoNT-AB. The BoNT-AB protect the host either by neutralizing BoNT, which then loses its toxic properties, or by only binding the BoNT. These BoNT–BoNT-AB complexes may retain their toxicity, but are, due to the linked BoNT-AB, easily recognized and phagocyted by accessory cells (clearing antibodies, Shankar *et al.*, 2007).

Some exogenic factors can facilitate the immune response. It is well known that certain lectins, such as wheat germ agglutinin, phytohemagglutinin, concanavalin A, the B-unit of cholera toxin or ricin, and others (e.g. components of wasp venom) may stimulate immune cells. Thus, these lectins may act as immune adjuvants enhancing the antibody concentration. Another factor stimulating the immune responses is the amount of antigen exposed to the immune system. In the case of exposure to BoNT-A the probability of stimulating the immune system increases with the dose of BoNT applied (Göschel *et al.*, 1997).

Product specificity of immune responses

The therapeutic use of proteins is always associated with immune reactions. Even drugs based on proteins of human origin such as insulin, human growth hormone, and erythropoietin may induce antibody formation (Kromminga & Schellekens, 2005). The factors which trigger immunogenicity are impurities, aggregation, formulation, and degradation (e.g. oxidation). Besides these product-specific factors, host-specific factors (e.g. host immune competence) can also determine the immunological response (Kromminga & Schellekens, 2005).

Botulinum toxin is a foreign protein and per se immunogenic. Only administration in extremely small quantities and with long intervals may prevent formation of BoNT-AB. Nevertheless, in a small number of patients, BoNT elicits BoNT-AB formation which can inactivate the BoNT. The formation of BoNT-AB in sufficient quantities effectively terminates BoNT therapy (Herrmann *et al.*, 2004).

In the following, factors influencing the immunogenic potential of different BoNT drugs are discussed. Although Botox, Dysport, CBTX-A and Xeomin are based on the same active substance, the 150 kDa BoNT-A protein, they contain a different set of other clostridial proteins. Moreover, they are formulated differently. These differences can influence the immune response to the BoNT-containing drugs.

It has long been known that the complexing proteins (especially the hemagglutinins) elicit antibodies in 40–60% of patients treated with the complex-containing products (Göschel *et al.*, 1997; Critchfield, 2002), whereas the proportion of patients with BoNT-AB remains small. Antibodies against the complexing proteins do not interfere with the neurotoxins, whereas BoNT-AB will neutralize the BoNT and thus cause BoNT-AB-induced therapy failure (Göschel *et al.*, 1997).

Whereas the non-toxic non-hemagglutinating protein is responsible for binding the neurotoxin into the complex, some of the other complexing proteins are hemagglutinins. They act as lectins with high specificity to galactose-containing glycoproteins or glycolipids. Other lectins are known to act as immune adjuvants. For example the cell binding subunit of ricin which resembles one of the *Clostridium botulinum* hemagglutinins (HA 1) stimulates the antibody production against a virus antigen (Choi *et al.*, 2006).

Concomitant administration of an adjuvant strongly facilitates the immune response against a single antigen (Critchfield, 2002). In an immunization experiment, Lee *et al.* (2006) showed that hemagglutinins act as adjuvants, enhancing the antibody titer against BoNT-B. They also demonstrated a hemagglutinin-induced increase of the production of interleukin 6 (a B-cell-activating cytokine).

However, Lee *et al.* (2005) used a formalin inactivated toxin (toxoid) in a dose 100 000 times exceeding therapeutic doses. In addition, Lee *et al.* (2005) injected in weekly intervals not reflecting therapeutic recommendations, as already discussed by Atassi (2006). Therefore, it is difficult to estimate the immunological role of the complexing proteins when therapeutic doses are applied even though hemagglutinins possess an immune adjuvant activity.

The amount of BoNT exposed to the immune system is also influenced by the specific activity of the BoNT used in the therapeutic preparation (Göschel *et al.*, 1997; Dressler & Hallett, 2006). In Botox approximately 40% of the original BoNT activity is lost during the manufacturing process, thus producing toxoid that cannot be used for therapeutic purposes but which still acts as an antigen (Hunt, 2007).

The specific activity of Dysport (1 U = 25 pg) is higher than that of Botox (1 U = 50 pg), which can be partly explained by the different size of the complex. Whereas Botox consists of the 900 kDa complex, Dysport contains the 300 kDa complex besides the 600 kDa complex (Hambleton, 1992). There is no information about the specific activity of the active substance before formulation; therefore, it is not known if there is any denatured neurotoxin in the final product. Despite the fact that Dysport has to be administered numerically in three times higher doses than Botox, the actual dose applied is probably lower because, due to a low concentration of albumin in this product, some of the toxin binds irreversibly to glass and plastic surfaces. This bound toxin will not reach the patient's tissue; thus, the dose applied is probably as low as a respective dose of Botox (Bigalke *et al.*, 2001).

The active substance of Dysport shows some impurities not related to the complexing proteins (Pickett *et al.*, 2005). It is notable that a flagellin is present, a protein which is known for its immune stimulatory properties (Honko *et al.*, 2006). It reacts with the Toll like receptor 5 and induces the maturation of dendritic cells which activate T-cells. It was shown that the addition of flagellin to tetanus toxoid in a vaccination experiment enhanced the antibody titer against tetanus toxin (Lee *et al.*, 2006). However, as discussed above for Botox, the doses of adjuvant proteins applied experimentally were much higher than the doses given therapeutically and also in this case difficulties arise about the assessment of the role flagellin plays in patients treated with Dysport.

The immunogenic potential of the BoNT-B vs. BoNT-A is not well investigated. In persons vaccinated with the pentavalent botulinum toxoid vaccine, the antibody titer against BoNT-A is markedly higher than the antibody titer against BoNT-B (Siegel, 1989). But the vaccine contains the toxins inactivated by treatment with formalin, which could influence their antigenic potential. It has to be considered that BoNT-B is not fully activated. The unnicked, non-activated proportion of BoNT-B (about 25%) is inactive and could act as a toxoid (Aoki, 2002). The specific activity of NeuroBloc/ Myobloc is remarkably higher (1 U = 11 pg) than the specific activity of the type A complex-containing products, but this is only true when mice are involved. If one considers that a substantially higher dose of NeuroBloc/Myobloc than the dose of the toxin A-containing products has to be injected to achieve a comparable therapeutic effect the specific activity in humans is much lower (estimated 40 fold; Dressler [2006]). This substantially increases the risk of developing antibodies. Therefore, more than 40% of de novo patients treated with NeuroBloc/ Myobloc for cervical dystonia developed complete antibody-induced therapy failure after only a few treatments (Dressler & Bigalke, 2004). In Table 4.1 the average protein load for the treatment of cervical dystonia is summarized (nanogram = ng (10^{-9} g), picogram = pg (10^{-12} g)).

The relatively high amount of BoNT-B administered with NeuroBloc/Myobloc explains why patients develop antibodies and become non-responders to BoNT-B after a few injections (Dressler & Hallett, 2006), whereas the percentage of patients who have developed antibodies against the neurotoxins in Botox and Dysport is much lower, approximately 1–3% (Kessler *et al.*, 1999). Information about the

Table 4.1. Doses of botulinum toxin for the treatment of cervical dystonia

	Botox	Dysport	Xeomin	NeuroBloc/Myobloc
Average dose of units	200	600	200	8000
Amount of administered clostridial protein (ng)	10	15	1	88
Calculated amount of neurotoxin* (ng)	2	5	1	22

Note:
*Based on the calculated proportion of the neurotoxin in Botox of approximately 20% (150 kDa/900 kDa) in Dysport of 33% (150 kDa/(300 kDa + 600 kDa)/2 and 25% in NeuroBloc/Myobloc (150 kDa/600 kDa).

immune response against Xeomin, a product lacking any impurities and complexing proteins, is not available yet because of the short period of time it has been on the market. If one considers, however, that the total load of foreign proteins is the lowest of the available products (Table 4.1) and, moreover, that this product lacks potential immune-stimulating proteins, one would expect that the already low number of secondary non-responders to BoNT-A-containing products might be decreased even to lower levels.

REFERENCES

Aoki, K. R. (2002). Immunological and other properties of therapeutic botulinum toxin serotypes. In M. F., Brin, J. Jankovic & M. Hallett, eds., *Scientific and Therapeutic Aspects of Botulinum Toxin*. Philadelphia: Lippincott, Williams & Wilkins, pp. 103–13.

Atassi, M. Z. (2006). On the enhancement of anti-neurotoxin antibody production by subcomponents HA1 and HA3b of Clostridium botulinum type B 16S toxin-haemagglutinin. *Microbiology*, **152**(Pt 7), 1891–5.

Bigalke, H. Wohlfarth, K., Irmer, A. & Dengler, R. (2001). Botulinum A toxin: Dysport improvement of biological availability. *Exp Neurol*. **168**(1), 162–70.

Choi, N. W., Estes, M. K. & Langridge, W. H. (2006). Ricin toxin B subunit enhancement of rotavirus NSP4 immunogenicity in mice. *Viral Immunol*, **19**(1), 54–63.

Critchfield, J. (2002). Considering the immune response to botulinum toxin. *Clin J Pain*, **18**(6 Suppl), S133–41.

Dressler, D. (2006). Pharmacological aspects of therapeutic botulinum toxin preparations. *Nervenarzt*, **77**(8), 912–21.

Dressler, D. & Bigalke, H. (2004). Antibody-induced failure of botulinum toxin type B therapy in de novo patients. *Eur Neurol*, **52**(3), 132–5.

Dressler, D. & Hallett, M. (2006). Immunological aspects of Botox, Dysport and Myobloc/NeuroBloc. *Eur J Neurol*, **13**(Suppl 1), 11–15.

Dressler, D., Lange, M. & Bigalke, H. (2005). The mouse diaphragm assay for detection of antibodies against botulinum toxin type B. *Mov Disord*, **20**, 1617–19.

Göschel, H., Wohlfarth, K., Frevert, J., Dengler, R. & Bigalke, H. (1997). Botulinum A toxin therapy: neutralizing and nonneutralizing antibodies–therapeutic consequences. *Exp Neurol*, **147**(1), 96–102.

Hambleton, P. (1992). Clostridium botulinum toxins: a general review of involvement in disease, structure, mode of action and preparation for clinical use. *J Neurol*, **239**(1), 16–20.

Herrmann, J., Geth, K., Mall, V., *et al.* (2004). Clinical impact of antibody formation to botulinum toxin in children. *Ann Neurol*, **55**, 732–5.

Honko, A. N., Sriranganathan, N., Lees, C. J. & Mizel, S. B. (2006). Flagellin is an effective adjuvant for immunization against lethal respiratory challenge with Yersinia pestis. *Infect Immun*, **74**(2), 1113–20.

Hunt, T. J. (2007). *Botulinum Toxin Composition*, US Patent application 2007/0025019.

Kessler, K. R., Skutta, M. & Benecke, R. (1999). Long-term treatment of cervical dystonia with botulinum toxin A: efficacy, safety, and antibody frequency. German Dystonia Study Group. *J Neurol*, **246**, 265–74.

Kromminga, A. & Schellekens, H. (2005). Antibodies against erythropoietin and other protein-based therapeutics: an overview. *Ann N Y Acad Sci*, **1050**, 257–65.

Lee, J. C., Yokota, K., Arimitsu, H., *et al.* (2005). Production of anti-neurotoxin antibody is enhanced by two subcomponents, HA1 and HA3b, of Clostridium botulinum type B 16S toxin-haemagglutinin. *Microbiology*, **151**(Pt 11), 3739–47.

Lee, S. E., Kim, S. Y., Jeong, B. C., *et al.* (2006). A bacterial flagellin, Vibrio vulnificus FlaB, has a strong mucosal adjuvant activity to induce protective immunity. *Infect Immun*, **74**(1), 694–702.

Paus, S., Bigalke, H. & Klockgether, T. (2006). Neutralizing antibodies against botulinum toxin a after a wasp sting. *Arch Neurol*, **63**(12), 1808–9.

Pickett, A., Shipley, S., Panjwani, N., O'Keeffe, R. & Singh, B. R. (2005). Characterization and consistency of botulinum type A toxin complex (Dysport) used for clinical therapy. *Neurotoxicity Res*, **9**, p. 46.

Shankar, G., Pendley, C. & Stein, K. E. (2007). A risk-based bioanalytical strategy for the assessment of antibody immune responses against biological drugs. *Nat Biotechnol*, **25**(5), 555–61.

Siegel, L. S. (1989). Evaluation of neutralizing antibodies to type A, B, E, and F botulinum toxins in sera from human recipients of botulinum pentavalent (ABCDE) toxoid. *J Clin Microbiol*, **27**(8), 1906–8.

Wohlfarth, K., Goschel, H., Frevert, J., Dengler, R. & Bigalke, H. (1997). Botulinum A toxins: units versus units. *Naunyn Schmiedebergs Arch Pharmacol*, **355**(3), 335–40.

Treatment of cervical dystonia

Reiner Benecke, Karen Frei and Cynthia L. Comella

Introduction

Cervical dystonia (CD), originally known as spasmodic torticollis and first described by Foltz in 1959, is a neurological syndrome characterized by abnormal head and neck posture due to tonic involuntary contractions in a set of cervical muscles (Foltz *et al.*, 1959). Myoclonic or tremulous movements are often superimposed in CD, producing a "tremor like" appearance – especially early in the disease state. The terms CD and spasmodic torticollis are not interchangeable: CD is the preferred term when referring to idiopathic focal dystonia of the neck. Spasmodic torticollis is now considered to be one of four types of CD. Cervical dystonia is classified into four types based on the principal direction of head posture: torticollis (abnormal rotation of the head to the right or to the left in the transverse plane); laterocollis (the head tilts toward the right or left shoulder); anterocollis (the head pulls forward with neck flexion); and retrocollis (the head pulls back with the neck hyperextended).

Cervical dystonia is slightly more common in females, with a male to female ratio of 1:1.2 (Kessler *et al.*, 1999). Onset is usually insidious, although in some patients the onset has been reported as sudden. Cervical dystonia may develop in patients of all age groups, but the peak age of onset is 41 years (Kessler *et al.*, 1999). Idiopathic CD usually progresses in severity over the first five years until it reaches a plateau, during which time the CD remains fairly constant and becomes a lifelong condition. Although remission can occur, it is rare and the dystonia usually returns after a period of time. The cervical component may also exist as part of a more extensive form of dystonia, in which the dystonia can spread to involve adjacent structures such as the face or the arm(s). When dystonia involves several contiguous body parts, it is considered segmental dystonia. When it involves several parts of the body that are not contiguous, such as the neck and foot, it is called multifocal, and when involving the majority of the body, it is referred to as generalized dystonia.

Characteristic traits of CD include transient relief from symptoms with a sensory trick or "geste antagoniste." A common form of a sensory trick in CD is placing the hand lightly on the cheek. This allows the head to return to a more normal posture. Resting the head against the headrest while driving or against a pillow while watching TV are examples of sensory tricks. Patients may obtain temporary relief from symptoms of CD in the morning hours following sleep; this is referred to as the "honeymoon" effect (Truong *et al.*, 1991). Stress can exacerbate symptoms of CD. Neck pain is common in CD and has been reported in 70–80% of affected patients (Van Zandijcke, 1995). Cervical dystonia is often a major source of disability. The pain appears

Manual of Botulinum Toxin Therapy, ed. Daniel Truong, Dirk Dressler and Mark Hallett. Published by Cambridge University Press.
© Cambridge University Press 2009.

to diffuse throughout the neck and shoulders with some radiation toward the side to which the head is twisted. Pain does not appear to be correlated with the degree of severity of CD, and is thought to involve central mechanisms in addition to pain arising from muscle spasms (Kutvonen et al., 1997). Degenerative disc disease seems to be accelerated in CD, which can aggravate the pain associated with this disorder. Depression, anxiety, and social phobia are also common associated conditions.

There are no diagnostic tests for CD. However, multichannel electromyography (EMG) may help to elicit the involved muscle patterns producing the particular posture. Electromyographic evidence of prolonged bursts of electrical activity that correlate with the involved musculature is helpful in diagnosing CD. Testing agonist/antagonist pairs of muscles allows the comparison of overall activity, which can also assist in distinguishing the most active muscles involved in producing the CD posture. Conventional brain magnetic resonance imaging (MRI) is usually normal; cervical MRI may show cervical muscle hypertrophy and cervical disc disease – this can be helpful but is not diagnostic.

Most often, the cause of CD is unknown. In the first part of the last century, CD was thought to be of psychogenic origin, although today an organic basis for the syndrome is well accepted. There are cases of hereditable forms of CD, such as DYT7, but the majority of hereditable dystonia types are variable in presentation and may include different forms of dystonia, such as blepharospasm, limb dystonia, and CD. Hereditable forms of dystonia generally have autosomal dominant transmission and incomplete penetrance. With the incomplete penetrance of these disorders, not all family members with the gene mutation will have dystonia. Moreover, affected family members may present with different signs/symptoms in different body regions – not all affected family members will have CD. Cervical dystonia is often a component of various secondary dystonias that manifest in a number of neurodegenerative diseases. Secondary causes of CD include neuroleptic medication exposure or trauma. A form of CD known as post-

traumatic CD may occur following a relatively mild trauma. This form usually begins within days of an incident, lacks the sensory trick response and tends to be more resistant to treatment with botulinum toxin (BoNT) (Truong et al., 1991; Frei et al., 2004). The role of trauma, however, remains controversial.

The clinical spectrum of abnormal head and neck posture is extremely variable. The reason for this is the wide variety of the dystonic muscle patterns within the 54 muscles affecting action on head and neck posture. Furthermore, muscles can be involved on one side or on both sides. Dystonic muscles can show a dominant tonic activity, myoclonic or tremulous activity often in complex mixtures. The extent of secondary changes in the muscles and connective and bony tissues may present differently from patient to patient and in their contribution to abnormal postures.

Intramuscular injections of BoNT are considered the first line of treatment in CD. Both botulinum toxin serotype A (BoNT-A) (old and new Botox®, Dysport®, Xeomin®) and serotype B (BoNT-B) (NeuroBloc®/Myobloc®) have been used. Medications such as the anticholinergic trihexyphenidyl (Artane®) and benztropine (Cogentin®) have some beneficial effects and can be used in more severe cases alongside BoNT injections. Other medications that have mild or limited usefulness include benzodiazepines, such as diazepam (Valium®) or lorazepam (Ativan®), and tricyclic antidepressants, such as amitriptyline (Elavil®) and nortriptyline (Pamelor®).

Surgical treatment with selective peripheral denervation has been reported in open studies to be helpful in some severe cases that do not respond to either oral medications or chemodenervation. Surgical myectomy has also been used; however, the dystonia tends to involve other muscles or continues to involve remnants of the resected muscles, thus producing less favorable results. Deep brain stimulation, with electrodes placed in the globus pallidus interna, has been successfully used for treatment of generalized dystonia. Although there have been less consistent results in treating CD with this method, improvements may be possible with further development of electrode placement and/or programming.

BoNT in CD

Botulinum toxin injections into the affected muscles remain the most effective treatment for CD. In 1985, Tsui and colleagues (Tsui *et al.*, 1985) published the results of BoNT-A injections into the neck muscles of 12 patients with CD, and followed a year later with a double-blind, placebo-controlled trial in 21 patients (Tsui *et al.*, 1986). Since then, several controlled trials have confirmed that BoNT-A injections improve CD (Blackie & Lees, 1990; Greene *et al.*, 1990; Lorentz *et al.*, 1991; Moore & Blumhardt, 1991), with only one exception (Gelb *et al.*, 1989). A number of open trials have clearly demonstrated the benefits of repeated neck muscle BoNT-A injections for up to 4 years in large numbers of patients (Blackie & Lees, 1990; Jankovic & Schwartz, 1990; Anderson *et al.*, 1992; Kessler *et al.*, 1999). In a double-blind study by Naumann and colleagues (Naumann *et al.*, 2002), 133 patients were injected with BoNT-A (Botox), produced from original and current bulk toxin sources, using a crossover design. The percentage improvement measured by Toronto Western Spasmodic Torticollis Rating Scale (TWSTRS) severity amounted to about 35% after injections of both toxin sources.

Three double-blind, placebo-controlled studies using BoNT-B (NeuroBloc) for treatment of CD have been performed. One study tested BoNT-B in unselected patients with CD (Lew *et al.*, 1997). Another study examined BoNT-B in patients who were responsive to BoNT-B injections, and compared placebo vs. BoNT-B 5000 (mouse) units vs. 10 000 units (Brashear *et al.*, 1999). A further study tested BoNT-B in patients who were BoNT-A resistant, comparing placebo vs. BoNT-B 10 000 units (Brin *et al.*, 1999). In all studies TWSTRS total scores significantly improved from baseline 2 weeks after BoNT-B, with the greater improvement observed in the 10 000 units group.

Table 5.1 provides a summary of the effects of BoNT-A and BoNT-B treatment in CD as published in a number of open and double-blind investigations (Tsui *et al.*, 1986; Gelb *et al.*, 1989; Stell *et al.*, 1989; Blackie & Lees, 1990; Greene *et al.*, 1990; Jankovic & Schwartz, 1990; Jankovic & Brin, 1991; Hambleton *et al.*, 1992; Benecke, 1993; Hatheway & Dang, 1994; Benecke, 1999; Kessler *et al.*, 1999; Naumann *et al.*, 2002; Benecke *et al.*, 2005). Studies are listed that evaluated responder rates and/or percentage improvements only.

Botulinum toxin therapy is indicated in all forms of CD. Worsening of CD while being treated with BoNT could be due to resistance of BoNT or the result of an actual increase in severity – often, wrong muscles have been injected. Treatment with BoNT should be initiated as early as possible, since secondary changes to the muscles involved (contractures) and of connective tissues, bony tissues, and cervical discs may occur with longstanding CD.

Botulinum toxin treatment results in the improvement of neck posture, muscle hypertrophy, and pain. The effect of BoNT begins 3–12 days after an injection and is sustained for approximately 3 months. Injections at 3-month intervals (or longer) are thought to reduce the risk of antibodies to the BoNT. Less experienced physicians should perform EMG recordings from sternocleidomastoid, splenius capitis, trapezius (upper portion), and levator scapulae muscles to confirm their clinical impression on the basis of head posture and muscle palpation – especially prior to the first BoNT treatment session. Needle EMG is needed for deeper muscles, but sometimes can even be useful for superficial muscles when they are close together. Electromyography may also be useful when response to BoNT treatment becomes unsatisfactory in order to determine whether injected muscles are denervated and to assist in identifying overactive muscles that may not have been injected. There may also be a change in the dystonic posturing of the head. Electromyography can assist in modifying injection pattern when this occurs.

The number of injection sites within a muscle ranges from one site in smaller muscles to eight sites in larger muscles. There is little evidence to assist in determining the optimum number

Table 5.1. Treatment effects of BoNT injections in CD

Study	Number of patients	Dose (units)	Responder (%) Dystonia	Responder (%) Pain	Scale	Improvement (%)
Botox (BoNT-A)						
Tsui et al., 1986[a]	19	100	63	89	Tsui	30
Gelb et al., 1989[a]	20	280	15	50	Tsui	20
Gelb et al., 1991[a]	28	280	32	64	Tsui	20
Greene et al., 1990[a]	34	240	74	?	GIR (0–3)	33
Jankovic & Schwartz, 1990[b]	195	209	90	93	GIR (0–4)	> 50
Comella et al., 1992[b]	52	374	71	86	TWSTRS	> 10
Naumann et al., 2002[b]	133	155	100*	100*	TWSTRS	> 10
Xeomin (BoNT-A)						
Benecke et al., 2005[b]	231	140	?	?	TWSTRS	40
Dysport (BoNT-A)						
Blackie & Lees, 1990[a]	19	960	84	75	Tsui	22
Stell et al., 1989[b]	10	1200	90	100	Tsui	47
Poewe et al., 1992[b]	37	632	86	84	Tsui	> 50
Wissel & Poewe, 1992[b]	180	594	85	85	Tsui	> 50
Kessler et al., 1999[b]	616	778	89	92	Tsui	> 60
NeuroBloc (BoNT-B)						
Lew et al., 1997[a]	27	10 000	77	83	TWSTRS	?

Note:
[a]Double-blind study, [b]open study,
TWSTRS = Toronto Western Spasmodic Torticollis Rating Scale, GIR = Global Improvement Rating.
*(comparative study of two Botox preparations only including responders – pain reduction 52%).

of injection sites. Although a study by Borodic and colleagues (Borodic et al., 1992) suggests that multiple injection sites may provide an improved result, this has not been adequately evaluated. Multiple injections with smaller doses might well also limit diffusion and reduce side effects. This might be particularly relevant in the neck, where dysphagia might result if there is excessive spread. Patients should be reexamined prior to each treatment. Muscle hypertrophy and involved muscle patterns may change over time, necessitating the alteration of injection sites over the course of repeated treatments. It is important to document the injected muscles as well as the dosage given. Upon follow up, this can help when adjusting injection patterns and dosage.

Neck muscles and their functions

Iliocostalis cervicis

The iliocostalis cervicis arises from the angles of the third, fourth, fifth, and sixth ribs, and is inserted into the posterior tubercles of the transverse processes of the fourth to sixth cervical vertebrae. The iliocostalis flexes the head laterally. When both iliocostalis cervicis are activated bilaterally they extend the neck dorsally (see Figure 5.1).

Interspinalis cervicis

These muscles lie between the spinosus processes of the cervical vertebrae. They assist in dorsal extension (see Figure 5.1).

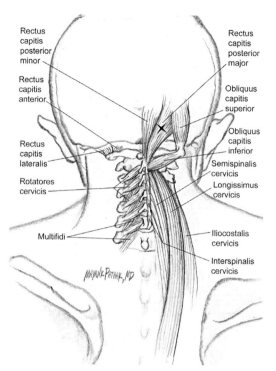

Figure 5.1 Most important neck muscles which play some role in retrocollis, but are usually not injected. The sign X denotes approximate injection site.

Intertransversarii cervicis

These muscles are placed in pairs, passing between the anterior and the posterior tubercles respectively to the transverse processes of two contiguous vertebrae. The anterior primary division of the cervical nerve separates the intertransversarii anteriores cervicis muscle from the posterior intertransversarii. They assist in the lateral and the dorsal flexion of the neck (see Figure 5.2).

Levator scapulae

The levator scapulae arises from the transverse processes of the first four cervical vertebrae and inserts into the medial border of the scapula. This muscle elevates the medial border of the scapula while rotating the lateral angle downward. Together with the rhomboid and trapezius, it pulls the scapula

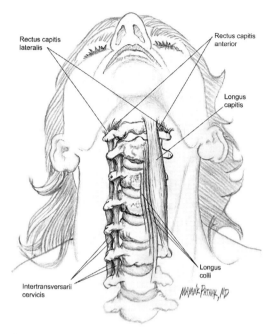

Figure 5.2 Juxta-vertebral muscles of the neck. The muscle longus colli is sometimes injected in anterocollis.

upward and medially, as well as tilts the neck ipsilaterally (see Figure 5.3).

Longissimus cervicis

The longissimus is located laterally to the semispinalis. It is the longest subdivision of the sacrospinalis that extends forward into the transverse processes of the posterior cervical vertebrae. Arising from long, thin tendons from the transverse processes of the upper four or five thoracic vertebrae, it is inserted into the posterior tubercles of the transverse processes of the cervical vertebrae from the second to the sixth. It tilts the head ipsilaterally. When the longissimus cervicis muscles are activated bilaterally, they extend the neck dorsally (see Figure 5.1).

Longus capitis

The longus capitis arises by four tendinous slips, from the anterior tubercles of the transverse processes

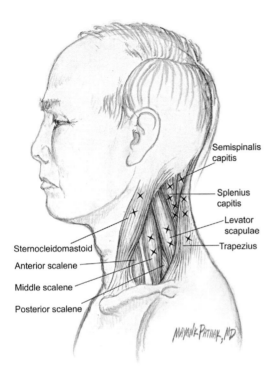

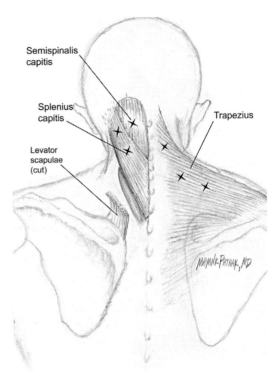

Figure 5.3 Muscles of importance for genesis and treatment of torticollis. The sternocleidomastoid muscle is injected contralaterally whereas the other muscles are injected on the ipsilateral side. The sign X denotes approximate injection site.

of the third, fourth, fifth, and sixth cervical vertebrae, and ascends, converging toward its fellow of the opposite side, to be inserted into the inferior surface of the basilar part of the occipital bone (see Figure 5.2).

Longus colli

The longus colli originates from the lower anterior vertebral bodies and transverse processes and inserts into the anterior vertebral bodies and transverse processes several segments above, flexing the head (see Figure 5.2).

Multifidi

The multifidus muscle fills up the groove on each side of the spinous processes of the vertebrae.

Figure 5.4 Superficial muscles of the neck. The sign X denotes approximate injection site.

It arises, in the cervical region, from the articular processes of the lower four vertebrae and inserts into the spinous process of one of the vertebrae above. It rotates the neck contralaterally. When both multifidi are activated they extend the neck (see Figure 5.1).

Obliquus capitis inferior

This muscle arises from the spinous process of the axis and inserts into the inferior and dorsal part of the transverse process of the atlas. It rotates the head and the first cervical vertebra ipsilaterally (see Figure 5.1).

Obliquus capitis superior

The obliquus capitis superior originates in the atlas mass, inserting into the lateral half of the inferior nuchal line of the occipital bone. At the atlanto-occipital joint, it extends and flexes the head ipsilaterally (see Figure 5.1).

Rectus capitis anterior

The rectus capitis anterior is a small muscle originating in the anterior base of the transverse process of the atlas and inserting into the occipital bone anterior to the foramen magnum, flexing the head. Furthermore, the rectus capitis anterior stabilizes the atlanto-occipital joint (see Figure 5.1).

Rectus capitis lateralis

The rectus capitis lateralis originates in the transverse process of the atlas and inserts into the jugular process of the occipital bone. It tilts the head laterally (see Figure 5.1).

Rectus capitis posterior major

This muscle arises from the spinous process of the axis, ascending into the lateral part of the inferior nuchal line of the occipital bone. As the two muscles of the two recti capitis posteriores majores pass upward and lateralward, they create a triangular space occupied by the recti capitis posteriores minores. The rectus capitis posterior major extends the head and rotates it to the same side (see Figure 5.1).

Rectus capitis posterior minor

The rectus capitis posterior minor is a muscle of triangular form and arises from the posterior arch of the atlas, inserting into the medial part of the occipital bone at, and below, the nuchal line. It extends the head (see Figure 5.1).

Rotatores cervicis

The rotatores cervicis arises from the transverse spinosus process and inserts into the above vertebrae, extending the neck and assisting in contralateral rotation (see Figure 5.1).

Anterior scalene

The scalene are lateral vertebral muscles that begin at the first and second ribs and pass up into the sides of the neck. There are three of these muscles. The anterior scalene originates in the anterior tubercles of the transverse processes, C3–C6, and inserts into the first rib. It elevates the ribs for respiration and rotates the head contralaterally. When both anterior scalene are contracted they flex the head forward (see Figure 5.3).

Middle scalene

The middle scalene arises from the transverse processes of all cervical vertebrae and inserts into the first rib (behind anterior scalene). It has the same function as the anterior scalene (see Figure 5.3).

Posterior scalene

This muscle arises from the posterior tubercles of the transverse processes, C5 and C6, and inserts into the second and/or third rib. The action of the posterior scalene is to elevate the second rib and tilt the neck to the same side (see Figure 5.3).

Semispinalis capitis

The semispinalis capitis originates in the transverse processes of the sixth thoracic vertebra and the seventh cervical vertebra, as well as the articular processes of the sixth to the fourth cervical vertebrae. It inserts between the superior and inferior nuchal lines of the occipital bone. The semispinalis capitis is often a cause of neck pain. Even though its main action is extension, restriction in this muscle can cause pain on rotation at the end of the range. It also rotates the head to the opposite side (see Figure 5.3).

Semispinalis cervicis

This muscle arises from the transverse processes of the upper five or six thoracic vertebrae. It inserts into the C2–C5 spinous processes. The semispinalis tilts the head to the same side and rotates the head to the contralateral side. Working together, the two semispinalis cervicis extend the head backward. The semispinalis capitis and cervicis, and longissimus capitis are commonly overused due to their role in supporting the head when leaning forward. They are often involved in headache pain (see Figure 5.1).

Splenius capitis

The splenius capitis originates in the process spinosus of the seventh cervical spine body and the first to third thoracic cervical body. It inserts into the mastoid process. This muscle turns and tilts the head ipsilaterally. Together, the two splenius capitis muscles extend the head backward (see Figure 5.4).

Splenius cervicis

This muscle arises from the spinosus processes of the third to sixth thoracic vertebrae. It is inserted, by tendinous fasciculi, into the posterior tubercles of the transverse processes of the upper three cervical vertebrae. This muscle turns the head ipsilaterally. When both splenius cervicis are activated, they extend the head backwards (see Figure 5.4).

Sternocleidomastoid

This muscle originates on the mastoid processes and inserts in two areas, one on the sternum and the other on the clavicle, hence the name sternocleidomastoid. It turns the head to the opposite side, and the chin upward to the opposite side. It also tilts the head to the same side (see Figure 5.3).

Trapezius

The trapezius originates from the occipital protuberante, the ligamentum nuchae and the processes spinosus, and inserts into the lateral third of the clavicular. The trapezius turns the head and neck

contralaterally. It also elevates the shoulder (see Figure 5.4).

Muscles involved in different subtypes of CD

Based on the presentation of the head position (see Figure 5.5), different muscles are involved. The anatomic localization, however, limits the muscles that can be treated. Tables 5.2 to 5.5 list the muscles which are anatomically involved and which are actually injected in torticollis (Table 5.2), in laterocollis (Table 5.3), in anterocollis (Table 5.4), and in retrocollis (Table 5.5).

Practical considerations for BoNT treatment of CD

The following questions must be answered before BoNT therapy of CD is considered:
1. Is the abnormal posture of the head and of the shoulder induced by dystonia or by another abnormality that only imitates CD?
2. Is the CD the primary cause of disability?
3. Does the patient have myasthenia gravis or other neuromuscular junction disorders?
4. Are there already secondary changes of muscles or connective and bony tissues?

Physical examination of the CD patient

A high level of patient cooperation during the physical examination is necessary. Patients must be requested to release any compensatory voluntary muscle activities in non-dystonic muscles, avoid the use of sensory tricks (geste antagoniste), and report accurately on pain severity. They should be asked to perform slow head movements in all common directions: evaluation of head posture is performed with the patient standing, walking slowly, and lying down. In a seated position, the

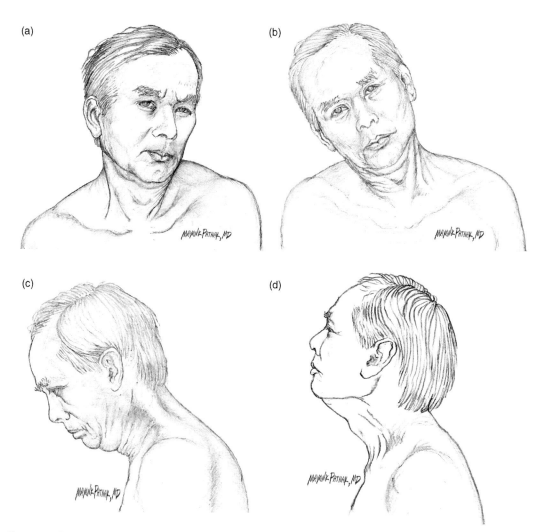

Figure 5.5 Illustration of postural abnormalities in pure forms of cervical dystonia: (a) Torticollis, (b) Laterocollis, (c) Anterocollis, (d) Retrocollis.

patient should be asked to demonstrate his/her favorite sensory trick (e.g. touching the chin with the right hand). Finally, patients should be asked to hold their heads in a neutral position, with assistance of antagonistic compensatory muscle activity, as long as possible.

Videotape documentation is always recommended as a means of documenting the examination.

Common CD rating scales include the TWSTRS and the Tsui scale. Such rating scales are not only recommended for clinical trials, but also for routine evaluation of CD and of BoNT treatment. They provide an objective detection of improvement of CD after BoNT injections, or lack of improvement in those patients who have developed antibodies.

Table 5.2. Muscles anatomically involved and muscles commonly injected in torticollis

Muscle name	Ipsilateral	Contralateral	Treated muscles
Splenius capitis and cervicis	X		X
Levator scapulae	X		X
Longissimus capitis and cervicis	X		X
Multifidi	X		
Rotatores cervicis	X		
Sternocleidomastoid		X	X
Anterior and middle scalene		X	X
Trapezius (upper part)		X	X
Semispinalis capitis and cervicis		X	X

Table 5.3. Muscles anatomically involved and muscles commonly injected in laterocollis

Muscle name	Ipsilateral	Contralateral	Treated muscles
Sternocleidomastoid	X		X
Trapezius	X		X
Middle and posterior scalene	X		X
Splenius capitis and cervicis	X		X
Longissimus capitis and cervicis	X		X
Multifidi	X		
Intertransversarii cervicis	X		

Table 5.4. Muscles anatomically involved and muscles commonly injected in anterocollis

Muscle name	Ipsilateral	Contralateral	Treated muscles
Sternocleidomastoid	X	X	X
Scaleni	X	X	X
Longus colli	X	X	X
Longus capitis	X	X	
Infrahyoid muscle	X	X	
Rectus capitis anterior	X	X	

BoNT injection procedure

Physicians should obtain written, informed consent from the patient. Possible adverse effects and procedure complications should be clearly explained to the patient, and the discussion documented in the patient's chart.

Muscle selection for treatment with BoNT is the next important step in developing an injection plan. Although there are 54 muscles that influence head and neck posture, as well as shoulder position, only a limited number of muscles are important to consider for injections. These muscles are the larger neck muscles that may be the most important factors in the abnormal postures.

The correct selection of doses for each individual muscle is the next step in the decision-making process, and perhaps the most difficult and most important part of BoNT treatment of CD. These decisions determine the success of treatment in

Table 5.5. Muscles anatomically involved and muscles commonly injected in retrocollis

Muscle name	Ipsilateral	Contralateral	Treated muscles
Levator scapulae	X	X	X
Splenius capitis and cervicis	X	X	X
Longissimus capitis and cervicis	X	X	X
Semispinalis capitis and cervicis	X	X	X
Iliocostalis cervicis	X	X	
Spinalis capitis and cervicis	X	X	
Rectus capitis posterior major and minor	X	X	
Rotatores cervicis	X	X	
Interspinalis cervicis	X	X	
Intertransversarii cervicis	X	X	

Table 5.6. Recommendations for total doses (units) in pure torticollis, laterocollis or combined forms in dependency on CD severity measured by the Tsui Score

Score	Botox	Xeomin	Dysport	NeuroBloc
12–15	200	200	800	10 000
9–12	150–200	150–200	600–800	7500–10 000
6–9	100–150	100–150	400–600	5000–7500
3–6	80–120	80–120	320–480	4000–6000

an individual patient. Some general comments regarding BoNT dosing are as follows:

1. Total and individual muscle doses may be higher in younger patients.
2. Women with small necks usually require smaller doses.
3. Men with larger necks or an athletic physique may require higher doses.
4. In cases of bilateral injections in the sternocleidomastoid and infrahyoid muscles, the dose per muscle is half of the regular dose.
5. In cases of bilateral injection into the splenius capitis and semispinalis capitis muscles, the individual dose per muscle should be reduced to 60% of the regular dose to prevent neck weakness.

The requirement of decreased doses in cases of bilateral injections results from increased severity and prevalence of side effects. Swallowing problems happen more frequently in cases of bilateral injections to the sternocleidomastoid and the infrahyoid muscles. Neck muscle weakness, which may cause problems with holding the head upright, is more frequent if injecting splenius capitis and semispinalis capitis muscles bilaterally.

Dose finding with the first injection treatment is more difficult than with subsequent treatments because the individual sensitivity of the muscles to the toxin and the probability of developing side effects are not known. In the case of an average patient (suffering from pure torticollis, laterocollis or a combination of these abnormal head postures), the recommended total dose depends on the severity of CD. In general, a lower dose is used initially in the newly diagnosed CD patient. Recommended total doses for the three products on the US market are given in Table 5.6. The total dose is divided into various portions, which are injected into individual dystonic muscles. Table 5.7 summarizes established dose ranges for the most important head and neck muscles. As can be derived from this table, there is an approximate relationship in doses between the four products on the market (Botox vs. Xeomin vs. Dysport vs. NeuroBloc/Myobloc = 1:1:4:50). Thus far, there is

Table 5.7. Recommended doses for individual muscles involved in CD

Muscle	Botox (units)	Xeomin (units)	Dysport (units)	NeuroBloc (units)
Sternocleidomastoid	20–50	20–50	0–200	1000–2500
Infrahyoid muscles	10–15	10–15	40–60	500–750
Anterior scalene	10–20	10–20	40–80	500–1000
Middle scalene	10–20	10–20	40–80	500–1000
Posterior scalene	10–20	10–20	40–80	500–1000
Levator scapulae	10–25	10–25	40–100	500–1250
Trapezius (upper portion)	20–50	20–50	80–200	1000–2500
Splenius capitis	50–100	50–100	200–400	2500–5000
Semispinalis capitis	15–30	15–30	60–120	750–1500

Note:
In bilateral injections of some muscles dose reduction is necessary (see text).

no evidence to support the superiority of one brand of BoNT-A (Botox, Xeomin, and Dysport).

In a recent study (Benecke *et al.*, 2005), a new BoNT-A free of complexing proteins (Xeomin) was compared with Botox in patients with CD by means of a double-blind, non-inferiority trial. This study showed that Xeomin is not inferior to Botox and has a similar safety profile.

Side effects of BoNT include hypersensitivity reactions, injection site infections, injection site bleeding or bruising, dry mouth, dysphagia, upper respiratory infection, neck pain, and headache. With bilateral posterior neck injections, neck weakness may occur, usually manifested by a feeling of instability when leaning forward or backward and often associated with pain. Dysphagia is associated with injections into the sternocleidomastoid muscle and is thought to be caused by the spread of the toxin locally. Transient muscle weakness may occur in muscles located adjacent to the injection site as a result of toxin diffusion.

To reduce the risk of developing resistance, a 3-month interval between injections is recommended. Prior to repeat injection, the patient should be asked to report on the effectiveness of the last injection, its time course and the type, severity, and duration of side effects. A clinical rating should be repeated and the actual scores be compared with those prior to and 4 weeks after the last injection.

Some patients will return prior to a waning effect of the toxin. In these cases, because the muscles are still denervated, it can be difficult to localize them for reinjection. If possible, these patients should be discouraged from receiving a repeat injection at that time, and be rescheduled for injection 2–4 weeks later when symptoms begin to appear. If the patient fulfills the criteria for a reinjection, total dose, dose per individual muscle, and selection of muscles to be injected must be reconsidered.

Making a change to the individual injection plan depends on the effectiveness and the side effects of the previous injection(s). The total dose should be decreased if severe side effects occur. If dysphagia occurs, the dose for the sternocleidomastoid muscle(s) should be decreased. If neck pain and/or neck weakness are prominent side effects, the dose for the splenius capitis muscle(s) should be reduced. The total dose should be increased when the peak effect (improvement) is less than 50–60%, or when the duration of the plateau phase is shorter than 4 weeks – provided side effects of clinical relevance do not occur. A change in the injection plan may need to be performed especially in cases where high-dose therapy and/or considerable side effects, in conjunction with only low or moderate effectiveness, occur. Selection of the muscles to be injected may have to be reconsidered, preferably with assistance of EMG.

The official recommendation from the manufacturers is to reconstitute 100 units Botox or 500 units Dysport in either 1 cc or 2.5 cc unpreserved NaCl solution, respectively. One hundred units of Xeomin are mostly dissolved in 2.0 cc NaCl solution. Neuro-Bloc does not require reconstitution, and is already in a solution of 5000 units/cc. Systematic studies dealing with any differences in effectiveness at various concentrations of Botox and Dysport are not available for treatment of CD; however, it is the experience of the authors that solutions of 400 units/cc, in the case of Dysport, and of 100 units/cc, in the case of Botox, may decrease the prevalence of side effects (Davis *et al.*, 1991; Bertrand, 1993; Kessler *et al.*, 1999). This observation may be due to a less pronounced diffusion of the toxins injected at lower volumes, especially in cases of injections into the sternocleidomastoid muscle.

Notes regarding muscle injections

Prior to sternocleidomastoid muscle injections, the patient should be asked to tonically activate the muscle by rotating their head against the hand of the physician or their own hand, placed at the opposite chin side. In this condition, the sternocleidomastoid muscle will become maximally prominent; furthermore, the safety of injection sites can be improved when the sternocleidomastoid muscle is held firmly with the physician's fingers while reaching behind the muscle. This maneuver is especially important in patients with obese necks. It is also recommended to concentrate the treatment on two injection sites in the upper third of the sternocleidomastoid muscle in order to reduce the incidence of dysphagia (Truong *et al.*, 1989).

Injections into the lateral neck muscles are best performed when the head is in a straight, neutral position. Injections into the trapezius muscles can be made easier when the patient is asked to elevate their shoulder. During injections into the hyoid muscles, the head is extended backwards. Injections are normally carried out with a 2–5 cc syringe and a 27 gauge hypodermic needle.

In summary, BoNT injections are effective treatments for abnormal posture, muscle hypertrophy and pain associated with CD. In order to obtain optimal results, the use of EMG and the knowledge of cervical anatomy are helpful in designing individualized injection patterns, which, in turn help patients with CD better manage the disorder.

REFERENCES

Anderson, T. J., Rivest, J., Stell, R., *et al.* (1992). Botulinum-toxin treatment of spasmodic torticollis. *J R Soc Med*, **85**, 524–9.

Benecke, R. (1993). Botulinum-Toxin A in der Behandlung der zervikalen Dystonien. In H. P. Richter & V. Braun, Eds., *Schiefhals. Behandlungskonzepte des Torticollis spasmodicus*. Berlin, Heidelberg, New York: Springer, pp. 63–78.

Benecke, R. (1999). Zervikale Dystonie. In R. Laskawi & P. Roggenkaemper, eds., *Botulinum-Toxin-Therapie imKopf-Hals-Bereich*. München: Urban und Vogel, pp. 171–212.

Benecke, R., Jost, W. H., Kanovsky, M. D., *et al.* (2005). A new botulinum toxin type A free of complexing proteins for treatment of cervical dystonia. *Neurology*, **64**, 1949–51.

Bertrand, C. M. (1993). Selective peripheral denervation for spasmodic torticollis: surgical technique, results, and observations in 260 cases. *Surg Neurol*, **40**, 96–103.

Blackie, J. D. & Lees, A. J. (1990). Botulinum toxin treatment in spasmodic torticollis. *J Neurol Neurosurg Psychiatry*, **53**, 640–3.

Borodic, G. E., Pearce, L. B., Smith, K. & Joseph, M. (1992). Botulinum a toxin for spasmodic torticollis: multiple vs single injection points per muscle. *Head Neck*, **14**, 33–7.

Brashear, A., Lew, M. F., Dykstra, D. D., *et al.* (1999). Safety and efficacy of NeuroBloc® (botulinum toxin type B) in type A-responsive cervical dystonia. *Neurology*, **53**, 1439–46.

Brin, M. F., Lew, M. F., Adler, M. D., *et al.* (1999). Safety and efficacy of NeuroBloc® (botulinum toxin type B) in type A-resistant cervical dystonia. *Neurology*, **53**, 1431–8.

Comella, C. L., Buchmann, A. S., Tanner, C. M., Brown-Toms, N. C. & Goetz, C. G. (1992). Botulinum toxin injection for spasmodic torticollis: increased magnitude of benefit with electromyographic assistance. *Neurology*, **42**, 878–82.

Davis, D. H., Ahlskog, J. E., Litchy, W. J. & Root, L. M. (1991). Selective peripheral denervation for torticollis: preliminary results. *Mayo Clin Proc*, **66**, 365–71.

Foltz, E. L., Knopp, L. M. & Ward, A. A. (1959). Experimental spasmodic torticollis. *J Neurosurg*, **16**, 55–72.

Frei, K., Pathak, M., Jenkens, S. & Truong, D. D. (2004). The natural history of posttraumatic cervical dystonia. *Mov Disord*, **12**, 1492–8.

Gelb, D. J., Lowenstein, D. H. & Aminoff, M. J. (1989). Controlled trial of botulinum toxin injections in the treatment of spasmodic torticollis. *Neurology*, **39**, 80–4.

Gelb, D. J., Yoshimura, D. M., Olney, R. K., Lowenstein, D. H. & Aminoff, M. J. (1991). Change in pattern of muscle activity following botulinum toxin injections for torticollis. *Ann Neurol*, **29**, 370–6.

Greene, P., Kang, U., Fahn, S., *et al.* (1990). Double-blind, placebo-controlled trial of botulinum toxin injections for the treatment of spasmodic torticollis. *Neurology*, **40**, 1213–8.

Hambleton, P., Cohen, H. E., Palmer, B. J. & Melling, J. (1992). Antitoxins and botulinum toxin treatment. *BMJ*, **304**, 959–60.

Hatheway, C. L. & Dang, C. (1994). Immunogenicity of the neurotoxins of Clostridium botulinum. In J. Jankovic & M. Hallett, eds., *Therapy with Botulinum Toxin*. New York: Dekker, pp. 93–107.

Jankovic, J. & Brin, M. F. (1991). Therapeutic uses of botulinum toxin. *N Engl J Med*, **324**, 1186–94.

Jankovic, J. & Schwartz, P. A. (1990). Botulinum toxin injections for cervical dystonia. *Neurology*, **40**, 277–80.

Kessler, K. R., Skutta, M. & Benecke, R. (1999). Long-term treatment of cervical dystonia with botulinum toxin A: efficacy, safety, and antibody frequency. *J Neurology*, **246**, 265–74.

Kutvonen, O., Dastidar, P. & Nurmikko, T. (1997). Pain in spasmodic torticollis. *Pain*, **69**(3), 279–86.

Lew, M. F., Adornato, B. T., Duane, D. D., *et al.* (1997). Botulinum toxin type B. A double blind, placebo-controlled, safety and efficacy study in cervical dystonia. *Neurology*, **49**, 701–7.

Lorentz, I. T., Subramaniam, S. S. & Yiannikas, C. (1991). Treatment of idiopathic spasmodic torticollis with botulinum toxin A: a double-blind study on twenty-three patients. *Mov Disord*, **6**, 145–50.

Moore, A. P. & Blumhardt, L. D. (1991). A double blind trial of botulinum toxin "A" in torticollis, with one year follow up. *J Neurol Neurosurg Psychiatry*, **54**, 813–6.

Naumann, M., Yakovleff, A. & Durif, F. (2002). A randomized, double-masked, crossover comparison of the efficacy and safety of botulinum toxin type A produced from the original bulk toxin and current bold toxin source for the treatment of cervical dystonia. *J Neurol*, **249**, 57–63.

Poewe, W., Schelosky, L., Kleedorfer, B., *et al.* (1992). Treatment of spasmodic torticollis with local injections of botulinum toxin. One-year follow-up in thirty-seven patients. *J Neurol*, **239**, 21–5.

Stell, R., Bronstein, A. M. & Marsden, C. D. (1989). Vestibulo-ocular abnormalities in spasmodic torticollis before and after botulinum toxin injections. *J Neurol Neurosurg Psychiatry*, **52**, 57–62.

Truong, D., Lewitt, P. & Cullis, P. (1989). Effects of different injection techniques in the treatment of torticollis with botulinum toxin. *Neurology*, **39**(Suppl), 294.

Truong, D., Dubinski, R., Hermanowicz, N., *et al.* (1991). Posttraumatic torticollis. *Arch Neurol*, **48**, 221–3.

Tsui, J. K., Eisen, A., Mak, E., *et al.* (1985). A pilot study on the use of botulinum toxin in spasmodic torticollis. *Can J Neurol Sci*, **12**, 314–16.

Tsui, J. K., Eisen, A., Stoesl, A. J., Calne, S. & Calne, D. B. (1986). Double-blind study of botulinum toxin in spasmodic torticollis. *Lancet*, **2**, 245–7.

Van Zandijcke, M. (1995). Cervical dystonia (spasmodic torticollis). Some aspects of the natural history. *Acta Neurol Belg*, **95**(4), 210–15.

Wissel, J. & Poewe, W. (1992). Dystonia–a clinical, neuropathological and therapeutic review. *J Neurol Transm Suppl*, **38**, 91–104.

6

Treatment of hemifacial spasm

Karen Frei and Peter Roggenkaemper

Hemifacial spasm (HFS) is characterized as involuntary irregular clonic or tonic movements of the facial muscles innervated by the seventh cranial nerve on one side of the face and is most often a result of vascular compression of the facial nerve at the root exit zone (Wang & Jankovic, 1998). Facial muscle twitches usually begin in the periocular region and can progress to involve the cheek and perioral muscles. Hemifacial spasm is usually unilateral; however, uncommonly, it can spread and affect the other side of the face. Atypical cases have been reported to initiate in the orbicularis oris and buccinator muscles and gradually spread upward to involve the orbicularis oculi (Ryu *et al.*, 1998). Muscles involved in HFS include the orbicularis oculi, frontalis (rarely), corrugator, nasalis, zygomaticus, risorius, orbicularis oris, and sometimes the platysma. (See Figure 6.1).

Hemifacial spasm appears to be more prevalent in females; commonly begins in the fifth decade and tends to have a fluctuating course. In contrast to essential blepharospasm, symptoms often continue during sleep and can provoke insomnia. Emotion and stress tend to exacerbate facial twitching. Although benign, HFS can be disabling due to social embarrassment and from excessive closure of one eye interfering with vision. Symptoms can progress over time and facial weakness can develop. Hypertension is thought to be a risk factor for the development of HFS (Oliveira *et al.*, 1999; Defazio *et al.*, 2000, 2003).

Hemifacial spasm is typically considered to be caused by vascular compression of the facial nerve at the root exit zone, which has been confirmed on imaging studies. The severity of compression correlates with severity of HFS symptoms (Banik & Miller, 2004). Vascular compression generally involves the AICA (anterior inferior cerebellar artery), PICA (posterior inferior cerebellar artery), the vertebral basilar artery, and the internal auditory artery which can be tortuous or ectatic. The offending vessel is usually ipsilateral to the facial nerve and side of the HFS. Occasionally, a contralateral vessel or a distal site from the root exit zone may be the source of the HFS (Ryu *et al.*, 1998). Non-vascular origins of HFS occur infrequently and consist of various forms of tumors and space occupying lesions occurring in the cerebellopontine angle.

Hemifacial spasm must be distinguished from other conditions involving the facial musculature including essential blepharospasm, facial myokymia, oromandibular dystonia, facial tic, masticatory spasm, post Bell's palsy synkinesis, and focal seizures. Essential blepharospasm usually occurs bilaterally at onset and concerns the eyes only (with the exception that it can be part of involvement of other facial muscles in Meige's syndrome). Essential blepharospasm is a form of dystonia and causes involuntary closure of the eyes by muscle spasm or without spasms in a special form called apraxia of eyelid opening. Bright light can exacerbate the condition

Manual of Botulinum Toxin Therapy, ed. Daniel Truong, Dirk Dressler and Mark Hallett. Published by Cambridge University Press. © Cambridge University Press 2009.

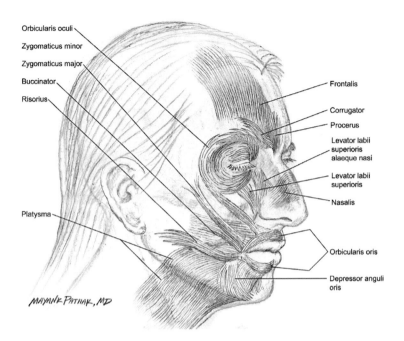

Orbicularis oculi
Zygomaticus minor
Zygomaticus major
Buccinator
Risorius
Platysma

Frontalis
Corrugator
Procerus
Levator labii superioris alaeque nasi
Levator labii superioris
Nasalis
Orbicularis oris
Depressor anguli oris

MAYANK PATHAK, MD

Figure 6.1 Facial muscles and botulinum toxin injection sites used for treatment of hemifacial spasm.

which subsides during sleep. Blepharospasm may (rarely) occur coexistent with HFS complicating the diagnosis. Facial myokymia is a fine rippling movement of the facial muscles. It is associated with an abnormality of the brain stem as can be seen in multiple sclerosis. Oromandibular dystonia is another form of dystonia involving only the lower facial muscles and it subsides during sleep similar to other dystonias. Facial tics tend to be multifocal and not unilateral, have more complex movements, and are usually associated with premonitory sensations and mild voluntary suppression. Masticatory spasm affects jaw closure with painful muscle contractions. Facial synkinesis generally involves a combination of facial movements such as eye closure while talking or chewing. Mild cases of synkinesis may be mistaken for HFS and orbicular synkinesis can be treated similar to HFS with botulinum toxin injections (Roggenkaemper *et al.*, 1994). Finally, focal seizures including epilepsia partialis continua may be erroneously diagnosed as HFS (Wang & Jankovic, 1998).

Diagnostic tests for HFS include a brain magnetic resonance imaging with attention to the cerebellopontine angle with and without contrast which will detect any space occupying lesion requiring neurosurgical intervention. Magnetic resonance angiography of the intracranial vessels may help to define the site of vascular compression. Electromyography can be useful in distinguishing non-vascular causes of HFS and an electroencephalograph may be able to detect epileptiform discharges characteristic of a focal seizure.

Treatment of HFS has included medications, botulinum toxin injections, and neurosurgery. Medications such as baclofen, clonazepam, carbamazepine, and phenytoin have been used to treat HFS. However, they tend not to be effective long term in HFS providing only transient relief. Microvascular decompression (Janetta's operation) has been useful for severe recalcitrant cases. Microvascular decompression involves placing surgical gauze in-between the facial nerve and compressing blood vessel. Success rates from microvascular decompression vary from 88% to 97% and a small percentage of patients may experience recurrence of HFS following surgery. Surgical complications include primarily hearing loss and facial weakness in addition to the accepted surgical risk of intracranial hemorrhage, stroke, and even death.

Botulinum toxin injections are the preferred treatment of HFS. They are successful in over 90% of patients and have better results than when used to treat essential blepharospasm in general. They can provide relief from symptoms without the adverse effects of neurosurgery. Currently botulinum toxins A and B are commercially available. Botulinum toxin A in the forms of Botox®, Dysport® and Xeomin®/Xeomeen® and botulinum toxin B (NeuroBloc®/Myobloc®) have all been used in the treatment of HFS. Contrary to botulinum treatment of spasmodic torticollis EMG recordings during injection are not necessary.

Side effects of botulinum toxin injections tend to be those associated with injections, such as erythema and ecchymosis of the region injected, dry eyes, mouth droop, ptosis, lid edema, and facial muscle weakness (Elston, 1986; Yoshimura *et al.*, 1992). The ptosis and facial muscle weakness tends to be transient and will resolve within 1–4 weeks. Ptosis could be due to local diffusion of the botulinum toxin affecting the levator palpabrea (Brin *et al.*, 1987). Onset of effect occurs within 3 days to 2 weeks generally with a peak effect at approximately 2 weeks. The beneficial effects of botulinum toxin injections are also transient with a mean duration of improvement of approximately 2.8 months (Yoshimura *et al.*, 1992). Between different patients there is a high variability of duration of the beneficial effect. The muscles injected to treat HFS tend to be the orbicularis oculi, corrugator, frontalis, risorius, buccinator, and depressor anguli oris (see Figure 6.1). The orbicularis oculi is composed of two parts: the pars palpebralis, which opens (with the help of the levator muscle) and closes the eyelid, and the pars orbitalis, which squeezes the eye shut. The pars palpebralis is composed of two parts: the preseptal and the pretarsal region (see Figure 6.2). The toxin is injected into four sites in the orbicularis oculi typically in the lateral and medial part of the upper and lower lid, as well as lateral from the middle of the lower lid. Injection into the brow area has an equally long

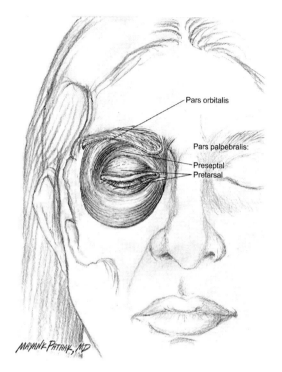

Figure 6.2 Orbicularis oculi anatomy and botulinum toxin injection sites used for treatment of hemifacial spasm.

duration of effect as into the pretarsal region but results in fewer side effects (Price *et al.*, 1997). Lower frequency of ptosis has been reported with injection either into the lateral (Jitpimolmard *et al.*, 1998) or into the pretarsal region than into the preseptal region of the orbicularis oculi (Cakmur *et al.*, 2002). In summary: at any rate the middle part of the upper lid has to be spared in order to prevent ptosis!

The orbicularis oris is avoided in order to prevent paralysis of the mouth producing further disability. The sites of injection should be decided with the patient's goals in mind. Occasionally, the preferred degree of control of the facial twitches occurs only at the expense of an ipsilateral upper lip droop of varying severity (Boghen & Lesser, 2000). In rare cases the platysma may need to be injected as well.

Total doses of botulinum toxin used per HFS treatment have been reported from 10 to 34 (mouse)

Table 6.1. Botulinum toxin doses used in the treatment of hemifacial spasm

	Frontalis	Corrugator	Orbicularis oculi	Zygomaticus major	Buccinator	Depressor angularis oris
Botox/Xeomin/ Xeomeen	10 u	1.0 u	15–20 u	1 u	2 u	1 u
Dysport	30 u	3 u	45–60 u	3 u	6 u	3 u
NeuroBloc/Myobloc	500 u	50 u	1000 u	50 u	100 u	50 u

Note:
*the new drug Xeomin/Xeomeen is considered to have the same dosage as Botox.
Source: Reproduced from Frei *et al.* (2006) with permission.

units of Botox (Flanders *et al.*, 1993; Mezaki *et al.*, 1999); for Dysport total doses used per treatment have been reported to range from 53 to 160 units (Elston, 1992; Yu *et al.*, 1992; Van den Bergh *et al.*, 1995; Jitpimolmard *et al.*, 1998) and for NeuroBloc/Myobloc doses ranging from 1250 units to 9000 units have been reported (Tousi *et al.*, 2004; Wan *et al.*, 2005). Table 6.1 lists the dosages of each toxin and the muscles commonly injected (Frei *et al.*, 2006).

After the coauthor's experience with 660 patients with HFS since 1985 the scheme in Figure 6.3 is proven to be effective with only few side effects, at least when beginning the treatment. In detail: injection points above the eyebrows are often not necessary. Two injection points along the lateral orbital rim which produce no side effects are very valuable and, as most of the patients suffer an involvement of the cheek area: around ten injection points (each with a low dose, strictly subcutaneously administered over a large area below the bony orbital rim) are effective, but prevent side effects such as drooping upper lip or of the corner of the mouth. In this technique you start with a low dose, which generally has of course less side effects, and a large number of patients consider this dose of 17.2 units Botox/Xeomin as sufficient over many years. In case of need you can, however, step by step increase the dose according to the experience of the patient with the last injection scheme, which

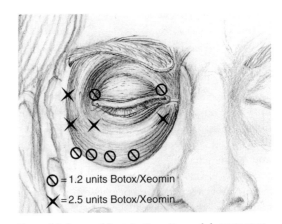

= 1.2 units Botox/Xeomin

= 2.5 units Botox/Xeomin

Figure 6.3 Proposal for injection sites and doses to start within treatment of hemifacial spasm.

has therefore to be meticulously documented in the files. And: in general it can be stated, that side effects get rarer and rarer with the experience of the treating doctor.

Injection pain can be reduced either with skin cooling using ice or EMLA® Cream (lidocaine 2.5% and prilocaine 2.5%) (Linder *et al.*, 2002; Soylev *et al.*, 2002). Treatment with botulinum toxin appears to remain effective over long-term use of several years (ranging from 4 to 20 years) and in most cases will not require dosage increase (Jitpimolmard *et al.*, 1998). If required, the dosage increase usually occurs within the first two years of treatment.

REFERENCES

Banik, R. & Miller, N. R. (2004). Chronic myokymia limited to the eyelid is a benign condition. *J Neuroophthalmol*, **24**(4), 290–2.

Boghen, D. R. & Lesser, R. L. (2000). Blepharospasm and hemifacial spasm. *Curr Treat Options Neurol*, **2**(5), 393–400.

Brin, M. F., Fahn, S., Moskowitz, C., *et al.* (1987). Localized injections of botulinum toxin for the treatment of focal dystonia and hemifacial spasm. *Mov Disord*, **2**, 237–54.

Cakmur, R., Ozturk, V., Uzunel, F., Donmez, B. & Idiman, F. (2002). Comparison of preseptal and pretarsal injections of botulinum toxin in the treatment of blepharospasm and hemifacial spasm. *J Neurol*, **249**, 64–8.

Defazio, G. B. A., Abbruzzese, G., Coviello, V., *et al.* (2000). Primary hemifacial spasm and arteria hypertension: a multicenter case-control study. *Neurology*, **54**(5), 1198–2000.

Defazio, G. M. D., Aniello, M. S., Masi, G., *et al.* (2003). Influence of age on the association between primary hemifacial spasm and arterial hypertension. *J Neurol Neurosurg Psychiatry*, **74**(7), 979–81.

Elston, J. S. (1986). Botulinum toxin treatment of hemifacial spasm. *J Neuro Neurosurg Psychiatry*, **49**, 827–9.

Elston, J. S. (1992). The management of blepharospasm and hemifacial spasm. *J Neurol*, **239**(1), 5–8.

Flanders, M., Chin, D. & Boghen, D. (1993). Botulinum toxin: preferred treatment for hemifacial spasm. *Eur Neurol*, **33**(4), 316–9.

Frei, K., Truong, D. D. & Dressler, D. (2006). Botulinum toxin therapy of hemifacial spasm: comparing different therapeutic preparations. *Eur J Neurol*, **13**(Suppl 1), 30–5.

Jitpimolmard, S., Tiamkao, S. & Laopaiboom, M. (1998). Long term results of botulinum toxin type A (Dysport) in the treatment of hemifacial spasm: a report of 175 cases. *J Neurol Neurosurg Psychiatry*, **64**(6), 751–7.

Linder, J. S., Edmonson, B. C., Laquis, S. J., Drewry, R. D., Jr. & Fleming, J. C. (2002). Skin cooling before periocular botulinum toxin A injection. *Ophthal Plast Reconstr Surg*, **18**, 441–2.

Mezaki, T., Kaji, R., Kimura, J. & Ogawa, N. (1999). [Treatment of hemifacial spasm with type A botulinum toxin (AGN 191622): a dose finding study and the evaluation of clinical effect with electromyography.] *No To Shinkei*, **51**(5), 427–32.

Oliveira, L. D., Cardoso, F. & Vargas, A. P. (1999). Hemifacial spasm and arterial hypertension. *Mov Disord*, **14**(5), 832–5.

Price, J., Farish, S., Taylor, H. & O'Day, J. (1997). Blepharospasm and hemifacial spasm. Randomized trial to determine the most appropriate location for botulinum toxin injections. *Ophthalmology*, **104**, 865–8.

Roggenkaemper, P., Laskawi, R., Damenz, W., Schroeder, M. & Nuessgens, Z. (1994). Orbicular synkinesis after facial paralysis: treatment with botulinum toxin. *Doc Ophthalmol*, **86**, 395–402.

Ryu, H., Yamamoto, S. & Miyamoto, T. (1998). Atypical hemifacial spasm. *Acta Neurochir* (*Wien*), **140**(11), 1173–6.

Soylev, M. F., Kocak, N., Kuvaki, B., Ozkan, S. B. & Kir, E. (2002). Anesthesia with EMLA cream for botulinum A toxin injection into eyelids. *Ophthalmologica*, **216**, 355–8.

Tousi, B., Perumal, J. S., Ahuja, K., Ahmed, A. & Subramanian, T. (2004). "Effects of botulinum toxin-B (BTX-B) injections for hemifacial spasm." *Parkinsonism Relat Disord*, **10**(7), 455–6.

Van den Bergh, P., Francart, J., Mourin, S., Kollman, P. & Laterre, E. C. (1995). Five-year experience in the treatment of focal movement disorders with low-dose Dysport botulinum toxin. *Muscle Nerve*, **18**(7), 720–9.

Wan, X. H., Vuong, K. D. & Jankovic, J. (2005). Clinical application of botulinum toxin type B in movement disorders and autonomic symptoms. *Chin Med Sci J*, **20**(1), 44–7.

Wang, A. & Jankovic, J. (1998). Hemifacial spasm: clinical findings and treatment. *Muscle Nerve*, **21**(12), 1740–7.

Yoshimura, D. M., Aminoff, M. J., Tami, T. A. & Scott, A. B. (1992). Treatment of hemifacial spasm with botulinum toxin. *Muscle Nerve*, **15**(9), 1045–9.

Yu, Y. L., Fong, K. Y. & Chang, C. M. (1992). Treatment of idiopathic hemifacial spasm with botulinum toxin. *Acta Neurol Scand*, **85**(1), 55–7.

7

Treatment of blepharospasm

Carlo Colosimo, Dorina Tiple and Alfredo Berardelli

Clinical features and pathophysiology

Primary blepharospasm is a common adult-onset focal dystonia, characterized by involuntary contractions of the periocular muscles resulting in forceful eye closure, and impairing normal opening and closing of the eyes (Marsden, 1976; Berardelli *et al.*, 1985). The severity of blepharospasm can vary from repeated frequent blinking, causing only minor discomfort, to persistent forceful closure of the eyelids leading to functional blindness (Figure 7.1). Blepharospasm can be caused by tonic or phasic contractions of the orbicularis oculi muscles and may also be associated with levator palpebrae muscle inhibition (apraxia of eyelid opening) or involuntary movements in the lower face or jaw muscles (Meige's syndrome). In most cases blepharospasm is considered primary and is only occasionally secondary to structural brain lesions or drug induced (Jankovic, 2006).

Neurophysiological recordings of the blink reflex have given important insight into the pathophysiology of blepharospasm. In patients with blepharospasm, the recovery cycle of the R2 component of the blink reflex is enhanced, presumably owing to a lack of brain stem interneuronal inhibition (Berardelli *et al.*, 1985, 1998). Blepharospasm is also associated with an abnormal responsiveness of the blink reflex to sensory stimuli. Recent studies with the technique of magnetic brain stimulation also suggest a loss of inhibition and increased plasticity in the central nervous system of patients with blepharospasm.

Anatomy of the periocular muscles

Knowledge of the anatomy of the upper facial muscles is essential for treating patients with blepharospasm. The muscle most commonly involved in blepharospasm is the orbicularis oculi, which is a sphincter muscle around the eye consisting of an orbital, preseptal, and pretarsal part (see Figure 6.2, Chapter 6). The orbital part originates in the medial part of the orbit and runs around the eye via the upper eye cover fold and lid and returns in the lower eyelid to the palpebral ligament. The preseptal or palpebral part originates in the palpebral ligament and runs above and below the eye to the lateral angle of the eye. The orbital and the preseptal muscles form concentric circles around the eye. The pretarsal part lies just around the palpebral margin.

Blepharospasm can also involve the levator palpebrae superioris. This muscle arises from the inferior surface of the sphenoid bone. From this point, it diverges anteriorly to insert into the skin of the upper eyelid and the superior tarsal plate. The levator palpebrae muscle elevates and retracts the upper eyelid. Other muscles that may also be affected in patients

Manual of Botulinum Toxin Therapy, ed. Daniel Truong, Dirk Dressler and Mark Hallett. Published by Cambridge University Press.
© Cambridge University Press 2009.

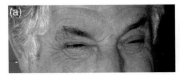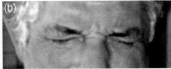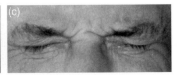

Figure 7.1 Example of a patient with severe chronic blepharospasm: a disabling spasm of the periocular muscles is observed.

with blepharospasm are the corrugator, the procerus, and the frontalis. The corrugator muscle originates at the inner orbit near the root of the nose and inserts into the skin of the forehead above the center of each eyebrow and pulls the eyebrows and skin from the center of each eyebrow to its inner corner medially and down. The procerus muscle originates in the fascia of the nasal bone and upper nasal cartilage, runs through the area of the root of the nose, and fans upward to insert in the skin in the center of the forehead between the eyebrows. It acts to pull the skin of the center of the forehead down, forming transverse wrinkles in the glabella region and bridge of the nose. It usually acts together with corrugator or orbicularis oculi or both. The frontalis muscle is a thin and quadrilateral muscle adherent to the superficial fascia. The frontalis muscle passes through and inserts into the bundles of the orbicularis oculi muscle on the superior border of the eyebrow at the middle and medial side of the upper eyelid. The frontalis muscle intermixes with the bundle of the orbicularis oculi muscle.

Botulinum toxin treatment techniques

In 1989 the US Food and Drug Administration approved botulinum toxin type A (BoNT-A, formulation Botox®) as a therapeutic agent in patients with blepharospasm, and European approval followed in 1994. Treatment of blepharospasm with BoNT-A is usually straightforward and easy. Four injections are usually given in the orbital or preseptal portion of the orbicularis oculi muscle, but the number of injections in the orbicularis oculi can be increased to include the lateral canthus. Injection in the middle of the upper lid should always be avoided in order not to cause ptosis. Botulinum toxin type A can also be injected into the pretarsal portion of the orbicularis oculi (Albanese *et al.*, 1996; Cakmur *et al.*, 2002) (see Figure 7.2a & b). In most patients pretarsal BoNT-A treatment achieves a significantly higher response rate and longer-lasting maximum response. Injection into the pretarsal part is more painful but produces fewer side effects. Botulinum toxin type A injected into the pretarsal portion of the orbicularis oculi muscle is considered the best method for treating involuntary eyelid closure due to contractions of this muscle and for treating apraxia of eyelid opening. Usually it is not worthwhile to use any preinjection anesthesia, even if in selected cases cold or anesthetic cream may be used. The total dose of BoNT-A injected per session (for both eyes together) ranges from 25 to 50 U (mouse units) Botox (standard dilution 50 mU per ml of saline) or 100 to 200 U Dysport® (standard dilution 200 U per ml of saline). In rare and selected patients with severe blepharospasm, refractory to standard treatment regimens, increasing the dose of BoNT-A up to 100 U (Botox) per session may be helpful. The mean treatment interval is around 3–4 months and appears strikingly constant in most treated patients. In patients with severe blepharospasm involving other nearby facial muscles the corrugator, procerus, and frontalis, can also be injected in addition to the orbicularis oculi. Different brands of BoNT-A, such as Dysport (Ipsen Ltd.) or Xeomin® (Merz Pharmaceuticals) lead to similar results, provided that a dose ratio of 1:4 (Botox/Dysport) and 1:1 (Botox/Xeomin) are utilized. Other botulinum toxin serotypes (B, C and F) have

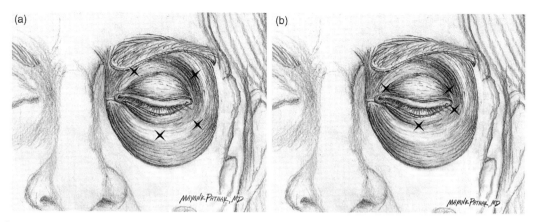

Figure 7.2 Comparison of (a) preseptal and (b) pretarsal injection points in blepharospasm.

proved substantially unhelpful and their use offers no advantage over standard treatment with BoNT-A (Colosimo *et al.*, 2003). Side effects after botulinum toxin injection, including ptosis, diplopia, dry eyes, epiphora, keratitis, lid edema, entropion/ectropion, and facial weakness, are transient and usually mild in experienced hands. Botulinum toxin type A is now recognized as the first-choice treatment for the symptomatic control of blepharospasm. Although few small randomized, controlled studies exist to support the use of BoNT-A in this indication (Jankovic & Orman, 1987), results from several open-label studies suggest that BoNT-A is highly effective, providing an improvement in 90–95% of the cases with very few side effects. In a study assessing the long-term efficacy of BoNT-A in the treatment of blepharospasm Calace *et al.* (2003) found no reduction in the efficacy after repeated treatments (range: 10–18 years, 10–41 treatments). A recent meta-analysis concluded that the efficacy of BoNT-A in blepharospasm should not be assessed in new placebo-controlled trials (Costa *et al.*, 2005). Future trials should only explore technical factors such as optimum treatment intervals and doses, different injection techniques, and the applicability of the various BoNT-A formulations (Ward *et al.*, 2006). Surgical treatments, such as facial nerve lysis and orbicularis oculi myectomy, once

used extensively in the treatment of blepharospasm, have been largely abandoned because BoNT-A is highly effective in most cases and without the frequent postoperative complications observed after surgery.

REFERENCES

Albanese, A., Bentivoglio, A. R., Colosimo, C., *et al.* (1996). Pretarsal injections of botulinum toxin improve blepharospasm in previously unresponsive patients. *J Neurol Neurosurg Psychiatry*, **60**, 693–4.

Berardelli, A., Rothwell, J. C., Day, B. L. & Marsden, C. D. (1985). Pathophysiology of blepharospasm and oromandibular dystonia. *Brain*, **108**(Pt 3), 593–608.

Berardelli, A., Rothwell, J. C., Hallett, M., *et al.* (1998). The pathophysiology of primary dystonia. *Brain*, **121**(Pt 7), 1195–212.

Cakmur, R., Ozturk, V., Uzunel, F., Donmez, B. & Idiman, F. (2002). Comparison of preseptal and pretarsal injections of botulinum toxin in the treatment of blepharospasm and hemifacial spasm. *J Neurol*, **249**, 64–8.

Calace, P., Cortese, G., Piscopo, R., *et al.* (2003). Treatment of blepharospasm with botulinum neurotoxin type A: long-term results. *Eur J Ophthalmol*, **13**, 331–6.

Colosimo, C., Chianese, M., Giovannelli, M., Contarino, M. F. & Bentivoglio, A. R. (2003). Botulinum toxin type B in blepharospasm and hemifacial spasm. *J Neurol Neurosurg Psychiatry*, **74**, 687.

Costa, J., Espirito-Santo, C., Borges, A., *et al.* (2005). Botulinum toxin type A therapy for blepharospasm. *Cochrane Database Syst Rev*, Jan 25(1), CD004900.

Jankovic, J. (2006). Treatment of dystonia. *Lancet Neurol*, **5**, 864–72.

Jankovic, J. & Orman, J. (1987). Botulinum A toxin for cranial-cervical dystonia: a double-blind, placebo-controlled study. *Neurology*, **37**, 616–23.

Marsden, C. D. (1976). Blepharospasm-oromandibular dystonia syndrome (Brueghel's syndrome). A variant of adult-onset torsion dystonia? *J Neurol Neurosurg Psychiatry*, **39**, 1204–9.

Ward, A. B., Molenaers, G., Colosimo, C. & Berardelli, A. (2006). Clinical value of botulinum toxin in neurological indications. *Eur J Neurol*, **13**(Suppl 4), 20–6.

8

Treatment of oromandibular dystonia

Francisco Cardoso, Roongroj Bhidayasiri and Daniel Truong

Oromandibular dystonia (OMD) is a form of focal dystonia that involves masticatory, lower facial, labial, and lingual musculature. The term "cranial dystonia" is used when OMD occurs in association with blepharospasm. This particular combination is often referred to as Meige's syndrome (for reviews see Bhidayasiri *et al.* [2006]).

Epidemiology, clinical features, and etiology

Oromandibular dystonia affects women more frequently than men and the prevalence was estimated to be 68.9 cases per 1 million Americans (for reviews see Bhidayasiri *et al.* [2006]). The range of mean age at onset varies from 50 to 60 years. The involvement of masticatory muscles in OMD may cause jaw-closing or -opening, lateral deviation, protrusion, retraction, or a combination. These movements often result in involuntary biting of the tongue, cheek, or lips and difficulty with speaking and chewing. Its appearance is often socially embarrassing and disfiguring. In patients with jaw-closing OMD, dystonic spasms of the temporalis and masseter muscles may result in clenching or trismus and grinding of the teeth or bruxism. On the other hand, the lateral pterygoids, anterior belly of the digastric muscle, and other submental muscles are commonly involved in jaw-opening dystonia, and contractions of these muscles may

lead to some degree of anterocollis. Oromandibular dystonia may be alleviated by different proprioceptive sensory inputs ("sensory trick"). These include touching the lips or chin, chewing gum, or biting on a toothpick. A recent study demonstrated that coexistence with dystonia in other regions and presence of sensory tricks are more common in jaw-opening than jaw-closing OMD. The contraction of mouth and pharynx muscles may cause involuntary vocalizations occasionally confounded with vocal tics. In addition to the dystonic symptoms, many patients with OMD complain of tension-type headache, dental wear, temporomandibular joint syndrome and, more rarely, temporomandibular joint dislocation resulting in upper airway collapse.

As with most forms of dystonia, most patients with OMD belong to the idiopathic category. However, tardive dystonia represents the most common cause of secondary OMD. While most patients with tardive OMD are more likely to have their dystonia confined to the oromandibular region, blepharospasm, cervical dystonia, and spasmodic dysphonia are more commonly associated with idiopathic OMD. On the other hand, the presence of akathisia, stereotypic movements in the limbs, or respiratory dyskinesias strongly suggests prior neuroleptic exposure (Tan & Jankovic, 2000). Less commonly, OMD can occur as an accompanying manifestation of neurodegenerative disorders, focal brain or brain stem lesions. Among degenerative illnesses, neuroacanthocytosis

Manual of Botulinum Toxin Therapy, ed. Daniel Truong, Dirk Dressler and Mark Hallett. Published by Cambridge University Press.
© Cambridge University Press 2009.

Table 8.1. Reports on treatment of oromandibular dystonia

Author	Year	Type of study	Number of patients	Duration of effect (weeks)	Toxin type	EMG guidance
Brin *et al.*	1987	Open	4	Not given	Botox	Yes
Jankovic & Orman	1987	Double	3	5.6*	Botox	No
Blitzer *et al.**	1989	Open	20	Not given	Botox	Yes
Hermanowicz & Truong	1991	Open	5	Not given	Botox	Yes
Van den Bergh *et al.*	1995	Open	5	27.0 ± 4.5	Dysport	Yes
Tan & Jankovic	1999	Open	162	16.4 ± 7.1	Botox	No
Laskawi & Rohrbach	2001	Open	6	14.0 ± 9.2	Botox	Yes
Wan *et al.*	2005	Open	12	13.8 ± 2.9	Myobloc	No

Note:
*Some patients previously described (Brin, 1994).
Source: Modified from Bhidayasiri *et al.* (2006) with permission.

is an important cause of OMD which needs to be ruled out whenever patients present with it combined with chorea, seizures, amyotrophy, and subcortical dementia. Recently attention has been devoted to OMD characterized by prominent lingua protrusion, a syndrome which can be caused by pantothenate kinase-associated neurodegeneration, Lesch-Nyhan syndrome, and anoxia (Schneider *et al.*, 2006).

Treatment options of oromandibular dystonia

Several studies suggest that OMD responds poorly to oral medications, which are commonly used to treat other forms of dystonia, including anticholinergics, tetrabenazine, baclofen or clonazepam (for reviews see Bhidayasiri *et al.* [2006]). Muscle afferent block by intramuscular injection of lidocaine and alcohol has shown to be helpful, but further experience and evaluation is needed to determine the long-term efficacy and benefit of afferent blockade (Yoshida *et al.*, 1998). Lastly, pallidal deep brain stimulation has been performed in a few patients with OMD-blepharospasm with positive results and may be considered as an option in some patients with intractable OMD (Bhidayasiri *et al.*, 2006).

The lack of a significant number of controlled trials has led authors of evidence-based reviews to state that, with the exception of jaw-closing dystonia, it is uncertain the role of botulinum toxin injections in the treatment of OMD (The National Institutes of Health Consensus Development, 1990; Bhidayasiri *et al.*, 2006). Nevertheless, many uncontrolled studies as well as clinical experience suggest that botulinum toxin is a reasonable first-line treatment for OMD regardless of its clinical presentation (Bhidayasiri *et al.*, 2006). Most of the reported literature on OMD has been open studies as seen in Table 8.1 but all have reported improvement with botulinum toxin. In a large prospective open study Tan and Jankovic (1999) reported a mean total duration of response up to 16.4 ± 7.1 weeks. Best response is obtained with jaw-closing OMD (Tan & Jankovic, 1999).

Dystonia is not a stereotyped disorder and its presentation in OMD is even more colorful. The treatment has to be individualized to accommodate the patients' needs and symptoms. Oromandibular dystonia can be subdivided into jaw-closing, jaw-opening, jaw deviation, lingual, pharyngeal, and mixed type. For the purpose of analyzing the muscle to be injected the function of each muscle needs to be understood. Tables 8.2 and 8.3, also adapted from a recent publication of Bhidayasiri *et al.* (2006), list the muscles and their respective function.

Table 8.2. Oral muscles and function

Muscle name	Function
Temporalis	Close the jaw
	Posterior fibers retract the mandible
	Move jaw to the same side
Masseter	Close the jaw by elevating the
	mandible
Medial pterygoid	Close the jaw
	Protrude the jaw
	Moving the jaw to the opposite side
Lateral pterygoid	Open the mouth
	Protrude the jaw
	Move the jaw to the opposite side
Digastric	Open the jaw
	Elevate the hyoid bone
Mylohyoid	Open the jaw
	Raise the floor of the mouth
Geniohyoid	Open the jaw
	Elevate and draw hyoid bone forward

Source: Modified from Bhidayasiri *et al.* (2006) with permission.

Table 8.3. Subtypes of oromandibular dystonia

Subtype	Muscle involved
Jaw-closing	Temporalis
	Masseter
	Medial pterygoid
Jaw-opening	Lateral pterygoid
	Mylohyoid
	Digastric
	Geniohyoid
Jaw deviation	Contralateral lateral pterygoid
	Contralateral medial pterygoid
	Ipsilateral temporalis

Source: Modified from Bhidayasiri *et al.* (2006) with permission.

Injection techniques

Because of the lack of controlled trials and the significant heterogeneity of clinical presentation of OMD, the discussion that follows, which is subdivided according to main clinical types, is primarily based on the clinical experience of the authors.

Jaw-closing oromandibular dystonia

For jaw-closing OMD, often the masseter is the initial muscle selected for denervation (Bhidayasiri *et al.*, 2006). If the response is not adequate other muscles which include temporalis and medial pterygoid, can be considered. Injection is individualized for each patient and electromyographic (EMG) guidance is optional to identify deep muscles which are not available to manual palpation since there is suggestion that comparable results could be obtained without EMG (Bhidayasiri *et al.*, 2006).

The masseter is a thick quadrilateral muscle consisting of three parts, superficial, intermediate, and deep, which arise from the zygomatic arch and insert into the angle and the lateral surface of the ramus of the mandible (Clemente, 1984) (Figure 8.1). It can be easily palpated by instructing the patient to clench the teeth. Very uncommonly EMG guidance is required to reach it. In this case, it is approached using a Teflon-coated needle connected to an EMG machine at 1 cm anterior to the posterior border of the ramus. The muscle discharge when the patient clenches the teeth also helps to localize the insertion and confirm that it is indeed not in the parotid gland, which extend from the ear to the masseter and partially covers the posterior part of the muscle. A good starting dose is 50 (mouse) units of Botox® or 100 units of Dyport®. Experience with Myobloc® is not available from the literature except in two non-English journals (Cardoso, 2003; Wan *et al.*, 2005). In our limited experience we have used 2500 units of Myobloc for each masseter muscle.

The medial pterygoid occupies the inner aspect of the ramus of the mandible opposite that of the masseter. It arises from the lateral pterygoid plate and the pyramical process of the palatine bone and inserts into the lower and back part of the medial surface of the ramus and angle of the mandible (Clemente, 1984) (Figure 8.2). Due to its deep location, its injection often requires EMG guidance. The medial pterygoid can be approached either intraorally or from below. When approach is from below the needle is inserted about 0.5–1 cm anterior to the angle of the mandible along the interior

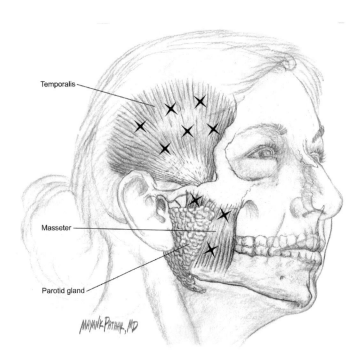

Temporalis

Masseter

Parotid gland

MAYANK PATHAK, MD

Figure 8.1 Lateral view of the masseter muscle. The sign X denotes approximate injection site.

aspect of the mandible and angled perpendicularly to the mandible until it can be verified by the EMG with the patient clenching the teeth. Care should be taken to avoid the facial artery which lies anteriorly. A good starting dose here is 20 units of Botox or 30 units of Dyport (Bhidayasiri *et al.*, 2006) or 1000 units of Myobloc.

The third muscle involved in the jaw closing is the temporalis muscle (Figure 8.1). This broad, radiating muscle arises from the temporal fossa. Its tendon inserts into the medial surface, apex, and anterior border of the coronoid process and the anterior border of the ramus of the mandible (Clemente, 1984). The temporalis closes the jaws and its posterior fibers retract the mandible. The temporalis is approached perpendicular to its plane and possibly high in the temporal fossa as the lower part of the temporalis is mostly tendon where the injection is painful. Due to its wide radiation pattern, three to four injections should be given. Recent recommended dose by the educational committee of "WE MOVE" is 40 units of Botox (www.wemove.org). The authors, however, opt for

a higher dose, 50 to 100 units. An early report used smaller doses (Bhidayasiri *et al.*, 2006). Starting dose for Dysport is about 100 units and adjusted according to patient's response (Van den Bergh *et al.*, 1995).

Jaw-opening oromandibular dystonia

The muscles involved in jaw opening include the lateral pterygoid, mylohyoid, digastric, geniohyoid, and platysma (Clemente, 1984). Opening of the jaws is performed primarily by the lateral pterygoid. In the beginning of the opening, it receives assistance from the submentalis complex which includes the mylohyoid, digastric, and geniohyoid (Clemente, 1984). The platysma may also play a minor role in the opening of the jaw. Most investigators reported injections of the lateral pterygoid in jaw-opening dystonia although others claim success with injection of the submentalis complexes only (Bhidayasiri *et al.*, 2006).

The lateral pterygoid is a short conical muscle and arises by two heads, a superior from the great wing of the sphenoid bone and an inferior from the

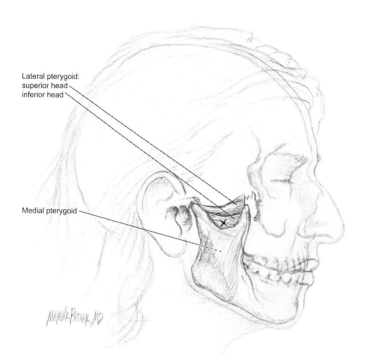

Lateral pterygoid:
superior head
inferior head

Medial pterygoid

Figure 8.2 View of the medial pterygoid muscle, showing its origin and insertion. The sign X denotes approximate injection site.

lateral surface of the lateral pterygoid plate of the sphenoid (Clemente, 1984) (Figure 8.2). The lateral pterygoid could be approached intraorally or laterally through the mandibular incisure. The entry point is about 35 mm from the external auditory canal and 10 mm from the inferior margin of the zygomatic arch. Using EMG guided technique, the needle is angled upward about 15 degrees to reach the inferior head of the lateral pterygoid. In close vicinity but more rostral is the pterygoid branch of the maxillary artery. The amount of toxin reported in literature ranges from 20 units to 40 units of Botox (Blitzer *et al.*, 1989; Laskawi & Rohrbach, 2001). There are limited experiences with Dysport and we recommend a starting dose of about 60 units and titrated up if needed.

The digastric muscle is part of the submentalis complex. It arises from the mastoid notch of the temporal bone and is attached to digastric fossa of the mandible (Figure 8.3). It is divided into the anterior and posterior belly by the middle tendon, which is attached to the hyoid bone (Clemente,

1984). Besides elevating the hyoid bone, the digastric pulls the chin backward and downward in opening the mouth in conjunction with the lateral pterygoid. In contrast to the posterior belly, which is crowded with many nerves, sympathetic trunk, arteries, and veins, the anterior belly is open to intervention. The geniohyoid arises from the hyoid bone and inserts into the inferior genial tubercle of the mandible. It elevates the hyoid bone and base of the tongue. With the hyoid bone fixed, it depresses the mandible and opens the mouth. The mylohyoid arises from the hyoid bone as well and is attached to the mylohyoid line on the mandible (Figure 8.3). It raises the floor of the mouth during swallowing. The mylohyoid elevates the hyoid bone, thereby pushing the tongue upward or causing protrusion of the tongue (Clemente, 1984). It assists in opening the mouth. Muscles of the submentalis complex may be fused together rendering them difficult to be separated from one another (Clemente, 1984). This muscle group can be palpated when the patient opens the mouth. It is approached

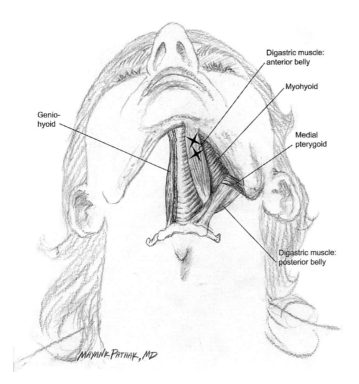

Figure 8.3 Inferior view of the floor of the mouth, showing the submentalis complex, including the digastric muscle. The sign X denotes approximate injection site.

about 1 cm from the mandible tip and injected slightly lateral from the midline (Figure 8.3). A good starting dose of Botox is 30 units. These units are divided and injected into the two locations on each side. Higher doses up to 200 units for the submentalis complex have been reported (Tan & Jankovic, 1999) but the risk of severe dysphagia is considerable. For Dysport, 90 units could be a good starting dose and for Myobloc about 500 units.

In some patients, injection of the platysma can give additional improvement. This muscle depresses the mandible and soft tissue of the lower face as well as tenses the skin of the neck. The platysma fascicles can be easily identified with visual inspection. Often the platysma is injected with 20 units of Botox, 60 units of Dysport, and for Myobloc about 1000 units.

Jaw-deviating oromandibular dystonia

The contralateral lateral pterygoid works in conjunction with the ipsilateral medial pterygoid to deviate

the mouth to opposite side. The temporalis pulls the jaw to the same side. The injections follow the above mentioned techniques (Figures 8.1 and 8.2).

Lingual oromandibular dystonia

The extrinsic muscles of the tongue include the genioglossus, hyoglossus, chondroglossus, styloglossus, and palatoglossus. Careful examination of the movements of the tongue is instrumental for successful treatment. The need to preserve functional activity limits the amount of toxin that can be used. As tongue thrusting is one of the movements often encountered in OMD, this movement is due to the action of the posterior fibers of the genioglossus, whereas the anterior fibers draw the tongue back into the mouth (Clemente, 1984). Suggested initial dose is 10 units of Botox, 30 units of Dysport respectively (Bhidayasiri et al., 2006). There is no known experience of Myobloc with this muscle but an initial therapy with 500 units may be reasonable.

The hyoglossus on the other hand depresses the tongue and draws down its side. Similar dose to the genioglossus is used here. One note of caution in injecting lingual muscles: the therapeutic window is quite narrow which means that doses slightly above the therapeutic level can induce disabling weakness associated with severe dysphagia.

Pharyngeal oromandibular dystonia

The pharyngeal muscles consist of the three constrictor muscles and the stylo-, salpingo-, and palatopharyngei. The three constrictors are superior, middle, and inferior constrictors. They exercise general sphincteric and peristaltic action in swallowing. Pharyngeal OMD often involves the constrictor pharynges. The patients often complain of choking and swallowing difficulty. Pharyngeal OMD often occurs with spasmodic dystonia. We have noted that sometimes after treatment of spasmodic dysphonia, there is also unexpected improvement of pharyngeal dystonia. As treatments of constrictor pharynges are almost invariably associated with dysphagia, injections of these muscles are seldom performed. Dosage often used is 10 units of Botox or 30 units of Dysport.

Conclusion

The development of botulinum toxin has markedly altered the treatment of focal dystonia, including OMD. The difference in potency between different commercially available toxins even when they are from the same class creates some confusion for the practicing. The lack of published material in OMD further complicates switching from one preparation to another. The dosages recommended in this chapter did not take into account the published literature suggesting the equivalence of Botox and Dysport, which has been reported to be between 1:2.5 and 1:6 (for review see Bhidayasiri *et al.* [2006]), as injections into the oral cavity are limited by side effects of the compound used.

ACKNOWLEDGMENTS

The authors thank Dr. Mauro César Quintão Cunningham, Débora Palma Maia, Antônio Lúcio Teixeira for their assistance during the preparation of the manuscript.

REFERENCES

Bhidayasiri, R., Cardoso, F. & Truong, D. (2006). Botulinum toxin in blepharospasm and oromandibular dystonia. *Eur J Neurol*, **13**(Suppl. 1), 21–9.

Blitzer, A., Brin, M. F., Greene, P. E. & Fahn, S. (1989). Botulinum toxin injection for the treatment of oromandibular dystonia. *Ann Otol Rhinol Laryngol*, **98**, 93–7.

Brin, M. F. (1994). Oromandibular dystonia: treatment of 96 patients with botulinum toxin type A. In J. Jankovic & M. Hallett, eds., *Therapy with Botulinum Toxin*. New York: Marcel Dekker, pp. 429–35.

Brin, M. F., Fahn, S., Moskowitz, C., *et al.* (1987). Localized injections of botulinum toxin for the treatment of focal dystonia and hemifacial spasm. *Mov Disord*, **2**, 237–54.

Cardoso, F. (2003). [Botulinum toxin type B in the management of dystonia non-responsive to botulinum toxin type A]. *Arq Neuropsiquiatr*, **61**, 607–10.

Clemente, C. (1984). Muscles and fasciae. In C. Clemente, ed., *Gray's Anatomy*. Philadelphia: Lea & Feabiger, pp. 429–605.

Hermanowicz, N. & Truong, D. D. (1991). Treatment of oromandibular dystonia with botulinum toxin. *Laryngoscope*, **101**, 1216–18.

Jankovic, J. & Orman, J. (1987). Botulinum A toxin for cranial-cervical dystonia: a double-blind, placebo-controlled study. *Neurology*, **37**, 616–23.

Laskawi, R. & Rohrbach, S. (2001). [Oromandibular dystonia. Clinical forms, diagnosis and examples of therapy with botulinum toxin]. *Laryngorhinootologie*, **80**, 708–13.

Schneider, S. A., Aggarwal, A., Bhatt, M., *et al.* (2006). Severe tongue protrusion dystonia: clinical syndromes and possible treatment. *Neurology*, **67**, 940–3.

Tan, E. K. & Jankovic, J. (1999). Botulinum toxin A in patients with oromandibular dystonia: long-term follow-up. *Neurology*, **53**, 2102–7.

Tan, E. K. & Jankovic, J. (2000). Tardive and idiopathic oromandibular dystonia: a clinical comparison. *J Neurol Neurosurg Psychiatry*, **68**, 186–90.

The National Institutes of Health Consensus
Development. (1990). Clinical use of botulinum toxins.
NIH Consensus Statement 8, 1–20.

Van den Bergh, P., Francart, J., Mourin, S., Kollmann, P. &
Laterre, E. C. (1995). Five-year experience in the
treatment of focal movement disorders with low-dose
Dysport botulinum toxin. *Muscle Nerve*, **18**, 720–9.

Wan, X. H., Vuong, K. D. & Jankovic, J. (2005). Clinical
application of botulinum toxin type B in movement
disorders and autonomic symptoms. *Chin Med Sci J*,
20, 44–7.

Yoshida, K., Kaji, R., Kubori, T., *et al.* (1998). Muscle
afferent block for the treatment of oromandibular
dystonia. *Mov Disord*, **13**, 699–705.

9

Treatment of focal hand dystonia

Chandi Prasad Das, Daniel Truong and Mark Hallett

Definition

Dystonic contractions are often aggravated by purposeful actions and may be specific to a particular task. A patient may have dystonia when using the hand for writing but not for other tasks such as eating or typing. Occupational dystonias are those that occur in individuals with a particular occupation requiring repetitive and excessive fine motor activity. Most of these dystonias are task specific and fall under the rubric of primary focal dystonias. The occupations especially prone to have focal task-specific dystonia are listed in Table 9.1.

In this chapter we discuss in detail writer's cramp and musician's cramp, the two most common occupational dystonias, followed by a brief mention of other focal occupational dystonias.

Pathogenesis

Although the exact cause of these focal dystonias is not yet elucidated, it seems that an interaction of proprioceptive, behavioral, genetic, gestural, environmental, and psychological factors plays a role. Excessive activation of antagonists, overflow into synergists, and prolongation of muscle activation are thought to reflect deficiency of premotor cortical network inhibition (Hallett, 2000, 2006a, b). Decreased levels of the inhibitory neurotransmitter gamma-aminobutyric acid (GABA) are present in

the contralateral sensorimotor cortex and lentiform nucleus in patients with writer's cramp (Levy & Hallett, 2002). Functional magnetic resonance imaging shows impaired activation of the primary sensorimotor and supplementary motor cortex during voluntary muscle relaxation and contraction (Oga et al., 2002). A genetic factor in the development of hand dystonia is possible, as up to 20% of patients with writer's cramp have family members with dystonia. It is likely that the disorder is mainly the consequence of repetitive activity on the background of a genetic predisposition (Hallett, 1998).

Writer's cramp

Writer's cramp was first reported amongst scribes in the eighteenth century under the term "Occupational Palsy," where some workers had disabling spasms of their hands only when performing their jobs (Solly, 1864). It is a focal task-specific hand dystonia seen in people whose profession involves excessive writing. The incidence of writer's cramp of 14 per 1 000 000 in Europe and 2.7 per 1 000 000 in Rochester Minnesota may represent underestimates because many patients do not seek medical attention (Nutt et al., 1988; ESDE et al., 2000). In support of this is a recent population-based study that found writer's cramp to be the most common focal dystonia (Das et al., 2007). Amongst the various forms of focal dystonias, writer's cramp is

Manual of Botulinum Toxin Therapy, ed. Daniel Truong, Dirk Dressler and Mark Hallett. Published by Cambridge University Press.
© Cambridge University Press 2009.

Table 9.1. Occupations prone to have dystonia

Excessive writers	Others
Students	Typists
Teachers	Telegraphers
Clerks	Computer operators
Musicians	Watchmakers
Pianists	Seamstresses
Horn player	Surgeons/Dentists
Clarinetists	Golfers
Guitarists	Fencing masters
Violinists	Cobblers
Flutists	Tailors
Saxophonists	Bookmakers

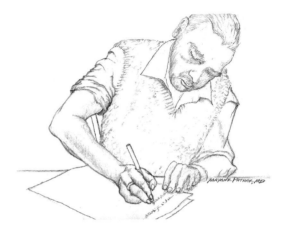

Figure 9.1 Arm abduction subtype. Arm abduction can occur while writing, which could be a primary writer's cramp or a compensatory mechanism to other types.

variably reported to be seen in 5–19% of cases (Duffey *et al.*, 1998; ESDE, 2000). In contrast to other focal dystonias, writer's cramp is seen more frequently in males (Soland *et al.*, 1996; Duffey *et al.*, 1998; ESDE, 1999). Patients with writer's cramp are able to conduct most of their normal activities without difficulty. In other tasks requiring activation of the same muscle group the hand appears normal and performs unremarkably.

Clinical subtypes

In "simple writer's cramp" other acts of dexterity, e.g. buttoning of clothes or handling of forks and knives, are unimpaired. Simple writer's cramp can be of flexion or extension type depending upon the type of abnormal finger movements. Rarely there may be a mixture of flexion in some finger(s) and extension in other(s). Some patients have difficulties with tasks other than writing as well and are said to have "dystonic writer's cramp," but the term "complex writer's cramp" may be more appropriate (Jedynak *et al.*, 2001). Simple writer's cramp can be a prelude to complex writer's cramp, but many patients' conditions remain simple. The posturing of the wrist may also be flexion or extension type. Commonly seen subtypes of writer's cramp include focal flexor, focal extensor, and generalized flexor of the fingers; similarly there may be generalized

flexion with or without finger flexion or extension of the wrist. Rarely, arm abduction occurs while writing, which could be a primary or a compensatory mechanism (Figure 9.1).

Disability in writer's cramp

When asked to write, dystonic muscle activity interferes with normal muscle activation patterns. Not infrequently muscle aching and pain may develop, largely as a consequence of the excessive muscle contractions. The development of pain usually does not correlate with the severity of writing impairment. Pain, however, correlates with the handicap score (Jedynak *et al.*, 2001). Frequently patients switch to writing with the non-dominant hand. Unfortunately, writer's cramp tends to develop in the non-dominant hand in about 10–15% of the patients. About half of the patients develop "mirror dystonia," i.e., they produce dystonic muscle activity in their dystonic hand when they are writing with the good hand (Jedynak *et al.*, 2001). Occasionally, writer's cramp is associated with other dystonias, most commonly cervical dystonia, especially in those having a hand tremor. Coexistence of writer's cramp with oromandibular dystonia is also seen.

Musician's focal dystonia

Musician's focal dystonia is localized to groups of muscles controlling fine movements of the digits or the embouchure muscles of wind instrumentalists (Tubiana, 2003). The dystonia consists of abnormal spasms or posturing of isolated muscle groups that may become apparent only during playing. Musicians often report incoordination while playing that is frequently accompanied by involuntary flexion or extension of fingers during music passages that emphasize rapid, forceful finger movements (Wilson *et al.*, 1993).

The "disobedient" fingers most often implicated are the two ulnar digits. These two fingers constitute the power grip part of the hand; they are not designed for the prolonged, rapid, highly complex movements demanded in musical performance (Newmark & Hochberg, 1987). However, the radial digits and thumb also may be involved, especially the thumb of the right hand in pianists. In violinists and viola players, the left side is more frequently involved. In wind instrumentalists, the hand supporting the instrument and doing the fingering at the same time is most often affected (e.g. left hand in flutists, right hand in clarinetists) (Figure 9.2a and b).

Sometimes the onset of symptoms is found to coincide with a period of intense musical activity and overuse, such as preparation for a competition, or obsessive practice in an attempt to increase the speed of a difficult passage. Usually the disorder does not progress beyond the focal task-specific problem, although it sometimes generalizes to other tasks or other parts of the body. The examination of the patient while playing his or her instrument is important for the diagnosis and for the therapeutic program. Sometimes it is possible to identify an abnormal movement of the fingers, involuntary flexion, "curling in" of one or two fingers, or, by contrast, involuntary extension of the "sticking fingers."

Treatment options

Writer's cramp

Of the several available options, use of botulinum toxin seems the most promising. Other methods may have some utility. A special type of ball pen having cylindrical shape and grip area that flares out at the bottom and is covered by a 2- to 3-mm thick, soft silicon rubber sleeve in the grip area is known to decrease fatigue in these patients. Sensory training by learning Braille reading and practicing for 30–60 minutes per day for up to one year also may provide benefit (Zeuner *et al.*, 2002;

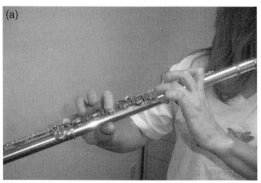
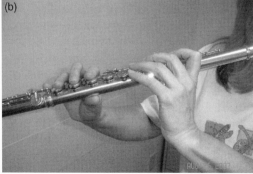

Figure 9.2 Musician hand. In wind instrumentalists, the hand supporting the instrument and doing the fingering at the same time is most often affected (e.g. left hand in flutists, right hand in clarinetists). (a) illustrates cramping in the second, third, and fourth fingers of the left hand. It also shows the wrist flexing out and away from the instrument. (b) is the correct hand position, showing a relaxed hand position and slight curving of the fingers and the wrist.

Zeuner & Hallett, 2003). Specific types of motor training may help (Zeuner et al., 2005). Limb immobilization via a plastic splint for 4–5 weeks has been proposed. Stereotactic nucleus ventrooralis (Vo) thalamotomy has shown benefit for up to 29 months in writer's cramp (Taira et al., 2003).

Botulinum toxin therapy

The first step in using botulinum toxin to treat hand dystonia is careful evaluation and selection of muscles for injection. The patient should be examined at rest and during movements that specifically activate the dystonia: writers should be observed while writing and musicians while playing their instruments. However, the complexity of such movements often makes it difficult to determine which movements are dystonic and which are part of the normal pattern for that activity. Patients should be asked to write without trying to compensate. Additionally, they can describe any abnormal pulling that they experience. It is often helpful also to have the patient perform other activities that may elicit the dystonia without associated movements or compensation. Writing with the non-dominant hand, which can evoke dystonia in the dominant, resting hand (mirror dystonia), is one such strategy. Mirror dystonia can be helpful to identify dystonic muscle activity and to distinguish dystonia from compensatory muscle activity (Singer et al., 2005). The injection site(s) of various muscles and hand/finger positions to activate the concerned muscles are depicted in sketches. The efficacy of treatment, however, depends more on the correct choice of muscle(s).

Botulinum toxin is effective in writer's cramp and other occupational dystonias (Karp et al., 1994; Karp, 2004). In the early study by Cohen et al. (1989), dose finding was aided by a booster dose at 2 weeks, but generally nowadays booster doses are not recommended. The onset of benefit starts approximately 1 week after injection, peaks at 2 weeks and lasts approximately 3 months. Recent studies have shown more than half of the patients with writer's cramp returned repeatedly for longer follow-up periods (Turjanski et al., 1996; Hsuing et al., 2002). A quantitative analysis by Wissel et al. (1996), using the Writer's Cramp Rating Scale (WCRS), performed on 31 patients showed a good response to botulinum toxin. The mean dose injected per session was 133.2 (mouse) units Dysport®. Of all 124 injection sessions during mean follow up of one year, 76% produced a good improvement. The most common side effect was weakness (72% of the follow-up visits). The WCRS scores and the speed of the pen movements showed significant improvement after treatment.

In a study of 53 patients, Karp et al. (1994) showed that patients with localized writer's cramp fared better and those with associated tremors were the worst off. In a prospective study on 47 patients, Djebbari et al. (2004) showed that those with a flexion and pronation of the forearm and those with thumb extension have a significantly better response on the Burke-Fahn-Marsden scale. An earlier placebo-controlled double-blind study by Tsui et al. (1993) also showed better outcome in those with wrist deviation. The restoration of normal motor function in focal task-specific dystonias is probably better when treatment is initiated as early as possible and when motor performance deterioration is still mild.

There are no head-to-head trials comparing efficacy of Botox® and Dysport in writer's cramp. There has been no study reported with NeuroBloc®/ Myobloc® or Xeomin®. Injection sites can be chosen clinically by muscle activation, eliciting mirror dystonia and by following localization points described in manuals of electrophysiology. However, botulinum toxin delivery is better ensured by use of specialized electromyographic (EMG) needles with a hollow core. The intended muscle or fascicle may be missed in up to 50% of attempts without use of EMG (Molloy et al., 2002). Electromyographic guidance is especially recommended where deeper muscles are targeted. Botulinum toxin is injected into one, two, or more sites depending on the dose to be injected and the muscle bulk. The dosage commonly used in various muscles of different preparations is summarized in Table 9.2.

Table 9.2. Dosage of botulinum toxin for various muscles in writer's cramp

Muscle	Botox or Xeomin units	Dysport units	Myobloc units
Flexor digitorum profundus (FDP)	20–40	60–120	750–2500
Flexor carpi ulnaris (FCU)	20–40	60–120	750–2500
Flexor digitorium superficialis (FDS)	25–50	75–50	1000–2500
Flexor carpi radialis (FCR)	25–50	75–50	1000–2500
Flexor pollicis longus (FPL)	10–20	30–50	500–1000
Extensor pollicis longus (EPL)	10–20	30–50	500–1000
Pronator teres (PT)	20–30	60–100	1000–1500
Lumbricals/extensor indicis proprius (EIP)	5–10	15–30	250–500
Extensor digitorium communis (EDC)	15–25	50–75	750–1250

Note:
Note that this is only a rough guide and that therapy must be individualized. Moreover, there is no certain fixed ratio between the toxin types (including Botox and Xeomin), and this might vary in different circumstances.

Writer's cramp subtypes

Botulinum toxin may be used to treat writer's cramp. For successful treatment, the hyperactive muscles should be known. Writer's cramp can be divided into subtypes based upon the hypothesized muscle group. The most common subtypes are:

    Focal flexor (finger) subtype
    Generalized flexor (finger) subtype
    Focal extensor (finger) subtype
    Generalized extensor (wrist) subtype
    Generalized flexor (wrist) subtype (with/without
      finger flexion)
    Arm abduction subtype.

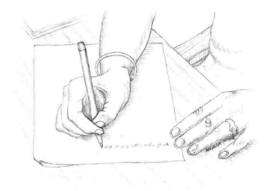

Figure 9.3 Focal flexor subtype.

Focal flexor subtype (Figure 9.3)

In the focal flexor subtype, up to two fingers may be involved. Often the thumb or the index finger flexes with the writing activities. Either the individual flexor pollicis longus or brevis are involved in the thumb flexion. Individual fascicles of the flexor digitorum superficialis (FDS) or profundus (FDP) can also be involved.

Flexor pollicis longus (FPL)
The FPL originates in the anterior surface of the middle half of the radius and inserts in the palmar surface of the distal phalanx of the thumb (Lee & DeLisa, 2000). The needle is inserted between the middle and the distal third of the forearm. The needle is verified by the patient flexing the distal phalanx of the thumb. Prior to needle insertion, the radial artery should be noted (Figure 9.4).

Flexor pollicis brevis (FPB)
The FPB has two heads. One head originates in the flexor retinaculum, trapezium, and trapezoid. The other one is from the second and third metacarpals. It inserts into the lateral side of the base of the proximal phalanx of the thumb. The needle is inserted into the medial half of the thenar eminence. The muscle is verified by the patient flexing the thumb (Figure 9.5) (Lee & DeLisa, 2000).

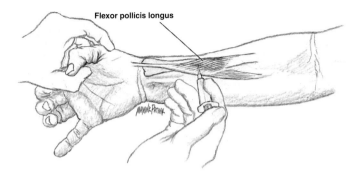

Flexor pollicis longus

Figure 9.4 Flexor pollicis longus (localization).

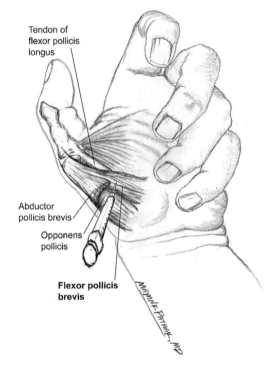

Tendon of flexor pollicis longus

Abductor pollicis brevis

Opponens pollicis

Flexor pollicis brevis

Figure 9.5 Flexor pollicis brevis (localization).

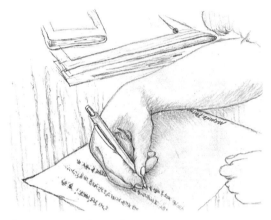

Figure 9.6 General wrist flexor.

Generalized flexor subtype (Figure 9.6 and Figure 9.7)

In the generalized flexor subtype the patient's hand has the tendency to flex after the start of the writing. The patient complains of pain and aching either on the palm or flexor forearm muscle group. The flexor carpi radialis and flexor carpi ulnaris are often involved. Commonly there are increased activations of the flexor muscle group of the fingers (FDS, FDP) and the palmaris longus (Figure 9.7). When severe, the pronator muscle group may also be activated, resulting in pronation of the hand.

Flexor digitorum superficialis (FDS)

The FDS originates from the medial epicondyle and coronoid process of the ulnar. It divides into four tendons and inserts into the middle phalanges of the second to fifth digit. With the patient's arm supinated, the needle is inserted at the mid forearm in the layer between the palmaris longus (PL) and flexor carpi ulnaris (FCU) (Lee & DeLisa, 2000). These two muscles are identified by following their tendons from the wrist. Each fascicle of the FDS can be identified by flexing the respective finger at the middle phalanx (Figure 9.8).

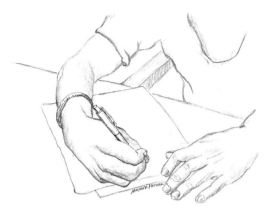

Figure 9.7 General wrist and finger flexor. The general wrist flexor may involve the flexor digitorum superficialis, flexor digitorum profundus, and palmaris longus as well to develop into general wrist and finger flexor. When severe, the pronator muscle group may also be activated, resulting in pronation of the hand.

Flexor digitorum profundus (FDP)

The FDP originates in the proximal anterior surface of the ulnar and the anterior interosseous membrane. It divides into four tendons and inserts into the palmar surface of the distal phalanges of the second to fifth finger. With the patient's hand supinated and the elbow flexed, the needle is inserted at the middle of the forearm, passing through the FCU and advanced tangentially toward the radial side. Each of the muscle fascicles can be identified by having the patient flex the distal phalanx of the second to fifth finger individually (Figure 9.9).

Palmaris longus (PL)

The PL muscle, which is medial to the flexor carpi radialis (FCR), originates in the medial epicondyle and inserts into the palmar aponeurosis and flexor retinaculum. The needle is inserted into the proximal upper third of the line between the middle of the wrist and the medial epicondyle (Figure 9.10). As this is a superficial muscle, caution must be taken to not insert the needle too deeply into the FDP.

Flexor carpi radialis (FCR)

This muscle originates in the medial epicondyle of the humerus and inserts at the second metacarpal bone. The needle is inserted at about a third of the distance from the medial epicondyle and the needle tip is verified by asking the patient to flex and adduct the wrist (Figure 9.11).

Flexor carpi ulnaris (FCU)

The FCU originates in the medial epicondyle of the humerus and inserts in the pisiform and hamate bone and the fifth metacarpal bone. The needle is inserted into the middle of the muscle. The needle tip is verified by the patient flexing with ulnar deviation of the wrist or by simply flexing and abducting the fifth finger (Figure 9.12).

Figure 9.8 Flexor digitorum superficialis (localization).

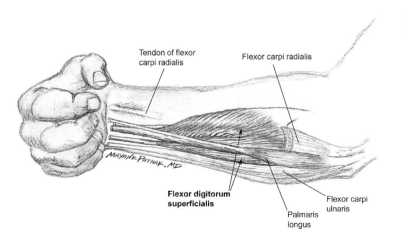

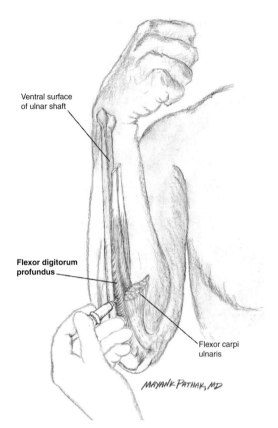

Figure 9.9 Flexor digitorum profundus (localization).

Pronator teres

The pronator teres originates in the medial epicondyle of the humerus and coronoid process of the ulna. It wraps around the radius and inserts into the lateral surface of the radius. With the patient in supine position and the forearm supinated, the needle is introduced medial to the cubital fossa about two fingers below the elbow. The position of the needle is verified by the patient pronating the forearm with slight elbow flexion (Figure 9.13).

Pronator quadratus

The pronator quadratus originates in the anteromedial aspect at the distal part of the ulna and inserts into the anteromedial aspect of the distal part of the radius (Figure 9.13). With the patient in supine position and the forearm pronated, the needle is inserted 3 cm proximal to the ulnar styloid close to the surface of the ulna. Another approach is from the dorsal surface of the distal forearm, the needle is advanced through the interosseous membrane to the pronator quadratus. Pronation of the forearm verifies the needle position.

Focal extensor subtype

In the focal extensor subtype often only the extensor pollicis longus (EPL) and extensor indicis proprius (EIP) are involved (Figure 9.14). With continuous use

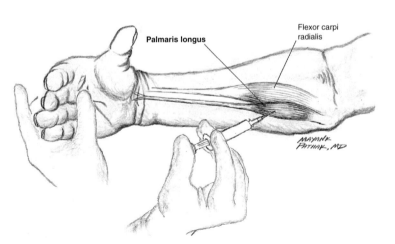

Figure 9.10 Palmaris longus (localization).

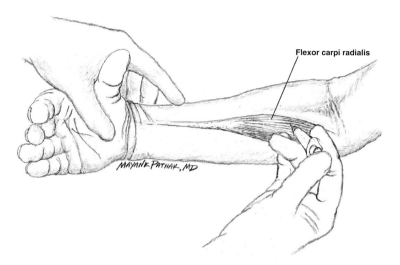

Figure 9.11 Flexor carpi radialis (localization).

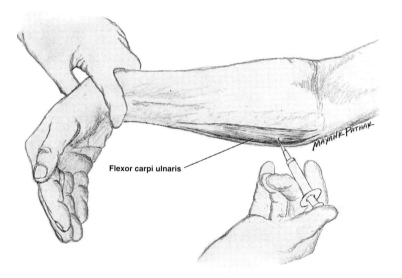

Figure 9.12 Flexor carpi ulnaris (localization).

of the dystonic hand, further worsening may lead to the generalized extensor subtype (Figure 9.15).

Extensor indicis proprius (EIP)

The EIP is often involved in the extensor subtype of writer's cramp. The patient extends the index finger while holding the pen with the others. The EIP originates in the dorsal surface of the ulna and inserts in the second finger. The muscle is approached with the hand pronated and the needle

inserted into the distal fourth of the forearm lateral to the radial side of the ulna (Figure 9.16). The needle is verified by extension of the index finger. Caution must be taken because if the needle is inserted too proximally, it will be in the EPL.

Extensor pollicis longus (EPL)

The EPL originates from the posterior surface of the middle third of the ulnar shaft and the posterior interosseous membrane (Figure 9.17). It inserts into

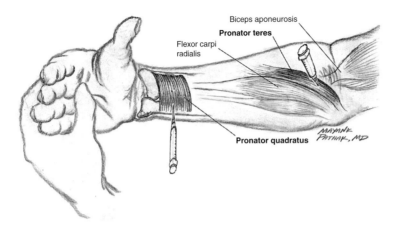

Figure 9.13 Pronator muscle group (localization).

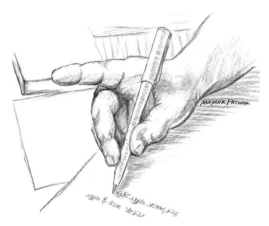

Figure 9.14 Focal extensor subtype.

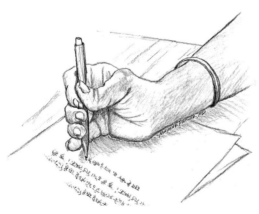

Figure 9.15 Generalized wrist extensor subtype.

the dorsal surface of the base of the distal phalanx of the thumb. The needle is inserted at the middle third of the forearm along the radial side of the ulna. The position of the needle is verified by the patient extending the thumb at the distal phalanx.

Generalized extensor subtype

In the generalized extensor subtype the hand extends with writing as seen in Figure 9.15, although different extensors are involved. The patient compensates by flexing the fingers to hold the pen. Intermittently different fingers will extend leading to dropping of the pen.

Extensor carpi radialis longus (ECRL)
The ECRL originates in the distal third of the lateral supracondylar ridge of the humerus and inserts in the dorsal surface and base of the second metacarpal bone. With the forearm pronated, the patient extends and slightly abducts the wrist radially, the needle is inserted 2–3 cm distal to the elbow joint. The position of the needle is verified by the patient extending the wrist toward the radial side (Figure 9.18).

Extensor carpi radialis brevis (ECRB)
The smaller ECRB originates from the lateral epicondyle of the humerus and radial collateral ligament of the elbow joint. It inserts in the dorsal surface of the base of the third metacarpal bone.

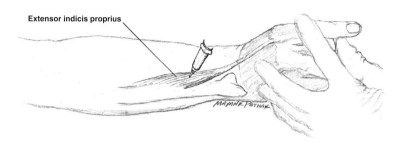

Figure 9.16 Extensor indicis proprius (localization).

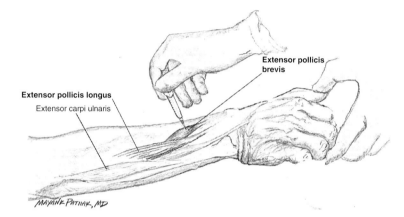

Figure 9.17 Extensor pollicis longus/brevis (localization).

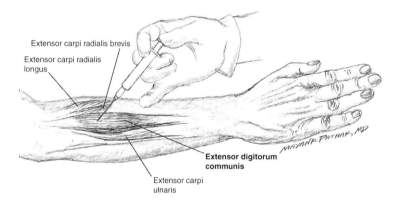

Figure 9.18 Extensor digitorum communis (localization).

For needle insertion the ECRB is slightly distal and lateral to the ECRL. Both ECRL and ECRB extend the wrist (Figure 9.18).

Extensor digitorum communis (EDC)
This muscle originates in the lateral epicondyle by a common extensor tendon and inserts with a central slip into the middle phalanges of fingers 2, 3, 4, 5 and two collateral slips to the terminal phalanges of the above four fingers. The needle insertion point is in the upper third on the line drawn between the lateral epicondyle and ulnar styloid (Figure 9.18). The position of the muscle can be verified by activating each finger separately while the other fingers

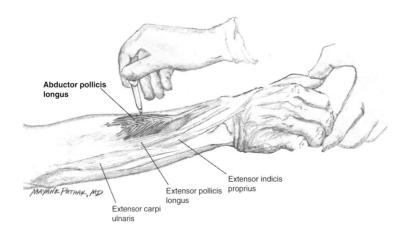

Figure 9.19 Abductor pollicis longus (localization).

form a fist. It extends and abducts at the wrist as well as extending the fifth finger.

Extensor carpi ulnaris (ECU)

The ECU muscle originates in the lateral epicondyle of the humerus and inserts at the base of the fifth metacarpal. It is activated by the forearm in the prone position slightly extended at the wrist with ulnar deviation. The needle is inserted at the junction of the upper and mid thirds of the forearm. Localization is confirmed by alternate activation and relaxation of the muscle (Figure 9.18).

Extensor indicis proprius (EIP)

The EIP can also be involved in the generalized extensor subtype of writer's cramp (already described on page 69).

Abductor pollicis longus (APL)

The APL is proximal to the EIP. Patients affected with APL and EIP spasms complain of involuntarily losing their pen when writing. The APL originates in the dorsal surface of the lower half of the ulna, posterior interosseus membrane, and the middle third of the radius. It inserts into the radial side of the base of the first metacarpal bone. The needle is inserted at the junction of the middle and lower third of the dorsal surface of the radial bone. Needle position is verified by the patient abducting or extending the thumb at the metacarpal joint (Figure 9.19).

Extensor pollicis longus (EPL)

Already described on p. 69.

Extensor pollicis brevis (EPB)

The EPB originates at the posterior surface of the radial shaft and the posterior interosseous membrane (Figure 9.17). It inserts at the dorsal surface of the base of the proximal phalanx of the thumb. The muscle is deep to the EPL. The needle is inserted at the junction of the lower and middle third of the posterior surface of the radial shaft. This thin muscle is verified by extension of the proximal phalanx.

Arm abduction subtype

In some patients, the upper arm may be abducted with attempted writing (Figure 9.1). These movements could be compensatory to accommodate the dystonic contraction of the generalized flexor subtype. Sometimes the abduction of the arm is the primary dystonic posture. In these cases the deltoid muscle is also involved.

Alternative methods for muscle localization

In the previous descriptions, we often noted that the muscle can be verified by voluntary contraction. This is not always the case, as patients can have difficulty isolating individual movement. Alternative methods for muscle verification include (1) passive movement of the joint with observation of needle movement, (2) stimulation through the needle with observation of movement, and (3) ultrasound.

Adverse effects of botulinum toxin

Excessive weakness of the target muscle is the most common side effect. In preliminary studies the improvement in writer's cramp was almost invariably accompanied by weakness. This weakness was considered necessary to produce improvement in writer's cramp. Weakness may impair non-writing tasks. A few patients may develop atrophy of the injected muscles after repeated injections; however, if injections are stopped, muscle strength will recover. Pain and bruising may also occur at the injection sites. Antibodies may develop against botulinum toxin, especially when larger doses are required. In this case botulinum toxin type A resistant patients may be treated with type B toxin.

Treatment of musicians' focal dystonia

Musicians' focal dystonia is difficult to treat and has uncertain results. Management requires a multidisciplinary approach. General sedatives and relaxants have been used with no obvious benefit. Anticholinergic drugs can be helpful in some cases but are difficult to tolerate.

Neurorehabilitation methods can be tried. One reasonable aim of treatment, given the task specificity of the disorder, is to establish a new sensorimotor program. Another aim would be to reprogram the original motor program. Different methods have been proposed to achieve these goals (Zeuner *et al.*, 2005). A rehabilitation program should include physical and psychological components (Candia *et al.*, 2002; Chamagne *et al.*, 2003). It consists of making a musician aware of their poor posture, deprogramming non-physiological postures and gestures to ensure that the patient understands the functional anatomy and biomechanics involved in their problems, and then teaching new movements that respect normal physiology.

Botulinum toxin is not as effective for musicians' focal dystonia as it is for writer's cramp. Musicians have proven notoriously difficult to treat with this modality and have shown a strong propensity to withdraw from treatment once they find that control of their instruments is not sufficiently improved, in part because of muscular weakness that follows botulinum toxin injection. One of the main problems with musicians is the need for improvement virtually to normal if they are going to play professionally, and this would only be rarely accomplished. Despite these considerations, botulinum toxin is the method of choice (Cole *et al.*, 1991). Approach to the different muscles is similar as with writer's cramp, but dosing should be conservative.

Other focal dystonias

Besides the most common occupational dystonias, some other less common occupational dystonias can be mentioned. Focal hand dystonia affecting golfers is termed "yips." Yips consists of involuntary movements occurring in the course of the execution of focused, finely controlled skilled motor activity (McDaniel *et al.*, 1989). The movements emerge particularly during "putting" and are less evident during "chipping" or "driving." It might worsen with anxiety and compensatory strategies such as changing hand preference, handgrip, and using a longer putter may ameliorate the symptoms. Recently, EMG studies have documented co-contractions of wrist flexors and extensors in golfers affected with yips, supporting the dystonic nature of this movement disorder. Spontaneous remissions may occur. Benzodiazepines are not helpful in the majority of cases. Botulinum toxin has not been systematically studied in golfers' dystonia.

Typists and telegraphers are also known to develop focal hand dystonia known as typist's cramp and telegrapher's cramp respectively. The affected telegraphers describe stiffness, spasm, cramp, tremor, and weakness. They also report that symptoms appear more in the afternoon than morning sessions, and on Friday more often than Sunday, suggesting a relationship with excessive work. Focal hand dystonia has also been described in cobblers, tailors, bookmakers, watchmakers, and doctors (surgeons/dentists), since these occupations also involve excessive and repetitive fine motor activity. The pathophysiology of these focal dystonias is likely to be the same as that of writer's cramp, though they have not been studied systematically. The treatment of these conditions also has not been established, but a program of neuromuscular rehabilitation and botulinum toxin is expected to be an appropriate course of action.

REFERENCES

Candia, V., Schafer, T., Taub, E., *et al.* (2002). Sensory motor retuning: a behavioral treatment for focal hand dystonia of pianists and guitarists. *Arch Phys Med Rehabil*, **83**, 1342–8.

Chamagne, P. (2003). Functional dystonia in musicians: rehabilitation. *Hand Clinics*, **19**, 309–16.

Cohen, L. G., Hallett, M., Geller, B. D. & Hochberg, F. (1989). Treatment of focal dystonias of the hand with botulinum toxin injections. *J Neurol Neurosurg Psychiatry*, **52**, 355–63.

Cole, R. A., Cohen, L. G. & Hallett, M. (1991). Treatment of musician's cramp with botulinum toxin. *Med Probl Perform Artists*, **6**, 137–43.

Das, S. K., Banerjee, T. K., Biswas, A., *et al.* (2007). Community survey of primary dystonia in the city of Kolkata, India. *Mov Disord*, **22**, 2031–6.

Djebbari, R., Dumontcel, S. T., Sangla, S., *et al.* (2004). Factors predicting improvement in motor disability in writer's cramp treated with botulinum toxin. *J Neurol Neurosurg Psychiatry*, **75**, 1688–91.

Duffey, O., Butler, A. G., Hawthorne, M. R. & Barnes, M. P. (1998). The epidemiology of the primary dystonias in the north of England. *Adv Neurol*, **78**, 12–15.

Epidemiological Study of Dystonia in Europe (ESDE) Collaborative Group. (1999). Sex related influences on the frequency and age of onset of primary dystonia. *Neurology*, **53**, 1871–3.

Epidemiological Study of Dystonia in Europe (ESDE) Collaborative Group. (2000). A prevalence study of primary dystonia in eight European countries. *J Neurol*, **247**, 787–92.

Hallett, M. (1998). Physiology of dystonia. *Adv Neurol*, **78**, 11–18.

Hallett, M. (2000). Disorder of movement preparation in dystonia. *Brain*, **123**, 1765–6.

Hallett, M. (2006a). Pathophysiology of dystonia. *Journal of Neural Transmission Suppl.* **70**, 485–8.

Hallett, M. (2006b). Pathophysiology of writer's cramp. *Hum Mov Sci*, **4–5**, 454–63.

Hsuing, G. Y., Das, S. K. & Ranawaya, R. (2002). Long term efficacy of botulinum toxin A in treatment of various movement disorders over a 10 year period. *Mov Disord*, **17**, 1288–93.

Jedynak, P. C., Tranchant, C. & Zegers Debeyl, D. (2001). Prospective clinical study of writer's cramp. *Mov Disord*, **16**, 494–9.

Karp, B. I. (2004). Botulinum toxin treatment of occupational and focal hand dystonia. *Mov Disord*, **19**(Suppl 8), S116–19.

Karp, B. I., Cole, R. A., Cohen, L. G., *et al.* (1994). Long term botulinum toxin treatment of focal hand dystonia. *Neurology*, **44**, 70–6.

Lee, H. & DeLisa, J. (2000). *Surface Anatomy for Clinical Needle Electromyography*. New York, NY: Demos Medical Publishing.

Levy, L. M. & Hallett, M. (2002). Impaired brain GABA in focal dystonia. *Ann Neurol*, **51**, 93–101.

McDaniel, K. D., Cummings, J. L. & Shain, S. (1989). The "yips": a focal dystonia of golfers. *Neurology*, **39**, 192–5.

Molloy, F. M., Shill, H. A., Kaelin–Lang, A. & Karp, B. I. (2002). Accuracy of muscle localization without EMG: implications for treatment of limb dystonia. *Neurology*, **58**, 805–7.

Newmark, J. & Hochberg, F. H. (1987). Isolated painless manual incoordination in 57 musicians. *J Neurol Neurosurg Psychiatry*, **50**, 291–5.

Nutt, J. G., Muenter, M. D., Aronson, A., Kurland, L. T. & Melton, L. J. (1988). Epidemiology of focal and generalised dystonia in Rochester Minnesota. *Mov Disord*, **3**, 188–94.

Oga, T., Honda, M., Toma, K., *et al.* (2002). Abnormal cortical mechanisms of voluntary muscle relaxation in patients with writer's cramp: an MRI study. *Brain*, **125**, 895–903.

Singer, C., Papapetropoulos, S. & Vela, L. (2005). Use of mirror dystonia as guidance for injection of botulinum toxin in writing dysfunction. *J Neurol Neurosurg Psychiatry*, **76**, 1608–9.

Soland, V. L., Bhatis, K. P. & Marsden, C. D. (1996). Sex prevalence of focal dystonias. *J Neurol Neurosurg Psychiatry*, **60**, 204–5.

Solly, S. (1864). Scrivener's palsy, or paralysis of writer's. *Lancet*, **2**, 709–11.

Taira, T., Harashima, S. & Hori, T. (2003). Neurosurgical treatment for writer's cramp. *Acta Neurochir*, **87**(Suppl), 129–31.

Tsui, J. K. C., Bhatt, M., Calne, S. & Calne, D. B. (1993). Botulinum toxin in the treatment of writer's cramp. A double blind study. *Neurology*, **43**, 183–5.

Tubiana, R. (2003). Musician's focal dystonia. *Hand Clinics*, **19**, 303–8.

Turjanski, N., Pirtosek, Z. & Quirk, J. (1996). Botulinum toxin in the treatment of writer's cramp. *Clin Neuropharmacol*, **19**, 314–20.

Wilson, F., Wagner, C. & Homberg, V. (1993). Biomechanical abnormalities in musicians with occupational cramp focal dystonia. *J Hand Ther*, **64**, 234–44.

Wissel, J., Kabus, C., Wenzel, R., *et al.* (1996). Botulinum toxin in writer's cramp: objective response evaluation in 31 patients. *J Neurol Neurosurg Psychiatry*, **61**, 172–5.

Zeuner, K. E. & Hallett, M. (2003). Sensory training as treatment for focal hand dystonia: a 1 year follow up. *Mov Disord*, **18**, 1044–7.

Zeuner, K. E., Bara-Jimenez, W., Noguchi, P. S., *et al.* (2002). Sensory training for patients with focal hand dystonia. *Ann Neurol*, **51**, 593–8.

Zeuner, K. E., Shill, H. A., Sohn, Y. H., *et al.* (2005). Motor training as a treatment in focal hand dystonia. *Mov Disord*, **20**, 335–41.

10

Botulinum toxin applications in ophthalmology

Peter Roggenkaemper and Alan B. Scott

Introduction

Justinus Kerner, a German medical doctor and poet, was the first to describe botulism in detail. He recognized the disease to be related to the consumption of poison in sausages, and described how these were improperly prepared. His description of the disease (Kerner 1822), including the paralysis of muscles and reduction of glandular function, was as accurate and complete as any today. He extracted the toxin, applied it in animals and considered the therapeutic value of the extracted poison, especially in motor overexcitability (for instance in chorea minor). However, it took around 150 years until botulinum toxin (BoNT) was first used for therapeutic measures. This was done by a coauthor of this chapter, who examined a number of chemical substances in order to find one which could lengthen an extrinsic eye muscle in order to have an alternative to squint operation. In animal tests BoNT proved to be the only substance that showed the desired paralytic effect and was locally and systemically well tolerated in a very low dose (Scott *et al.*, 1973). The first patients were treated in 1978 (Scott, 1980). Meanwhile, it is evident that this method is safe but cannot replace surgery for most strabismus cases, because the long-term effect is not stable in many patients (Figure 10.1).

Besides strabismus – as you see in this book – BoNT has emerged as an important or even first-line treatment for many medical disorders as well as for cosmetic indications. Around the eye/orbit a number of diseases can be treated: predominantly essential blepharospasm and hemifacial spasm (for both BoNT is the first choice treatment, see Chapters 7 and 6 respectively); to lengthen retracted lids and to overcome double vision in Graves' disease; to reduce oscillopsia and improve vision in nystagmus; to produce protective ptosis in case of lagophthalmos or corneal diseases; to reduce tearing by injections into the lacrimal gland; and to treat special cases of spastic entropion.

BoNT treatment of strabismus

General

Physical realignment of the eyes is often needed in strabismus treatment to remove diplopia, to align the eyes to allow development of binocular function, and for cosmesis. Botulinum toxin injection was developed as an alternative to surgery to treat small angles (Figure 10.2), to treat infantile esotropia, to reduce antagonist contracture in acquired paralytic strabismus, and for patients who decline surgery. In the eye muscle system an interval of 3–4 months of reduced abnormal activity is not the goal as it is in blepharospasm and many other disorders. Instead, the induced paralysis acts to alter eye position and hence alter eye muscle lengths for

Manual of Botulinum Toxin Therapy, ed. Daniel Truong, Dirk Dressler and Mark Hallett. Published by Cambridge University Press.
© Cambridge University Press 2009.

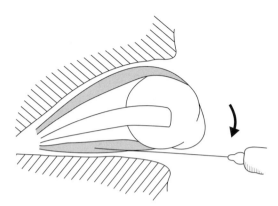

Figure 10.1 Extraocular muscle injection, schematically.

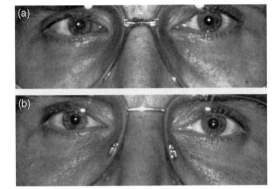

Figure 10.2 (a) Small angle esotropia. (b) Same patient 3 months after botulinum toxin injection of the medial rectus muscle.

a period of 2–3 months. The muscles respond to this change by sarcomeric adaptation, actual lengthening of the injected muscle and shortening of the antagonist, just as do skeletal muscles. (Scott, 1994) In general, about 40% of cases are corrected to within 10 prism diopters at one year with one injection, about 65% corrected with an average of 1.6 injections.

Indications

Botulinum toxin injections in extraocular muscles are useful for both normal and restrictive strabismus.

Sixth nerve paralysis is a frequent indication: the medial rectus is injected to reduce contracture.

There is often a good effect on double vision. In patients who have a good prognosis, e.g. a diabetic or hypertensive origin of the paresis, BoNT can provide earlier rehabilitation. In cases with more severe paresis where a long recovery time is anticipated, the contracture of the medial rectus and the increase of esotropia can be prevented. Functional as well as cosmetic results are available compared to the cases without BoNT injection. In cases of permanent paralysis, an operation such as a transposition procedure is necessary, but BoNT can improve contracture of the medial rectus and thereby avoid surgical recession and its concomitant reduction of range of motion. In addition the anterior ciliary artery supply is left intact, reducing or eliminating the problem of anterior segment ischemia.

Botulinum toxin is also useful in certain cases of third and fourth nerve paresis: see special literature (McNeer et al., 1999).

A number of strabismus specialists are treating children with infantile esotropia, acquired esotropia, intermittent exotropia, and strabismus in cerebral palsy. Results approach those of surgery and the brief general anesthesia is an added advantage.

In case of adult strabismus BoNT injection is especially valuable in frequently operated patients, who fear further operation without adequate long-term success. There are often rewarding results in post retinal detachment strabismus and post-cataract strabismus especially with smaller strabismic angle and normal binocular vision. Botulinum toxin injection is useful as a postoperative adjustment of those post squint surgery cases in which the intended goal has not been achieved or in which a further surgical procedure may threaten the vascularity of the anterior segment. Diplopia from strabismus in chronic myasthenia and in progressive external ophthalmoplegia is an additional indication. For a discussion of the place of BoNT use in the above mentioned specific strabismus cases see McNeer et al. (1999).

In addition to the well-documented indications mentioned above, the authors use BoNT injection in adults who desire strabismus correction, but who respond with diplopia to preoperative prism

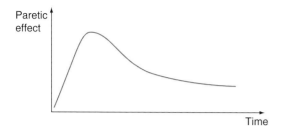

Figure 10.3 Paretic effect of extraocular muscle injection over time, schematically. Maximum effect 10–14 days after injection.

adaptation or forced duction tests. The eye position to be achieved by an operation can be temporarily tested with respect to double vision during the period of overcorrection around one week after BoNT injection (Figure 10.3). It was shown that there is adaptation of suppression or habitation to double vision in 80% of cases (Nuessgens & Roggenkaemper, 1993).

Use of electromyography (EMG)

Teflon insulated injection needles that record only from the tip localize the site of injection in the active muscle. These and an EMG amplifier are important tools for use in eye muscle injection. Practiced injectors do well without EMG for the previously unoperated medial rectus, but for vertical muscles, for cases with unusual muscles such as Graves' disease, and in previously operated cases, EMG guidance is very helpful. The sharp sound of individual motor units indicates correct penetration of the muscle; this is easily appreciated and differentiated from the general hum of nearby muscle. Injection under direct vision after a small conjunctival opening is also good practice. Electromyography is of occasional use also to locate muscles that have been displaced and to determine if a weak muscle is partly or wholly denervated (Figures 10.4, 10.5, and 10.6).

Dosage

For comitant strabismus of 15–30 prism diopters the initial dose is 2.5 (mouse) units Botox®; for

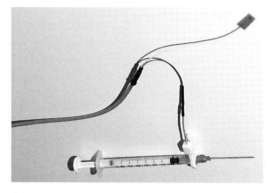

Figure 10.4 Bipolar wire for EMG recording. One pole is connected to the special injection needle.

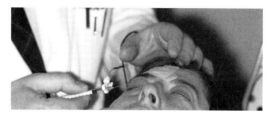

Figure 10.5 Before injection, functioning of the equipment is tested by recording the electric activity of the orbicularis muscle.

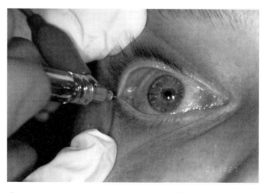

Figure 10.6 Injection of the right lateral rectus muscle.

larger deviations 5.0 units Botox. (Other toxin formulations could also be used, but we have less experience with them. All subsequent dosing in this chapter will also refer to Botox.) While most muscles respond well to this dosage scheme, occasional persons require much more toxin to be effective. We increase the dose by about 50% if an initial dose was inadequate as measured by the degree of induced paralysis and the resulting correction. For medial rectus injection in partial lateral rectus paresis, a dose of 1.0–1.5 units is appropriate.

The intended volume with some extra should be loaded into a 1.0 cc tuberculin syringe, the electrode needle firmly attached, and the excess ejected to assure patency of the needle and absence of leak at the needle/hub. For multiple muscles, multiple syringes are good, as it is often impossible to view the gradations on the syringe for partial volume injection. The EMG amplitude diminishes as the bolus of fluid pushes the muscle fibers away from the injection site, a sign of a good insertion. Leave the needle in place 30–60 seconds after injection to allow the injection bolus to dissipate in the muscle – otherwise it runs back out the needle tract, as we have shown with dyed solution in animals.

Anesthesia

Proparacaine 1% drops are followed 30 seconds later by an alpha-agonist such as Alphagan® or epinephrine 0.1%. Three additional proparacaine drops are placed at intervals of one minute. Where there is scar tissue from prior muscle surgery, injection of 100–200 μl of lidocaine beneath the conjunctiva is helpful.

Medial rectus

The patient gazes at a target slightly into abduction with the fellow eye. Avoiding blood vessels, the electrode tip is inserted 8–10 mm from the limbus and advanced straight back to a position behind the equator of the eye. Gaze is then slowly brought to moderate adduction to activate the muscle, rotating the needle and syringe to keep the electrode tip in position relative to the muscle. Some muscle activity is usually heard at this point, but the needle should be advanced until a sharp motor unit sound is produced. Botulinum toxin diffuses about 15 mm

from the point of injection, and so does not need to be placed far back in the muscle.

Lateral rectus

This is treated similarly, recognizing that the needle must be first directed backward behind the equator of the eye, then angled medially 40 degrees or so.

Inferior rectus

This is done very much as for horizontal muscles. Keeping on the orbital side of the muscle to avoid penetrating the globe, the needle will often penetrate the inferior oblique. Continue on through the inferior oblique, directing the needle medially about 23 degrees along the line of the inferior rectus. There is a step up in the orbital floor 15 mm from the orbital apex and the electrode will often hit against that – angling superiorly will put it directly in the inferior rectus. Injection through the lower lid is easier in thyroid eye disease. The electrode is inserted at the midpoint of the lid, about 8 mm from the lid margin. Penetration through the inferior oblique is usual.

Inferior oblique

This is injected through the conjunctiva, aiming for a point slightly temporal to the lateral border of the inferior rectus at about the equator of the eye. With the eye in far up-gaze, the inferior oblique is highly innervated and its insertion is moved forward, making the muscle accessible.

Superior rectus and superior oblique

These are seldom injected, as prolonged and severe ptosis always results as an effect of diffusion of toxin from the target muscle.

Complications, adverse outcomes

Overflow from diffusion of toxin causes transient vertical deviation and ptosis especially after medial rectus injection in 5–10% of cases; 1–2% of these persist over 6 months. Undercorrection is the most frequent adverse outcome. Consider reinjection at a higher dose if the earlier injection was not fully paralytic. Progressive correction of large deviations is possible by multiple injections.

Endocrine disorders

Endocrine myopathy

Although only 15% of the authors' patients achieved a permanent result, BoNT injection into the involved (thickened) eye muscles is very useful to diminish double vision and anomalous head position in cases where the angle of squint is not yet stable. After injection the passive motility restriction becomes better, and patients feel less tension around the eye. This disease is suitable for the beginner in eye muscle injection technique, because the eye muscles are thickened and easier to hit. In a number of cases it was not possible to get appropriate EMG signals, but even without these the injections were effective. Injection of the inferior rectus can also easily be performed transcutaneously, as mentioned above (Figures 10.7 and 10.8).

Lid retraction in endocrine myopathy

The injection of BoNT (initially 5 or 7.5 units of Botox) into the anterior part of the levator muscle and Mueller's muscle is a valuable method for treatment of lid retraction in a mild or unstable situation as an alternative to the lid lengthening operation. The transcutaneous injection technique used initially, with injection under the orbital roof similar to the technique used for protective ptosis, often gave an over-effect with ptosis. Therefore the authors propose the following subconjunctival technique used by Uddin and Davies (2002), which gives an effect lasting around 3 months, with rare ptosis or double vision: after topical anesthetic drops, the upper lid is everted on a Desmarre retractor, and an injection is made into the center

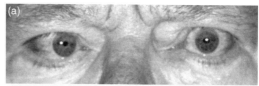
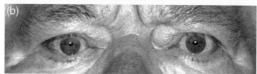

Figure 10.7 (a) Endocrine myopathy of the right medial rectus muscle. (b) Same patient 3 weeks after botulinum toxin injection into the affected muscle.

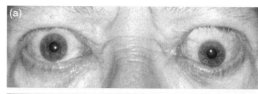
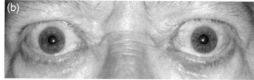

Figure 10.8 (a) Endocrine myopathy of the left inferior rectus muscle. (b) Same patient 4 weeks after injection of this muscle.

of the levator aponeurosis above the upper tarsal rim, and a second injection made into the lateral third of the levator (Figure 10.9).

Protective ptosis

To close the eye in order to protect the cornea or to promote corneal healing, injection of BoNT into the levator palpebrae will last several months. Injection can be done through the upper lid, keeping to the orbital roof and then angling downward until one hears the sound of the levator, or by turning the upper lid and injecting the insertion of the levator.

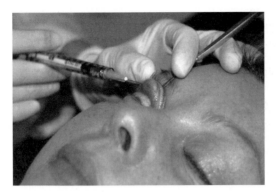

Figure 10.9 Technique of lengthening levator and Mueller's muscle in upper eyelid retraction (Graves' disease).

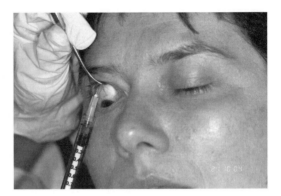

Figure 10.11 Protective ptosis: transconjunctival injection.

Another useful indication for BoNT injection of the levator is temporary lagophthalmos from seventh cranial nerve paresis; e.g., in cases after neurosurgical intervention in the cerebellopontine angle because of acoustic neurinoma. Reinjection may be required until the facial nerve has recovered (Figure 10.12).

Orbital injection for nystagmus

For chair- or bed-bound patients with vision of 20/80 or less the recovered ability to recognize persons, read, and see TV can be very dramatic. It is only realistic to treat one (the better) eye because it is impossible to have both sides paralyzed symmetrically to avoid double vision. Ambulation is severely compromised by the spatial distortion of the induced paralysis, so this is not practical for mild nystagmus. The syringe is loaded with 20–25 units Botox without EMG, the needle is inserted through the lower lid to a point behind the eye as for retrobulbar anesthesia. Place this slightly low in the orbit to reduce the chance of diffusion to the levator with consequent ptosis. Injection of the horizontal muscles for apparent horizontal nystagmus will often reveal a significant residual vertical or torsional component, so orbital injection is preferred. Unlike eye muscle injections that are expected to have a long duration, orbital injection

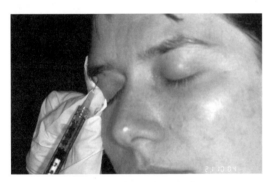

Figure 10.10 Protective ptosis: transcutaneous injection.

Paresis of the superior rectus from diffusion is variable; it is probably dose related and may be less with injection into the levator above the tarsus, as described above (Adams *et al.*, 1987; Naik *et al.*, 2007).

The authors always use the high amount of 20 units Botox because of some failures with less: 10 units are distributed into three sites with a 30 gauge needle transcutaneously, and 10 units transconjunctively by lifting the upper lid with a Desmarre hook but not turning the lid) (Figures 10.10 and 10.11). For this application EMG is not necessary, the effect is relatively sure to be achieved. Diplopia has not been a problem, probably because in injecting the anterior part of the levator the superior rectus was not reached or the superior rectus was only affected when the ptosis was present.

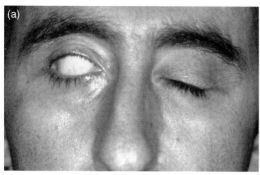 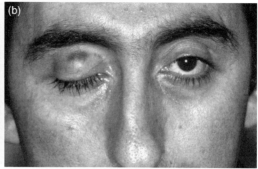

Figure 10.12 (a) Patient with transient lagophthalmos after operation in the cerebellopontine angle because of acoustic neurinoma. Intense Bell's phenomenon during attempt to close the eyes. (b) Same patient after injection of the levator muscle.

for nystagmus will require repetition at intervals of 4–6 months.

Lacrimal gland injection

Botulinum toxin injection of the lacrimal gland is the first choice treatment for the abnormal lacrimation in so-called crocodile tears, i.e., excess tearing during eating caused after proximal facial nerve injury by misrouting to the lacrimal gland of autonomic nerve fibers originally supplying the salivatory gland. Botulinum toxin suppression of lacrimal function is useful also in other situations with excessive tearing such as cases of blocked tear duct.

At first injections were done transcutaneously. However, it has been shown that the incidence of the side effects of ptosis and incomplete lid closure is reduced by injection through the conjunctiva. The following injection technique is recommended (Meyer, 1995; Riemann *et al.*, 1999): firstly, topical anesthetic eye drops are applied several times; the patient gazes in the direction away from the eye to be injected; the temporal part of the upper lid is lifted by a finger so that the palpebral part of the lacrimal gland is visible; the injection of 2.0–2.5 units Botox is done using a 30 gauge needle directed temporarily between the secretory orifices (Figure 10.13). The effect of this procedure lasts 4–6 months; reinjection in the same way is possible. Interestingly,

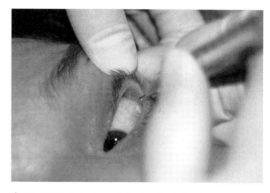

Figure 10.13 Injection of the lacrimal gland.

the reduction of lacrimal function did not produce symptoms of dryness or corneal irritation in our patients; perhaps the accessory tear gland function is sufficient to prevent that.

Treatment of entropion

Botulinum toxin injections can be valuable in cases of involutional (senile) and spastic entropion (not in cases of cicatricial or congenital entropion). The pathophysiology of the involutional form, the most common type of entropion, is explained as follows: the subcutaneous tissues and overlying skin of the lid becomes atonic and less adherent to the orbicularis muscle with age. Therefore during lid closure a part of the orbicularis can override the upper end of the tarsus and by this move the eyelashes against the cornea.

Long-term good results in this condition can be achieved by an operation. In some cases (for instance if it is not clear if the disease will be permanent or in the case of patients being long-term confined to bed at home or in an old-age asylum) BoNT injections can free the patients from their severe discomfort due to the rubbing of the eyelashes to the cornea.

We inject similar to the technique of Clarke 10–12.5 I. U. BoNT subcutaneously in 3 mm distance from the border of the eyelid with a very fine needle, spread over the full length of the lower lid (Clarke & Spalton, 1988). The beneficial effect will last around 3 months, then the easily performed procedure can be repeated again and again.

REFERENCES

Adams, G. G., Kirkness, C. M. & Lee, J. P. (1987). Botulinum toxin A induced protective ptosis. *Eye*, **1**, 603–8.

Clarke, J. R. & Spalton, D. J. (1988). Treatment of senile entropion with botulinum toxin. *Br J Ophthalmol*, **72**, 361–2.

Kerner, J. (1822). *Das Fettgift oder die Fettsäure und ihre Wirkungen auf den thierischen Organismus, ein Beytrag zur Untersuchung des in verdorbenen Würsten giftig wirkenden Stoffes*. Stuttgart, Tübingen: Cotta.

McNeer, K. W., Magoon, E. H. & Scott, A. B. (1999). Chemodenervation therapy. In A. L. Rosenbaum & A. P. Santiago, eds., *Clinical Strabismus Management*. Philadelphia: WB Saunders Co, pp. 423–32.

Meyer, M. (1995). Krokodilstraenen und gustatorisches Schwitzen. In *Botulinum-Toxin-Forum 1995*. Hamburg: Wissenschaftsverlag Wellingsbuettel.

Naik, M. N., Gangopadhyay, N., Fernandes, M., Murthy, R. & Honavar, S. G. (2007). Anterior chemodenervation of levator palpebrae superioris with botulinum toxin type-A (Botox®) to induce temporary ptosis for corneal protection. *Eye*, 2007 May 18 [Epub ahead of print].

Nuessgens, Z. & Roggenkaemper, P. (1993). Botulinum toxin as a tool for testing the risk of postoperative diplopia. *Strabismus*, **1**, 181–6.

Riemann, R., Pfennigsdorf, S., Riemann, E. & Naumann, M. (1999). Successful treatment of crocodile tears by injection of botulinum toxin into the lacrimal gland: a case report. *Ophthalmology*, **106**, 2322–4.

Scott, A. B. (1980). Botulinum toxin injection into extraocular muscles as an alternative to strabismus surgery. *J Pediatr Ophthalmol Strabismus* **7**, 21–5.

Scott, A. B. (1994). Change of eye muscle sarcomeres according to eye position. *J Pediatr Ophthalmol Strabismus*, **31**, 85–8.

Scott, A. B., Rosenbaum, A. L. & Collins, C. C. (1973). Pharmacologic weakening of extraocular muscles. *Invest Ophthalmol*, **112**, 924–7.

Uddin, J. M. & Davies, P. D. (2002). Treatment of upper eyelid retraction associated with thyroid eye disease with subconjunctival botulinum toxin injection. *Ophthalmology*, **109**, 1183–7.

11

Botulinum toxin therapy of laryngeal muscle hyperactivity syndromes

Daniel Truong, Arno Olthoff and Rainer Laskawi

Introduction

Spasmodic dysphonia is a focal dystonia characterized by task-specific, action-induced spasm of the vocal cords. It adversely affects the patient's ability to communicate. It can occur independently, as part of cranial dystonia (Meige's syndrome), or in other disorders such as in tardive dyskinesia.

Clinical features

There are three types of spasmodic dysphonia: the adductor type, the abductor type, and the mixed type.
- Adductor spasmodic dysphonia (ADSD) is characterized by a strained-strangled voice quality and intermittent voice stoppage or breaks due to overadduction of the vocal folds, resulting in a staccato-like voice.
- Abductor spasmodic dysphonia (ABSD) is characterized by intermittent breathy breaks, associated with prolonged abduction folds during voiceless consonants in speech.
- Patients with the mixed type have presentations of both.

Symptoms of spasmodic dysphonia begin gradually over several months to years. The condition typically affects patients in their mid 40s and is more common in women (Adler *et al.*, 1997; Schweinfurth *et al.*, 2002).

Spasmodic dysphonia may coexist with vocal tremor. Patients with ADSD show evidence of phonatory breaks during vocalization. The vocal breaks typically occur during phonation associated with voiced speech sounds (Sapienza *et al.*, 2000).

Stress commonly exacerbates speech symptoms; while they are absent during laughing, throat clearing, coughing, whispering, humming, and falsetto speech productions (Aronson *et al.*, 1968). The voice tends to improve when the patient is emotional.

Treatment options for ADSD

The efficacy of botulinum toxin in the treatment of spasmodic dysphonia has been proven in a double-blind study (Truong *et al.*, 1991). On average, patients treated for ADSD with botulinum toxin experience a 97% improvement in voice. Side effects included breathiness, choking, and mild swallowing difficulty (Truong *et al.*, 1991; Brin *et al.*, 1998). The duration of benefit averages about 3–4 months depending on the dose used.

Muscles injected with botulinum toxin in ADSD

- Treatment of ADSD involves mostly injection of botulinum toxin into the thyroarytenoid muscles.
- Findings of fine wire electromyography (EMG) revealed that both the thyroarytenoid and the

Manual of Botulinum Toxin Therapy, ed. Daniel Truong, Dirk Dressler and Mark Hallett. Published by Cambridge University Press.

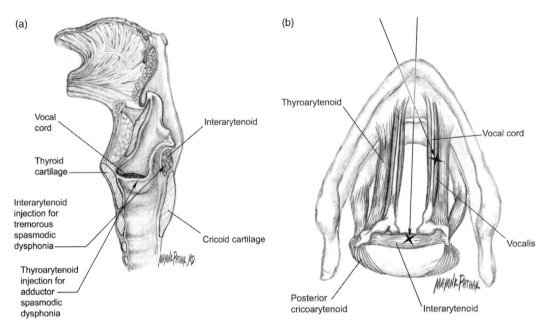

(a)

Vocal cord

Interarytenoid

Thyroid cartilage

Interarytenoid injection for tremorous spasmodic dysphonia

Cricoid cartilage

Thyroarytenoid injection for adductor spasmodic dysphonia

(b)

Thyroarytenoid

Vocal cord

Vocalis

Posterior cricoarytenoid

Interarytenoid

Figure 11.1 Anatomy of laryngeal muscles relevant for botulinum toxin injections (a) Saggital view showing the laryngeal structure. The arrows denote the direction for injection into the thyroarytenoid muscle for adductor spasmodic dysphonia and into the interarytenoid muscle for the tremorous spasmodic dysphonia. (b) Superior view showing the laryngeal structure and the above-mentioned technics looking from superior angle. The sign X denotes approximate injection site.

lateral cricoarytenoid muscle may be affected in ADSD, although the involvement of thyroarytenoid was more predominant.

- Thyroarytenoid and lateral cricoarytenoid muscles were equally involved in tremorous spasmodic dysphonia.
- The interarytenoid muscle may be involved in some patients in both ADSD and tremorous spasmodic dysphonia (Klotz *et al.*, 2004).
- Successful injections of botulinum toxin into the ventricular folds indicated the involvement of the ventricular muscles in ADSD (Schönweiler *et al.*, 1998).

Botulinum toxin can be injected into the thyroarytenoid muscle, either unilaterally or bilaterally. Unilateral injection may result in fewer adverse events such as breathiness, hoarseness, or swallowing difficulty after the injection (Bielamowicz *et al.*, 2002), but the strong voice intervals are also reduced.

The patient may experience breathiness for up to 2 weeks, followed by the development of a strong voice. After an effective period of a few months, the spasmodic symptoms slowly return as the clinical effect of botulinum toxin wears off. The duration of effect is dose related.

Injection techniques

Botulinum toxin is injected intramuscularly. Different techniques of injection have been proposed, including the percutaneous approach (Miller *et al.*, 1987), the transoral approach (Ford *et al.*, 1990), the transnasal approach (Rhew *et al.*, 1994), and point touch injections (Green *et al.*, 1992).

Percutaneous technique

A Teflon-coated needle connected to an EMG machine is inserted through the space between the cricoid and thyroid cartilages and pointing toward the thyroarytenoid muscle (Figure 11.1a and b). The localization of the needle is verified by

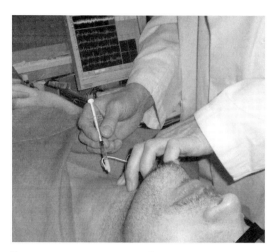

Figure 11.2 Transcutaneous technique of injection. Injection should be done using EMG control.

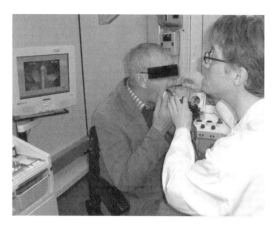

Figure 11.3 Situation during transoral application via 90°-video-endoscopy.

high-frequency muscle discharges on the EMG when the patient performs a long "/i/" (Miller *et al.*, 1987). The toxin is then injected (Figure 11.2).

For patients with excessive gag reflex, 0.2 cc of 1% lidocaine can be injected either through the cricothyroid membrane or underneath into the airway. The resulting cough would anesthetize the undersurface area of the vocal cord as well as the endotracheal structures, enabling the patients to tolerate the gag reflex (Truong *et al.*, 1991).

Transoral technique

In the transoral approach, the vocal folds are indirectly visualized and the injections are performed using a device originally designed for collagen injection. Indirect laryngoscopy is used to direct the needle in an attempt to cover a broad area of motor end plates (Figures 11.3 and 11.4) (Ford *et al.*, 1990).

Large waste of the toxin due to the large dead volume of the long needle is a drawback of this technique.

In patients who cannot tolerate the gag reflex a direct laryngoscopic injection can be performed under short total anesthesia (Figure 11.5).

Transnasal technique

In the transnasal approach, botulinum toxin is injected though a channel running parallel to the laryngoscope with a flexible catheter needle. This technique requires prior topical anesthesia with lidocaine spray (Rhew *et al.*, 1994). The location of botulinum toxin injection is lateral to the true vocal fold in order to avoid damaging the vocal fold mucosa.

In the point touch technique, the needle is inserted through the surface of the thyroid cartilage halfway between the thyroid notch and inferior edge of the thyroid cartilage. The botulinum toxin is given once the needle is passed into the thyroarytenoid muscle (Green *et al.*, 1992).

For injections into the ventricular folds a transoral or transnasal approach is required (Figure 11.4). Because EMG signals cannot be received from the ventricular muscle a percutaneous technique is not recommended.

Botulinum toxin doses

Doses of botulinum toxin used for the treatment of spasmodic dysphonia vary depending on the particular brand of toxin used (see Table 11.1). In general although there are correlations between the doses, the appropriate dose for a given toxin is dictated by the possible side effects caused by

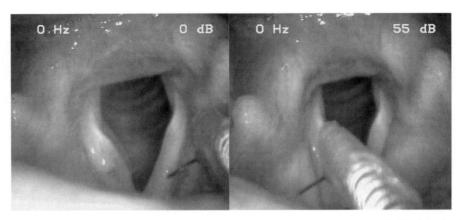

Figure 11.4 Endoscopic view during transoral botulinum toxin application (see Figure 11.3). Left side: injection into the left vocal fold. Right side: injection into the right ventricular muscle (ventricular fold).

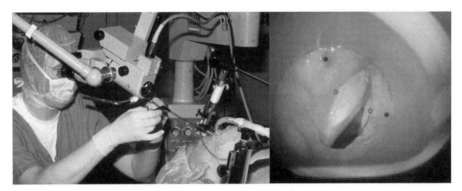

Figure 11.5 Injection during microlaryngoscopy with short general anesthesia (see left side). Normally the patients get no tracheal tube and the injection is done in a short apnea. Right side: microscopical view of the larynx during microlaryngoscopy, the dots mark the typical injection points.

Table 11.1. Approximate dose relationship between toxins for spasmodic dysphonia

Botox®	Dysport®	Xeomin®	NeuroBloc®/Myobloc®
1	4	1	50

the effects of the toxin on the adjacent organs or muscles.

In the early literature, the doses of botulinum toxin (Botox®) used for ADSD ranged from 3.75 to 7.5 (mouse) units for bilateral injections (Brin *et al.*, 1988, 1989; Truong *et al.*, 1991) to 15 units for uni-lateral injections (Miller *et al.*, 1987; Ludlow *et al.*,

1988). Later literature and common practice have recommended the use of lower doses (Blitzer & Sulica, 2001). We recommend starting with 0.5 units of Botox/Xeomin® or 1.5 units of Dysport® or 200 units of NeuroBloc®/Myobloc® when injected bilaterally and to adjust the dose as needed. Our estimated average dose is 0.75 units Botox/Xeomin or 2 to 3 units (Dysport) or 300 units of NeuroBloc/Myobloc.

Beneficial effects last about 3–4 months in patients treated with Botox, Dysport and Xeomin and about 8 weeks with NeuroBloc/Myobloc (Adler *et al.*, 2004b) but may be longer with higher dose (Guntinas-Lichius, 2003). In patients who received type B after

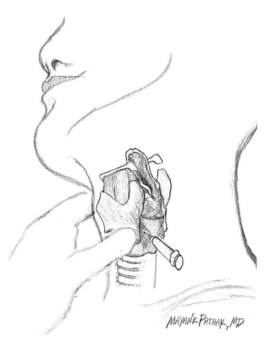

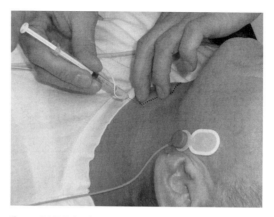

Figure 11.7 Injection into the posterior cricoarytenoid muscle using a lateral approach in a patient.

Figure 11.6 Anterolateral view of the larynx and posterior cricoarytenoid muscle with the thyroid lamina rotated forward and to the other side.

A failure the duration was only about 2 months despite higher doses up to 1000 units per cord.

Botulinum toxin treatment of ABSD

Injection technique and muscles injected

With the thyroid lamina rotated forward, the needle is inserted behind the posterior edge and directed toward the posterior cricoarytenoid muscle. Location is verified by maximal muscle discharge when patients perform a sniff (Figures 11.6 and 11.7) (Blitzer *et al.*, 1992).

The average onset of effect is 4 days and duration of benefit is 10.5 weeks.

Adverse effects included exertional wheezing and dysphagia.

In another approach, the needle is directed along the superior border of the posterior cricoid lamina

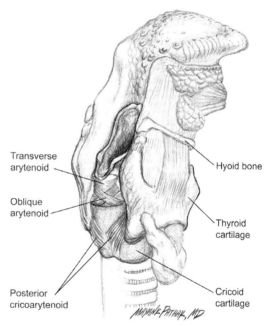

Figure 11.8 Dorsolateral view showing the anatomy of posterior cricoarytenoid, oblique arytenoids and transverse arytenoid muscles.

and between the arytenoid cartilages. For anatomic reasons, the toxin is injected at a high location and allowed to diffuse down into the muscle for therapeutic effects (Figure 11.8).

Table 11.2. Doses of various botulinum toxin products

Diagnosis and treatment technique	Botox	Xeomin	Dysport	NeuroBloc/Myobloc
ADSD unilateral injections	5–15 units	5–15 units	15–45 units	250–500 units
ADSD bilateral injections	0.5–3 units	0.5–3 units	1.5–9 units	100–250 units
ABSD unilateral injections	15 units	15 units	45 units	Not known
ABSD bilateral injections	1.25–1.75 units	1.25–1.75 units	4.5–6 units	Not known
Vocal tremor	2.5 units	2.5 units	7.5 units	100–250 units
Laryngeal spasmodic dyspnea	2.5 units	2.5 units	7.5 units	100–250 units

Source: Modified from Truong and Bhidayasiri (2006) with permission.

A refined technique with the needle penetrating through the posterior cricoid lamina into the posterior cricoarytenoid muscle seems to be simpler and has the advantage of direct injection into the muscle (Meleca *et al.*, 1997).

Between 2 and 4 units of Botox or Xeomin, or 12 units of Dysport on one side, and 1 unit of Botox or 3 units of Dysport on the opposite side are used. If a higher dose is required for each side, the injection of the opposite side should be delayed for about 2 weeks to avoid compromising the airway.

Spasmodic laryngeal dyspnea

Spasmodic laryngeal dystonia results in laryngopharyngeal spasm primarily during respiration. Patients' breathing problems are even improved with speaking (Zwirner *et al.*, 1997). Dyspnea is caused by an intermittent glottic and supraglottic airway obstruction from both laryngeal and supralaryngeal/pharyngeal muscle spasms. Treatment includes injections with botulinum toxin into the thyroarytenoid and ventricular folds (Zwirner *et al.*, 1997). These improvements last from 9 weeks to 6 months.

Vocal tremors

Essential tremor patients also demonstrate tremors of the voice.

Intrinsic laryngeal muscles are tremulous during respiration and speech with the thyroarytenoid muscles most often involved (Koda & Ludlow, 1992).

Patients reported subjective reduction in vocal effort and improvement in voice tremors following injection with botulinum toxin into the vocal cord (Adler *et al.*, 2004a).

Improvement may occur with treatment of the lateral cricoarytenoid and interarytenoid muscle as well (Klotz *et al.*, 2004).

For the treatment of vocal tremors, the thyroarytenoid muscles are often injected using a technique similar to that used for ADSD.

The average doses used are about 2 units of Botox or Xeomin, or 8 units of Dysport. For NeuroBloc/Myobloc about 200 units would be needed.

REFERENCES

Adler, C. H., Edwards, B. W. & Bansberg, S. F. (1997). Female predominance in spasmodic dysphonia. *J Neurol Neurosurg Psychiatry*, **63**, 688.

Adler, C. H., Bansberg, S. F., Hentz, J. G., *et al.* (2004a). Botulinum toxin type A for treating voice tremor. *Archives of Neurology*, **61**, 1416–20.

Adler, C. H., Bansberg, S. F., Krein-Jones, K. & Hentz, J. G. (2004b). Safety and efficacy of botulinum toxin type B (Myobloc) in adductor spasmodic dysphonia. *Mov Disord*, **19**, 1075–9.

Aronson, A. E., Brown, J. R., Litin, E. M. & Pearson, J. S. (1968). Spastic dysphonia. II. Comparison with essential (voice) tremor and other neurologic and psychogenic dysphonias. *J Speech Hear Disord*, **33**, 219–31.

Bielamowicz, S., Stager, S. V., Badillo, A. & Godlewski, A. (2002). Unilateral versus bilateral injections of botulinum toxin in patients with adductor spasmodic dysphonia. *J Voice*, **16**, 117–23.

Blitzer, A. & Sulica, L. (2001). Botulinum toxin: basic science and clinical uses in otolaryngology. *Laryngoscope*, **111**, 218–26.

Blitzer, A., Brin, M. F., Stewart, C., Aviv, J. E. & Fahn, S. (1992). Abductor laryngeal dystonia: a series treated with botulinum toxin. *Laryngoscope*, **102**, 163–7.

Brin, M. F., Fahn, S., Moskowitz, C., *et al.* (1988). Localized injections of botulinum toxin for the treatment of focal dystonia and hemifacial spasm. *Adv Neurol*, **50**, 599–608.

Brin, M. F., Blitzer, A., Fahn, S., Gould, W. & Lovelace, R. E. (1989). Adductor laryngeal dystonia (spastic dysphonia): treatment with local injections of botulinum toxin (Botox). *Mov Disord*, **4**, 287–96.

Brin, M. F., Blitzer, A. & Stewart, C. (1998). Laryngeal dystonia (spasmodic dysphonia): observations of 901 patients and treatment with botulinum toxin. *Adv Neurol*, **78**, 237–52.

Ford, C. N., Bless, D. M. & Lowery, J. D. (1990). Indirect laryngoscopic approach for injection of botulinum toxin in spasmodic dysphonia. *Otolaryngol Head Neck Surg*, **103**, 752–8.

Green, D. C., Berke, G. S., Ward, P. H. & Gerratt, B. R. (1992). Point-touch technique of botulinum toxin injection for the treatment of spasmodic dysphonia. *Ann Otol Rhinol Laryngol*, **101**, 883–7.

Guntinas-Lichius, O. (2003). Injection of botulinum toxin type B for the treatment of otolaryngology patients with secondary treatment failure of botulinum toxin type A. *Laryngoscope*, **113**, 743–5.

Klotz, D. A., Maronian, N. C., Waugh, P. F., *et al.* (2004). Findings of multiple muscle involvement in a study of 214 patients with laryngeal dystonia using fine-wire electromyography. *Ann Otol Rhinol Laryngol*, **113**, 602–12.

Koda, J. & Ludlow, C. L. (1992). An evaluation of laryngeal muscle activation in patients with voice tremor. *Otolaryngol Head Neck Surg*, **107**, 684–96.

Ludlow, C. L., Naunton, R. F., Sedory, S. E., Schulz, G. M. & Hallett, M. (1988). Effects of botulinum toxin injections on speech in adductor spasmodic dysphonia. *Neurology*, **38**, 1220–5.

Meleca, R. J., Hogikyan, N. D. & Bastian, R. W. (1997). A comparison of methods of botulinum toxin injection for abductory spasmodic dysphonia. *Otolaryngol Head Neck Surg*, **117**, 487–92.

Miller, R. H., Woodson, G. E. & Jankovic, J. (1987). Botulinum toxin injection of the vocal fold for spasmodic dysphonia. A preliminary report. *Arch Otolaryngol Head Neck Surg*, **113**, 603–5.

Rhew, K., Fiedler, D. A. & Ludlow, C. L. (1994). Technique for injection of botulinum toxin through the flexible nasolaryngoscope. *Otolaryngol Head Neck Surg*, **111**, 787–94.

Sapienza, C. M., Walton, S. & Murry, T. (2000). Adductor spasmodic dysphonia and muscular tension dysphonia: acoustic analysis of sustained phonation and reading. *J Voice*, **14**, 502–20.

Schweinfurth, J. M., Billante, M. & Courey, M. S. (2002). Risk factors and demographics in patients with spasmodic dysphonia. *Laryngoscope*, **112**, 220–3.

Schönweiler, R., Wohlfarth, K., Dengler, R. & Ptok, M. (1998). Supraglottal injection of botulinum toxin type A in adductor type spasmodic dysphonia with both intrinsic and extrinsic hyperfunction. *Laryngoscope*, **108**, 55–63.

Truong, D. & Bhidayasiri, R. (2006). Botulinum toxin in laryngeal dystonia. *Eur J Neurol*, **13**(Suppl 1), 36–41.

Truong, D. D., Rontal, M., Rolnick, M., Aronson, A. E. & Mistura, K. (1991). Double-blind controlled study of botulinum toxin in adductor spasmodic dysphonia. *Laryngoscope*, **101**, 630–4.

Zwirner, P., Dressler, D. & Kruse, E. (1997). Spasmodic laryngeal dyspnea: a rare manifestation of laryngeal dystonia. *Eur Arch Otorhinolaryngol*, **254**, 242–5.

12

The use of botulinum toxin in otorhinolaryngology

Rainer Laskawi and Arno Olthoff

Various disorders in the ear, nose, and throat (ENT) field are suited for treatment with botulinum toxin (BoNT). They can be divided into two general groups:

1. Disorders concerning head and neck muscles (movement disorders)
2. Disorders caused by a pathological secretion of glands located in the head and neck region.

Table 12.1 summarizes the diseases relevant to otolaryngology. The focus in this chapter lies on indications that are not reviewed in other chapters. Thus, laryngeal dystonia, hemifacial spasm, blepharospasm, and synkinesis following defective healing of the facial nerve will not be covered here.

Dysphagia and speech problems following laryngectomy

Some patients are unable to achieve an adequate speech level for optimal communication after laryngectomy. One of the causes is spasms of the cricopharyngeal muscle. In this condition BoNT can reduce the muscle activity and improve the quality of speech (Chao et al., 2004). Swallowing disorders in neurological patients can result from a disturbed coordination of the relaxation of the upper esophageal sphincter (UES) and can lead to pulmonary aspiration. The cricopharyngeal muscle is a sphincter between the inferior constrictor muscle and the cervical esophagus and is primarily innervated by the vagus nerve.

Twenty (mouse) units of Botox® (100 units of Dyport®; 1000 units of NeuroBloc®/Myobloc® [BoNT-B]; [conversion factors see Table 12.2]) were injected into each of three injection points under general anesthesia (Figure 12.1). This procedure can be used as a test prior to a planned myectomy or as a single therapeutic option that has to be repeated.

In cases of dysphagia caused by spasms or insufficient relaxation of the UES, injection of BoNT as described can improve the patients' complaints (example see Figure 12.2). The patient should be evaluated for symptoms of concomitant gastroesophageal reflux to avoid side effects such as "reflux-laryngitis." In cases of gastroesophageal reflux, the etiology and treatment should be clarified prior to initiation of BoNT therapy.

Palatal tremor

Repetitive contractions of the muscles of the soft palate (palatoglossus and palatopharyngeus muscles, salpingopharyngeus, tensor, and levator veli palatini muscles) lead to a rhythmic elevation of the soft palate. This disorder has two forms, symptomatic palatal tremor (SPT) and essential palatal tremor (EPT). Symptomatic palatal tremor can cause speech and also swallowing disorders due

Manual of Botulinum Toxin Therapy, ed. Daniel Truong, Dirk Dressler and Mark Hallett. Published by Cambridge University Press.
© Cambridge University Press 2009.

Table 12.1. Diseases treated with BoNT-A in otorhinolaryngology

Movement disorders	Disorders of the autonomous nerve system
Facial nerve paralysis	Gustatory sweating, Frey's syndrome
Hemifacial spasm	Hypersalivation, sialorrhea
Blepharospasm, Meige's syndrome	Intrinsic rhinitis
Synkinesis following defective healing of the facial nerve	Hyperlacrimation, tearing
Oromandibular dystonia	
Laryngeal dystonia	
Palatal tremor	
Dysphagia	

Note:
Diseases printed in italics are not reviewed in this chapter.

Table 12.2. Approximate conversion factors for various preparations containing BoNT-A and BoNT-B. One unit of Botox® has been chosen as the reference value. These reference values may vary with different indications in part due to possible side effects

Preparation	Conversion factor/units reference value: 1 unit Botox® equivalent dose
Botox®	1
Dysport®	3–5
Xeomin®	1
NeuroBloc®	50

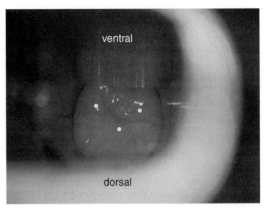

Figure 12.1 Intraoperative aspect prior to injection of BoNT into the cricopharyngeal muscle. The dots mark the injection sites. Twenty units of Botox are injected at each point.

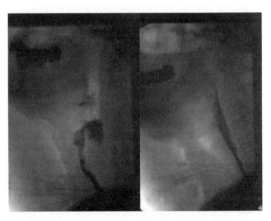

Figure 12.2 Patient with severe swallowing disorder caused by irregular function of the UES. The left illustration shows aspiration during swallowing. Following BoNT injection of 3 × 20 units Botox, pharyngo-esophageal passage is normalized (right side).

to a velopharyngeal insufficiency. Most patients suffering from EPT complain of "ear clicking." This rhythmic tinnitus is caused by a repetitive opening and closure of the orifice of the Eustachian tube. A particular sequel of pathological activity of soft palate muscles is the syndrome of a patulous Eustachian tube (PET). These patients suffer from "autophonia" caused by an open Eustachian tube due to the increased muscle tension of the paratubal muscles (salpingopharyngeus, tensor, and levator veli palatini muscles) (Olthoff *et al.*, 2007).

For the first treatment session, the injection of 5 units of Botox (uni- or bilaterally) (25 units of Dysport; 250 units of NeuroBloc/Myobloc) into the soft palate (see Figures 12.3 and 12.4) is adequate

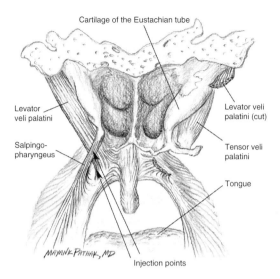

Figure 12.3 Dorsal view of the nasopharynx and soft palate (modified after Tillmann, 1997 with permission). The arrows mark the possible sites of Botox injections for the treatment of palatal tremor.

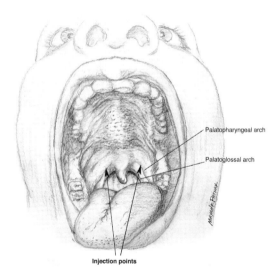

Figure 12.4 Transoral view of injection sites in palatal tremor patients.

in most cases. If necessary, this can be increased to 15 units of Botox (75 units of Dysport; 750 units of NeuroBloc/Myobloc) on each side. The application is normally performed transorally (transpalatinal

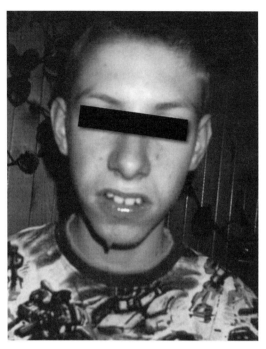

Figure 12.5 Clinical picture of a patient with a neuropediatric disorder (postinfectious encephalopathy) unable to swallow his saliva. Drooling is obvious from patient's mouth.

or via postrhinoscopy) under endoscopic control. For the treatment of PET, the salpingopharyngeal fold should be used as a landmark (Figure 12.3). To optimize the detection of the target muscle, injection under electromyographic control is recommended. To avoid side effects such as iatrogenic velopharyngeal insufficiency the treatment should be started with low doses as described above.

Hypersalivation, sialorrhea

Hypersalivation can be caused by various conditions such as tumor surgery, neurological and pediatric disorders (Figure 12.5), and disturbances of wound healing following ENT surgery.

Hypersalivation also is of relevance for a number of reasons in patients suffering from head and

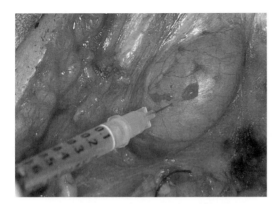

Figure 12.6 Intraoperative injection of 15 units of Botox into the submandibular gland during laryngectomy demonstrating the anatomical situation of the gland in the submandibular fossa.

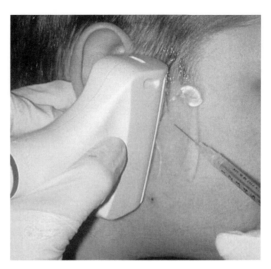

Figure 12.7 Technique of BoNT-A-injection into the parotid and submandibular glands (same technique). We prefer to inject both glands with 7.5 units of Botox into each of the three points of each parotid gland and with 15 units of Botox into each submandibular gland. Ultrasound-guided injection is recommended.

neck cancers. Some of these patients are unable to swallow their saliva because of a stenosis of the UES caused by scar formation after tumor resection. In other patients, there are disturbances of the sensory control of the "entrance" of supraglottic tissues of the larynx allowing passage of the saliva into the larynx. This may lead to continuous aspiration and aspiration pneumonia. In a third group of patients, complications of impaired wound healing after extended surgery can occur, such as fistula formation following laryngectomy. Saliva is a very aggressive agent and can inhibit the normal healing process.

Both the parotid and submandibular glands are of interest in this context. The parotid gland is the largest of the salivary glands. It is located in the so-called parotid compartment in the pre- and subauricular region with a large compartment lying on the masseter muscle. The gland also has contact with the sternocleidomastoid muscle. The submandibular gland (Figure 12.6) lies between the two bellies of the digastric muscle and the inferior margin of the mandible that form the submandibular triangle. The gland is divided into two parts – the superficial lobe and the deep lobe – by the mylohyoid muscle.

We inject 22.5 units of Botox into each parotid gland under ultrasound guidance at three locations (Ellies *et al.*, 2004) (see Figures 12.7 and 12.8). Each submandibular gland is treated with 15 units of Botox at one or two sites (see Figure 12.9). Injection of BoNT-A has been shown to be effective in reducing saliva flow (Figure 12.10). Side effects such as local pain, diarrhea, luxation of the mandible, and a "dry mouth" are quite rare.

Gustatory sweating, Frey's syndrome

Gustatory sweating is a common sequel of parotid gland surgery (Laskawi & Rohrbach, 2002). The clinical picture is characterized by extensive production of sweat in the lateral region of the face. The sweating can be intense and become a cause of a serious social stigma. Botulinum toxin has become the first-line treatment (Laskawi & Rohrbach, 2002).

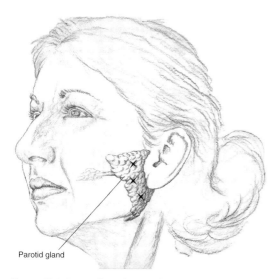

Figure 12.8 Fronto-lateral view of the left parotid gland with typical injections sites for BoNT. The sign X denotes approximate injection site.

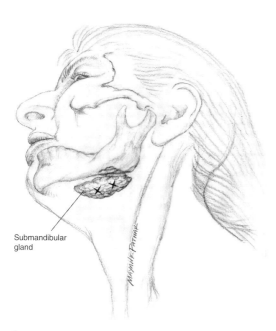

Figure 12.9 Latero-caudal view of the left submandibular gland with typical injections sites for BoNT. The sign X denotes approximate injection site.

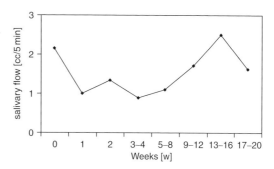

Figure 12.10 The effect of BoNT injection on saliva flow in patients with hypersalivation (Ellies *et al.*, 2004 with permission). Pretreatment status returns after 12 weeks.

For an optimal outcome the affected area should be marked with Minor's test (Figure 12.11). First, the face is divided into regional "boxes" using a waterproof pen (Figure 12.11). The affected skin is covered with iodine solution before starch powder is applied. The sweat produced by masticating an apple induces a reaction between the iodine solution and the starch powder resulting in an apparent deep blue color (Laskawi & Rohrbach, 2002).

Botulinum toxin is injected intracutaneously (approximately 2.5 units Botox [12.5 units of Dysport, 125 units of NeuroBloc/Myobloc/4 cm^2]) (Figure 12.11). Side effects are rare, and with no conceivable sequelae, such as dryness of the skin or eczema in some patients.

The total required dose depends on the extent of the affected area and up to 100 units of Botox (500 units of Dysport; 5000 units of NeuroBloc/Myobloc) can be necessary. The duration of improvement persists longer than that seen in patients with movement disorders (Laskawi & Rohrbach, 2002), and some patients have a symptom-free interval of several years.

Rhinorrhea, intrinsic rhinitis

In the last few years BoNT has been used in intrinsic or allergic rhinitis (Özcan *et al.*, 2006). The main

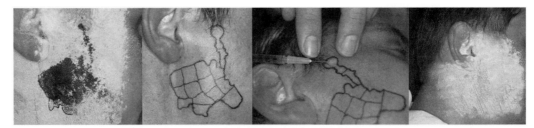

Figure 12.11 Treatment of gustatory sweating (Frey's syndrome) with BoNT. *Left picture*: Patient with extensive gustatory sweating following total parotidectomy. The affected area is marked by Minor's test showing a deep blue color. *Second picture from left*: The affected area is marked with a waterproof pen and divided into "boxes" to guarantee that the whole plane is treated. *Second picture from right*: Intracutaneous injections of BoNT are performed. One can see the white colour of the skin during intracutaneous application of BoNT-A. *Right picture*: Patient eating an apple 2 weeks after BoNT treatment. The marked area which was sweating prior to treatment is now completely dry.

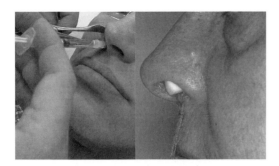

Figure 12.12 Sponges soaked with BoNT-A solution and placed in both nasal cavities (right side of the picture). The alternative possibility is the transnasal *injection* into the middle and lower turbinate (left side of the picture).

symptom in these disorders is extensive rhinorrhea with secretions dripping from the nose.

There are two approaches for applying BoNT in these patients: it can either be injected into the middle and lower nasal turbinates, or applied with a sponge soaked with a solution of BoNT-A (Figure 12.12). For the injection 10 units of Botox (50 units of Dysport; 500 units of NeuroBloc/Myobloc) are injected into each middle or lower turbinate. With the other technique, the sponge is soaked with a solution containing 40 units of Botox and one is applied into each nostril.

The effect of the injections has been demonstrated in placebo-controlled studies (Özcan *et al.*, 2006). Nasal secretion is reduced for about 12 weeks (Figure 12.13). Side effects such as epistaxis or nasal crusting are uncommon.

Hyperlacrimation

Hyperlacrimation can be caused by stenoses of the lacrimal duct, misdirected secretory fibers following a degenerative paresis of the facial nerve (crocodile tears) or mechanical irritation of the cornea (in patients with lagophthalmus).

The application of BoNT is useful in reducing pathological tearing in these patients (Whittaker *et al.*, 2003; Meyer, 2004). The lacrimal gland is located in the lacrimal fossa in the lateral part of the upper orbit and is divided into two sections. Usually 5–7.5 units of Botox (25–37.5 units of Dysport; 250–375 units of NeuroBloc/Myobloc) are injected into the pars palpebralis of the lacrimal gland, which is accessible under the lateral upper lid (Figure 12.14). Medial injection may result in ptosis as a possible side effect. The reduction of tear production lasts about 12 weeks (see Figure 12.15) (Meyer, 2004).

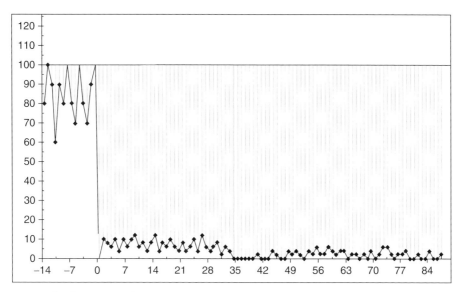

Figure 12.13 Example of a patient with extensive intrinsic rhinitis. BoNT-A has been applied with sponges. The consumption of paper handkerchiefs (number shown on vertical axis) is reduced dramatically after BoNT-A application for a long period (horizontal axis).

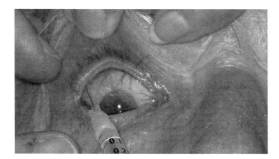

Figure 12.14 Technique of injection into the pars palpebralis of the lacrimal gland. With the patient looking strongly in the medial direction; the upper lid is lifted, a little "lacrimal prominence" becomes evident. Entering here in a lateral direction, the gland tissue can be approached easily.

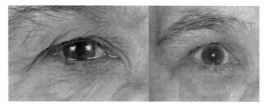

Figure 12.15 Patient with extensive tearing caused by a stenosis of the lacrimal duct after resection of a malignant tumor of the right maxilla. Left side: Pretreatment, Right side: Posttreatment.

REFERENCES

Chao, S. S., Graham, S. M. & Hoffman, H. T. (2004). Management of pharyngoesophageal spasm with Botox. *Otolaryngol Clin North Am*, **37**, 559–66.

Ellies, M., Gottstein, U., Rohrbach-Volland, S., Arglebe, C. & Laskawi, R. (2004). Reduction of salivary flow with botulinum toxin: extended report on 33 patients with drooling, salivary fistulas, and sialadenitis. *Laryngoscope*, **114**, 1856–60.

Laskawi, R. & Rohrbach, S. (2002). Frey's syndrome: treatment with botulinum toxin. In O. P. Kreyden, R. Böni & G. Burg, eds., *Hyperhidrosis and Botulinum Toxin in Dermatology*. Basel: Karger.

Meyer, M. (2004). Störungen der Tränendrüsen. In R. Laskawi & P. Roggenkämper, eds., *Botulinumtoxintherapie im Kopf-Hals-Bereich*. München: Urban und Vogel.

Olthoff, A., Laskawi, R. & Kruse, E. (2007). Successful treatment of autophonia with botulinum toxin: case report. *Ann Otol Rhinol Laryngol*, **116**, 594–8.

Özcan, C., Vayisoglu, Y., Dogu, O. & Gorur, K. (2006). The effect of intranasal injection of botulinum toxin A on the symptoms of vasomotor rhinitis. *Am J Otolaryngol*, **27**, 314–18.

Tillmann, B. (2005). *Atlas der Anatomie des Menschen*. Berlin: Springer-Verlag, p. 180.

Whittaker, K. W., Matthews, B. N., Fitt, A. W. & Sandramouli, S. (2003). The use of botulinum toxin A in the treatment of functional epiphora. *Orbit*, **22**, 193–8.

13

Spasticity

Mayank S. Pathak and Allison Brashear

Introduction

Spasticity is part of the upper motor neuron syndrome produced by conditions such as stroke, multiple sclerosis, traumatic brain injury, spinal cord injury, or cerebral palsy that affect upper motor neurons or their efferent pathways in the brain or spinal cord. It is characterized by increased muscle tone, exaggerated tendon reflexes, repetitive stretch reflex discharges (clonus), and released flexor reflexes (great toe extension; flexion at the ankle, knee, and hip) (Lance, 1981). Late sequelae may include contracture, pain, fibrosis, and muscle atrophy. Chemodenervation by intramuscular injection of botulinum toxin can reduce spastic muscle tone, normalize limb posture, ameliorate pain, and may improve motor function and prevent contractures.

Reduction of muscle tone, as measured by the Ashworth scale and by changes in range of motion after treatment with botulinum toxin, is best documented in the upper limbs (Brashear et al., 2002; Childers et al., 2004; Suputtitada & Suwanwela, 2005). In the lower limbs, muscle tone improvements are modest, with best results achieved from treatment below the knee.

Improvement of motor function has been noted in some studies, using measures such as the Barthel index, dressing, analyses of gait parameters such as walking speed, and the performance of other standardized tasks (Sheean, 2001; Brashear et al., 2002). In summary, motor function may be improved in a select subgroup of patients who retain selective motor control and some degree of dexterity in important distal muscles, require injection of relatively few target muscles, and especially if combined with other interventions such as physical therapy (Bhakta et al., 2000; Sheean, 2001).

Preparation and dosing

Dilution

Botox® is customarily diluted with 1–4 cc of preservative-free normal saline per 100 (mouse) unit vial, Dysport® with 2.5 cc per vial, and NeuroBloc®/Myobloc® is pre-diluted (Table 13.1).

Maximum doses

Although there are no absolutes, the usual dose maximums found in the literature for a single injection session are also presented in Table 13.1. Higher doses in a single session may increase the risk of both local and diffuse side effects and adverse reactions (Dressler and Benecke, 2003; Francisco, 2004).

Individual muscle doses

The dose of toxin for individual muscles depends mainly on their size and the degree of spastic

Manual of Botulinum Toxin Therapy, ed. Daniel Truong, Dirk Dressler and Mark Hallett. Published by Cambridge University Press.
© Cambridge University Press 2009.

Table 13.1. Dilutions and maximum dose/session of botulinum toxins

Neurotoxin	Dilution (cc saline)	Maximum dose
Botox	1–4+	400 U/limb
		600 U/session
Dysport	2.5 usual,	1500 U/upper limb
	10 reported	2000 U/lower limb
		2000 U/session
NeuroBloc/	Pre-diluted	10 000 U/upper limb
Myobloc		17 500 U/session

Sources: (Hesse *et al.*, 1995; Hyman *et al.*, 2000; Brashear *et al.*, 2003, 2004; Francisco, 2004; Suputtitada & Suwanwela, 2005; WE MOVE Spasticity Study Group, 2005a, b).

contraction. Consideration must also be made of the total number of muscles to be injected and the maximum recommended dose per injection session of the particular toxin preparation used. Employing these considerations, Table 13.2 gives the dose ranges usually employed for individual muscles in clinical practice.

Guidance techniques

Palpation and anatomical landmarks may be used to place injections. However, the use of various guidance techniques increases precision and may improve safety, decrease side effects, and possibly increase efficacy (O'Brien, 1997; Traba Lopez and Esteban, 2001; Childers, 2003; Monnier *et al.*, 2003). Guidance is recommended for injecting cervical muscles and deep pelvic or small limb muscles; it is optional for larger easily palpated muscles. The principal guidance techniques are: electromyography (EMG), electrical stimulation, ultrasound, and fluoroscopy.

In EMG guidance, injection is made through a cannulized, Teflon-coated monopolar hypodermic needle attached to an EMG machine. If able, the patient is asked to voluntarily contract the target

muscle. When the bare needle tip is within the target muscle belly, the crisp staccato of motor units firing close to the tip should be heard and sharp motor units with short rise times seen on the video monitor. If the needle tip is outside the muscle or in a tendinous portion, only a distant rumbling will be heard, and dull indistinct motor units seen. Tapping the tendon or passively moving the joint may elicit motor units in paralyzed patients.

In patients who are either paralyzed or unable to follow commands, low-amperage electrical stimulation directly through the bare tip of the insulated hypodermic needle may be used to produce visible contraction in the target muscle (O'Brien, 1997; Childers, 2003; Chin *et al.*, 2005). The needle is repositioned until contractions may be reproduced by the lowest stimulation intensities.

Ultrasonography has been used to guide injections in the urinary system and salivary glands and is being assessed for skeletal muscles. (Berweck *et al.*, 2002; Westhoff *et al.*, 2003). Fluoroscopy is utilized mainly for injection of deep pelvic girdle muscles in nerve entrapment and pain syndromes (Raj, 2004).

Injection placement

Smaller muscles generally require only one injection site anywhere within the muscle belly. Larger, longer, or wider muscles are best injected at two to four sites. Injection placement near the motor nerve insertion or endplate region is unnecessary, usually requires repeated repositioning of the needle under electrical stimulation or EMG guidance (Traba Lopez & Esteban, 2001), is painful, and any advantage in efficacy appears minimal.

Spasticity patterns

The most common pattern of spasticity in the upper limb involves flexion of the fingers, wrist, and elbow, adduction with internal rotation at the

Table 13.2. Recommended botulinum toxin doses for individual muscles and groups

Muscle	Botox (units)	Dysport (units)	NeuroBloc (units)	# Injection sites
SHOULDER				
Pectoralis major & minor	50–150	150–300	2500–7500	2–4
Latissimus dorsi	50–150	150–300	2500–7500	2–4
Teres major	25–50	75–150	1500–2500	1–2
UPPER LIMB				
Flexors				
Biceps/brachialis	25–100	100–300	1500–5000	2–4
Brachioradialis	25–50	75–150	1000–2500	1
Flexor carpi radialis	25–50	75–150	1000–2500	1
Flexor carpi ulnaris	25–75	72–250	1500–5000	2–3
Flexor digitorum superficialis	25–50	75–200	1000–2500	2–4
Flexor digitorum profundus	20–50	75–150	750–2500	1–2
Flexor pollicis longus	10–20	30–60	500–1000	1
Thenar adductors and flexors of Thumb	5–10	20–40	250–500	1
Extensors				
Triceps	50–100	100–250	250–750	2–3
Extensor carpi ulnaris	10–30	30–100	50–150	1–2
Extensor carpi radialis	10–30	30–100	50–150	1–2
Extensor digitorum communis	10–20	30–60	50–100	1–2
LOWER LIMB				
Iliopsoas	75–150	250–500	5000–7500	1–2
Adductor Group				
Magnus, longus, & brevis	100–300	500–1000	5000–7500	3–6
Quadriceps Group				
Rectus femoris, vastus medialis, vastus lateralis, sartorius	100–300	500–1000	5000–7500	3–6
Hamstring Group				
Biceps femoris long head, biceps femoris short head, semitendinosus, semimembranosus	100–300	500–1000	5000–7500	3–6
Triceps Surae				
Medial & lateral gastrocnemius, soleus	100–200	250–1000	5000–7500	3–4
Tibialis posterior	50–100	150–250	2500–5000	1–2
Extensor hallucis longus	25–75	75–200	1000–2500	1
Tibialis anterior	25–75	75–200	1000–2500	1–2

Note:
Number of different injection sites in any given muscle that the neurotoxin dose is usually spread.
Source: (WE MOVE Spasticity Study Group, 2005a, b; Pathak *et al.*, 2006).

shoulder, and sometimes thumb curling across the palm or fist (Mayer *et al.*, 2002) (Figure 13.1). Wrist or elbow extension is less common. There may sometimes be a combination of metacarpophalangeal flexion and proximal interphalangeal extention.

The most common pattern of spasticity in the lower limb involves extension at the knee, plantar-flexion at the ankle, and sometimes inversion of the foot (Mayer *et al.*, 2002) (Figure 13.1). This pattern is seen unilaterally in stroke. It occurs bilaterally

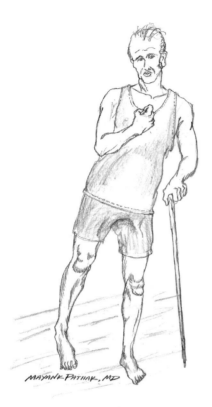

Figure 13.1 Common pattern of spasticity in upper and lower limbs.

in cerebral palsy and some spinal cord lesions, producing a "toe-walking pattern." Other patterns of spasticity in the lower limbs include "scissoring" adduction at the hip joints, along with flexion or extension at the knees, and spastic extension of the great toe (Mayer *et al.*, 2002).

It is important to distinguish plantarflexion posture caused by spastic contraction of the calf muscles from flaccid "drop foot" caused by paresis of the tibialis anterior and other dorsiflexor muscles. Drop foot classically occurs with peroneal nerve palsy or lumbar radiculopathy, and occasionally after stroke. Botulinum toxin is not indicated in flaccid drop foot, and ankle-foot orthotic splints are usually sufficient to bring the foot and ankle to neutral position.

Extensor posturing at the knee also requires careful consideration before injection because quadriceps

strength is important in maintaining weight-bearing stance during walking, and some degree of residual spasticity may be helpful. Additionally, the large powerful muscles of the proximal lower limb require high doses of botulinum toxin approaching recommended maximums, and most patients will benefit more from the application of this dose elsewhere.

Treatment guide

Note: in the following figures, target muscles are printed in bold lettering and lines with arrowheads represent approximate injection vectors.

The upper limb

Flexion at the proximal interphalangeal joints

Inject flexor digitorum superficialis (Figure 13.2).

The flexor digitorum superficialis muscle is involved in the clenched hand posture. The muscle is often treated in conjuction with the flexor digitorum profundus. Insert the needle obliquely approximately one-third of the distance from the antecubital crease to the distal wrist crease. Advance toward the radius, passing through fasicles for each of the fingers as the bolus is injected. Activate the muscle by having the patient flex the fingers. Confirmation of needle placement can be performed using EMG or electrical stimulation.

Flexion at distal interphalangeal joints

Inject flexor digitorum profundus (Figure 13.3).

The flexor digitorum profundus muscle is involved in the clenched hand. This muscle is often treated in conjunction with the flexor digitorum superficialis. Flexor digitorum profundus lies against the ventral surface of the ulna. Insert the needle along the ulnar edge of the forearm one-third of the distance from the antecubital crease to the distal wrist crease and direct it across the ventral surface of the ulnar shaft. After advancing through

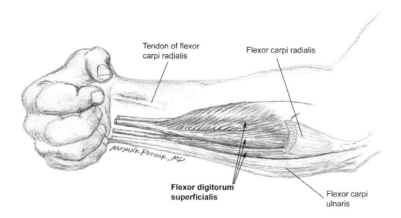

Figure 13.2 Injection of flexor digitorum superficialis.

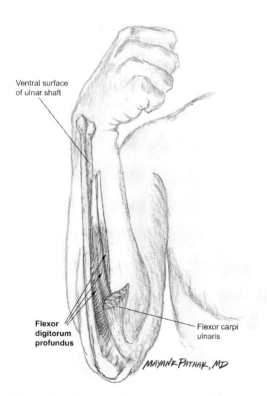

Figure 13.3 Injection of flexor digitorum profundus.

a thin section of the flexor carpi ulnaris, the first fibers of the flexor digitorum profundus entered will be those for the fifth and fourth digits. Activate them by having the patient flex the distal phalanges

of these fingers. Deeper fibers flex the distal phalanges of the third and second digits.

Thumb curling

Inject adductor pollicis and other thenar muscles (Figure 13.4), and flexor pollicis longus (Figure 13.5).

Thumb curling may present with the clenched hand or alone. A curled thumb can prevent a patient from having an effective grasp and may also get caught during activities of daily living such as dressing.

Adductor pollicis spans the web between the first two metacarpals. It may be approached from the dorsal surface by going through the overlying first dorsal interosseus muscle; or, more commonly, from the palmar side. Three other thenar muscles can be injected with insertion in the palmar surface over the proximal half of the first metacarpal. The needle will first encounter abductor pollicis brevis, which may be injected if required, followed by the deeper opponens pollicis, activated by flexion of the first metacarpal in opposing the thumb against the fifth digit. Flexor pollicis brevis lies medial and adjacent to abductor pollicis brevis and may be reached by partially withdrawing the needle and directing it toward the base of the second digit; it is activated by flexion of the metacarpophalangeal joint.

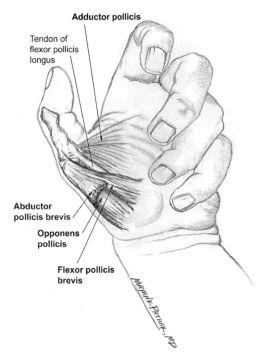

Adductor pollicis

Tendon of
flexor pollicis
longus

Abductor
pollicis brevis

Opponens
pollicis

Flexor pollicis
brevis

Figure 13.4 Injection of thenar muscles.

Flexor pollicis longus is approached by inserting the needle in the middle third of the ventral forearm, adjacent to the medial border of the brachioradialis, and directing it toward the ventral surface of the radius. The radial pulse may be palpated and avoided. Once contact with bone is made, withdrawing the tip a few millimeters will place it in the muscle belly, which is activated by flexion of the interphalangeal joint.

Wrist flexion

Inject flexor carpi ulnaris and flexor carpi radialis (Figure 13.6).

The flexed wrist may present with the flexed elbow and/or flexed hand, or alone. Persistent flexion of the wrist may cause pain and often interferes with a useful grasp regardless of involvement of the finger flexors.

Flexor carpi ulnaris is approached directly at the medial border of the forearm midway between the antecubital and distal wrist creases. Activate

Figure 13.5 Injection of flexor pollicis longus.

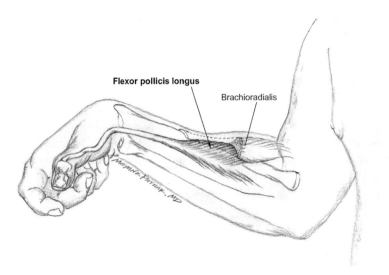

Flexor pollicis longus

Brachioradialis

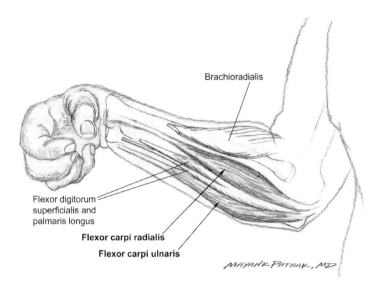

Figure 13.6 Injection of wrist flexors.

this superficial muscle by having the patient flex the wrist with slight ulnar deviation.

Flexor carpi radialis lies along the ventral surface of the forearm just medial to the midline. Localize it by first having the patient flex the wrist, then follow the line of the tendon from its insertion at the wrist toward the lateral edge of the biceps aponeurosis, where its fibers of origin may be palpable. The muscle is superficial, and injection is made four to five fingerbreadths distal to the antecubital crease.

Elbow flexion

Inject biceps and brachialis muscles (Figure 13.7).

The elbow may be flexed alone or in combination with the flexed hand and/or wrist. The flexed elbow may be exacerbated by walking and contribute to gait abnormalities, interfere with functional activities such as reaching and lifting, and impair activities of daily living such as dressing and eating.

Biceps is approached from the ventral arm surface. Divide the toxin dose between the short

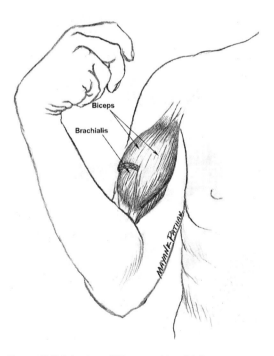

Figure 13.7 Injection of biceps and brachialis.

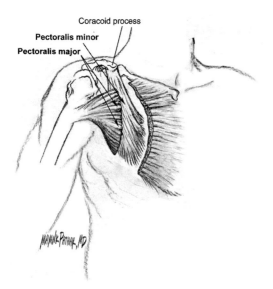

Figure 13.8 Injection of pectoralis major and minor.

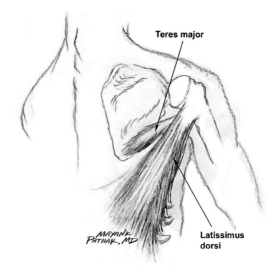

Figure 13.9 Injection of latissimus dorsi and teres major.

(medial) and long (lateral) heads. The brachialis lies lateral and deep to both heads of the biceps. Inject it by advancing the needle further toward the ventral surface of the humerus. Activate these muscles by having the patient flex the elbow against resistance.

Adduction and internal rotation at the shoulder

Inject pectoralis major and minor (Figure 13.8), with optional injection of latissimus dorsi and teres major (Figure 13.9).

Overactivity of the shoulder muscles may limit the patient in movements used in such routine activities as reaching, dressing, and eating.

Palpate the pectoralis insertion fibers at the anterior axillary fold and insert the needle parallel to the chest wall to minimize the risk of pneumothorax. Activate these muscles by having the patient press the palms together. Pectoralis major is superficial; advance through it to reach pectoralis minor. Distribute the dose among several sites. Latissimus

dorsi and teres major may both also cause shoulder adduction. They are accessible below the posterior axillary fold.

The lower limb

Plantarflexion spasm

Inject the lateral gastrocnemius, medial gastrocnemius (Figure 13.10), and soleus (Figure 13.11), with optional injection of the tibialis posterior (Figure 13.12).

Plantarflexion is a typical posture of the spastic limb and interferes with fitting of splints and placement of the foot flat in activities such as walking and transfers. Care must be taken to distinguish this spastic posture from flaccid "drop foot" as discussed previously.

Lying superficially in the calf, the lateral and medial heads of the gastrocnemius should be injected separately. When the tip is inside the muscle belly, the syringe will wiggle back and forth as the muscle is stretched and relaxed by passively

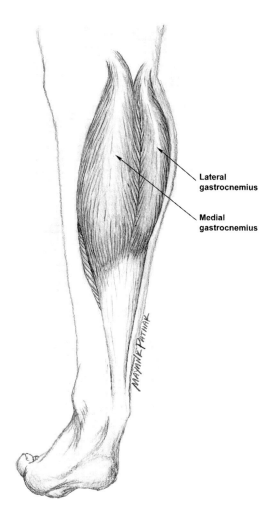

Lateral
gastrocnemius

Medial
gastrocnemius

Figure 13.10 Injection of lateral and medial gastrocnemii.

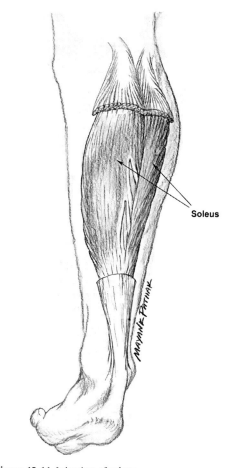

Soleus

Figure 13.11 Injection of soleus.

rocking the foot at the ankle with the knee extended. Soleus is best reached by advancing the needle through the medial gastrocnemius. Check the position of the needle tip by first flexing the knee to minimize movement of the gastrocnemii, then passively rocking the foot at the ankle until movement of the syringe is seen. All of these muscles are activated by having the patient plantarflex.

The tibialis posterior is an often overlooked contributor to foot plantarflexion and inversion, a posture noted in the spastic and dystonic foot. Those

patients with the tibialis posterior involved may walk on the side of the foot or be unable to wear shoes or orthotics. Because the tibialis posterior lies deep and is difficult to localize, we recommend guidance by electrical stimulation or EMG and the use of a 50 mm injection needle. Approaching through the tibialis anterior can be painful for patients whose muscles are in involuntary spasm, and inadvertent injection into the tibialis anterior may cause foot drop, exacerbating the plantarflexion. We prefer a medial approach, slipping the needle behind the medial border of the tibia, advancing along its posterior surface through the

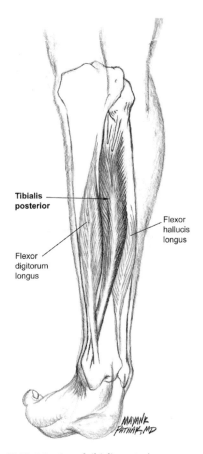

Figure 13.12 Injection of tibialis posterior.

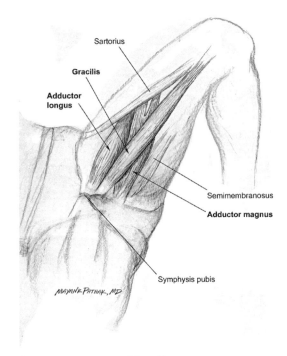

Figure 13.13 Injection of the adductor group.

smaller flexor digitorum longus and into the tibialis posterior. Injection into either of the two adjacent muscles, the flexor digitorum longus or flexor hallucis longus, will not be problematic and may also ameliorate plantarflexion posturing.

Adductor spasms

Inject the adductor group (Figure 13.13).

Patients with overactive adductor muscles will present with difficulty with personal hygiene and dressing.

Approach the adductor muscles with the patient supine, thighs flexed and abducted at the hips,

and knees flexed. The muscles are best found proximally in the anteromedial thigh approximately a handbreadth distal to the groin fold, where they are superficial and the separations (in anterior to medial progression) of the adductor longus and gracilis are palpable. The adductor brevis lies deep to longus. Adductor magnus may be injected by advancing deep through the gracilis, or entered directly just posterior to the posterior edge of the gracilis.

Extensor posturing at the knee

Inject the qadriceps group (Figure 13.14).

Patients with involvement of the quadricep group may have difficulty with relaxing the thigh making it difficult to balance, walk or fit in a wheelchair. For patients in whom quadriceps injection is warranted, the rectus femoris, vastus lateralis, and

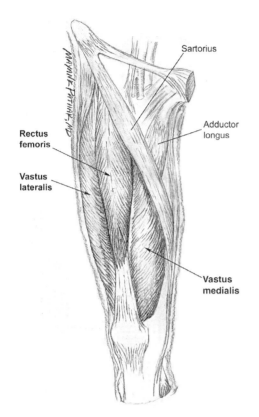

Figure 13.14 Injection of the quadriceps group.

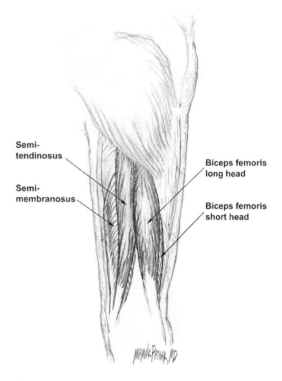

Figure 13.15 Injection of hamstring muscles.

vastus medialis are readily approached in the anterior thigh. The rectus femoris and vastus lateralis are injected halfway between the patella and the groin fold. The vastus medialis is best found more distally.

Knee flexion spasm

Inject the hamstring muscles (Figure 13.15).

Patients with overactive hamstrings may present with pain. Spasticity in these muscles will make bending the knee difficult and may result in difficulty with sitting or walking. These large muscles are palpable in the posterior thigh of most patients and approaches are straightforward. Semitendinosus and semimembranosus are medial in the posterior

thigh, while biceps femoris long and short heads are lateral.

Toe extension

Inject the extensor hallucis longus (Figure 13.16).

Patients with involvement of the great toe extensor may present with excessive wear to the top of the shoe or abrasions to the great toe. Patients or caregivers may have difficulty applying footwear or splints. Locate this muscle by palpating its tendon just lateral to the tendon of the tibialis anterior and following it proximally about one-third of the way up the tibia. At this level, its muscular belly lies one fingerbreadth lateral to the tibia. Activate by having the patient extend the toe. Avoid injection into the belly of the tibialis anterior, which may result in foot drop.

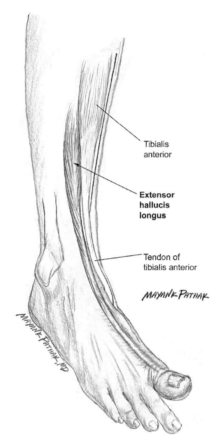

Figure 13.16 Injection of extensor hallucis longus.

REFERENCES

Berweck, S., Feldkamp, A., Francke, A., *et al.* (2002). Sonography-guided injection of botulinum toxin A in children with cerebral palsy. *Neuropediatrics*, **33**, 221–3.

Bhakta, B. B., Cozens, J. A., Chamberlain, M. A. & Bamford, J. M. (2000). Impact of botulinum toxin type A on disability and carer burden due to arm spasticity after stroke: a randomised double blind placebo controlled trial. *J Neurol Neurosurg Psychiatry*, **69**, 217–21.

Brashear, A., Gordon, M. F., Elovic, E., *et al.* (2002). Intramuscular injection of botulinum toxin for the treatment of wrist and finger spasticity after a stroke. *N Engl J Med*, **347**, 395–400.

Brashear, A., McAfee, A. L., Kuhn, E. R. & Ambrosius, W. T. (2003). Treatment with botulinum toxin type B for upper-limb spasticity. *Arch Phys Med Rehabil*, **84**, 103–7.

Brashear, A., McAfee, A. L., Kuhn, E. R. & Fyffe, J. (2004). Botulinum toxin type B in upper-limb poststroke spasticity: a double-blind, placebo-controlled trial. *Arch Phys Med Rehabil*, **85**, 705–9.

Childers, M. K. (2003). The importance of electromyographic guidance and electrical stimulation for injection of botulinum toxin. *Phys Med Rehabil Clin N Am*, **14**, 781–92.

Childers, M. K., Brashear, A., Jozefczyk, P., *et al.* (2004). Dose-dependent response to intramuscular botulinum toxin type A for upper-limb spasticity in patients after a stroke. *Arch Phys Med Rehabil*, **85**, 1063–9.

Chin, T. Y., Nattrass, G. R., Selber, P. & Graham, H. K. (2005). Accuracy of intramuscular injection of botulinum toxin A in juvenile cerebral palsy: a comparison between manual needle placement and placement guided by electrical stimulation. *J Pediatr Orthop*, **25**, 286–91.

Dressler, D. & Benecke, R. (2003). Autonomic side effects of botulinum toxin type B treatment of cervical dystonia and hyperhidrosis. *Eur Neurol*, **49**, 34–8.

Francisco, G. E. (2004). Botulinum toxin: dosing and dilution. *Am J Phys Med Rehabil*, **83**, S30–7.

Hesse, S., Jahnke, M. T., Luecke, D. & Mauritz, K. H. (1995). Short-term electrical stimulation enhances the effectiveness of Botulinum toxin in the treatment of lower limb spasticity in hemiparetic patients. *Neurosci Lett*, **201**, 37–40.

Hyman, N., Barnes, M., Bhakta, B., *et al.* (2000). Botulinum toxin (Dysport) treatment of hip adductor spasticity in multiple sclerosis: a prospective, randomised, double blind, placebo controlled, dose ranging study. *J Neurol Neurosurg Psychiatry*, **68**, 707–12.

Lance, J. W. (1981). Disordered muscle tone and movement. *Clin Exp Neurol*, **18**, 27–35.

Mayer, N. H., Esquenazi, A. & Childers, M. K. (2002). Common patterns of clinical motor dysfunction. In N. H. Mayer & D. M. Simpson, eds., *Spasticity: Etiology, Evaluation, Management and the Role of Botulinum Toxin*. New York: WE MOVE, pp. 16–26.

Monnier, G., Parratte, B., Tatu, L., *et al.* (2003). [EMG support in botulinum toxin treatment]. *Ann Readapt Med Phys*, **46**, 380–5.

O'Brien, C. F. (1997). Injection techniques for botulinum toxin using electromyography and electrical stimulation. *Muscle Nerve Suppl*, **6**, S176–80.

Pathak, M. S., Nguyen, H. T., Graham, H. K. & Moore, A. P. (2006). Management of spasticity in adults: practical application of botulinum toxin. *Eur J Neurol*, **13**(Suppl 1), 42–50.

Raj, P. P. E. (2004). Treatment algorithm overview: BoNT therapy for pain. *Pain Pract*, **4**, S60–4.

Sheean, G. L. (2001). Botulinum treatment of spasticity: why is it so difficult to show a functional benefit? *Curr Opin Neurol*, **14**, 771–6.

Suputtitada, A. & Suwanwela, N. C. (2005). The lowest effective dose of botulinum A toxin in adult patients with upper limb spasticity. *Disabil Rehabil*, **27**, 176–84.

Traba Lopez, A. & Esteban, A. (2001). Botulinum toxin in motor disorders: practical considerations with emphasis on interventional neurophysiology. *Neurophysiol Clin*, **31**, 220–9.

WE MOVE Spasticity Study Group. (2005a). BTX-A Adult Dosing Guidelines. WE MOVE. www.mdvu.org/library/dosingtables/btxa_adg.html.

WE MOVE Spasticity Study Group. (2005b). BTX-B Adult Dosing Guidelines. WE MOVE. www.mdvu.org/library/dosingtables/btxb_adg.html.

Westhoff, B., Seller, K., Wild, A., Jaeger, M. & Krauspe, R. (2003). Ultrasound-guided botulinum toxin injection technique for the iliopsoas muscle. *Dev Med Child Neurol*, **45**, 829–32.

14

The use of botulinum toxin in spastic infantile cerebral palsy

Ann Tilton and H. Kerr Graham

Introduction

Cerebral palsy is not a specific disease but a group of clinical syndromes, caused by a non-progressive injury to the developing brain that results in a disorder of movement and posture that is permanent but not unchanging. It is the most common cause of physical disability affecting children in developed countries. The incidence is steady in most countries at approximately 2/1000 live births. The location, timing, and severity of the brain lesion are extremely variable, which results in many different clinical presentations. Despite the static nature of the brain injury, the majority of children with cerebral palsy develop progressive musculoskeletal problems such as spastic posturing and muscle contractures (Koman *et al.*, 2004).

Classification

Cerebral palsy may be classified according to the cause of the brain lesion (when this is known), and the location of the brain lesion as noted on imaging such as magnetic resonance imaging or computerized tomography scan. Clinically more useful classification schemes are based on the type of movement disorder, the distribution of the movement disorder (Box 14.1), and the gross motor function of the child.

It is important to correctly characterize the movement disorder because different movement disorders can be managed by different interventions.

Spasticity is the most common movement disorder, affecting between 60% and 80% of children with cerebral palsy (Figure 14.1). Spasticity is defined as hypertonia in which one or both of the following signs are present:

- resistance to externally imposed movement increases with increasing speed of stretch and varies with the direction of joint movement
- resistance to externally imposed movement rises rapidly above a threshold speed or joint angle.

When focal, spasticity is often managed by injections of botulinum toxin (BoNT). When severe or generalized, spasticity may be managed by selective dorsal rhizotomy or intrathecal baclofen.

Dystonia is characterized by involuntary sustained or intermittent muscle contractions that cause twisting and repetitive movements, abnormal postures, or both. Focal dystonia may also be treated with BoNT.

Athetosis, or intermittent writhing movement, is also very common. It is sometimes influenced by oral medications, and when severe by intrathecal baclofen pump, but never by selective dorsal rhizotomy.

Ataxia is less common in cerebral palsy, and is difficult to treat successfully.

In addition to the positive features of cerebral palsy such as spasticity and dystonia, there are also

Manual of Botulinum Toxin Therapy, ed. Daniel Truong, Dirk Dressler and Mark Hallett. Published by Cambridge University Press. © Cambridge University Press 2009.

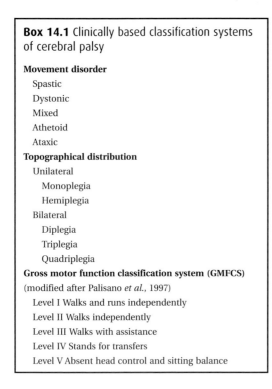

Box 14.1 Clinically based classification systems of cerebral palsy

Movement disorder
  Spastic
  Dystonic
  Mixed
  Athetoid
  Ataxic
Topographical distribution
  Unilateral
    Monoplegia
    Hemiplegia
  Bilateral
    Diplegia
    Triplegia
    Quadriplegia
Gross motor function classification system (GMFCS)
(modified after Palisano *et al.*, 1997)
  Level I Walks and runs independently
  Level II Walks independently
  Level III Walks with assistance
  Level IV Stands for transfers
  Level V Absent head control and sitting balance

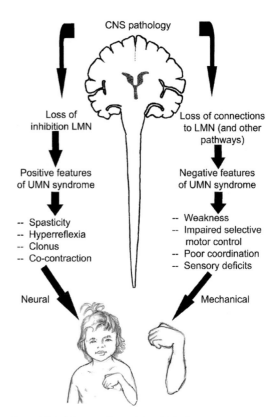

Figure 14.1 Scheme of spasticity. LMN, lower motor neuron; UMN, upper motor neuron.

negative features – principally weakness and loss of selective motor control. In the long term, weakness and difficulty in controlling muscles ("negative features") have a much greater impact on gross motor function than the various forms of muscle over-activity ("positive features"). Nevertheless, spasticity has been implicated in the development of fixed deformities which can further impair function and quality of life in the child or adolescent affected by cerebral palsy.

Topographical distribution and anatomical approach to management

Understanding the topographical distribution of symptoms, and recognizing the common clinical patterns of muscle overactivity, forms the basis for development of management strategies. We review these patterns as the basis for intervention with BoNT and other therapies, before turning to injection techniques.

As indicated in Box 14.1, involvement may be uni-lateral, either monoplegic or hemiplegic; or bilateral, diplegic, paraplegic or quadriplegic. Spastic diplegia usually refers to individuals with minimal involvement of the upper limbs but bilateral lower limb involvement. Spastic quadriplegia refers to individuals with involvement of all four limbs, with the upper limbs sometimes more affected than the lower limbs. However, the differentiation between spastic diplegia and spastic quadriplegia is not clear cut and it is more clinically useful to classify bilateral cerebral palsy according to gross motor function as noted above.

Unilateral cerebral palsy: spastic hemiplegia

In hemiplegia, motor pathway involvement on one side of the brain leads to contralateral motor

(a)   (b)

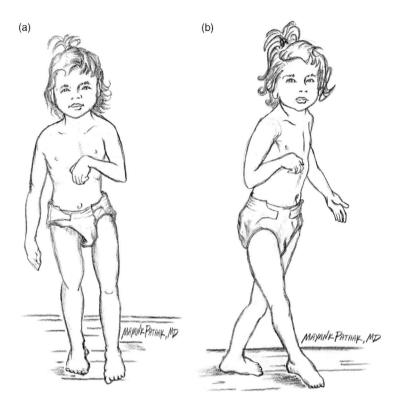

Figure 14.2 Spastic hemiplegia coronal (a) and sagittal (b) views. Muscles that are commonly overactive in spastic hemiplegia are biceps, brachialis, adductor pollicis, flexor carpi ulnaris, flexor carpi radialis pronator teres, gastrocnemius, soleus, tibialis posterior.

symptoms (Figure 14.2a, 2b). The most common movement disorder is spastic but mixed spastic and dystonic types are also very common. Sometimes the upper limb has mainly a dystonic movement disorder and the lower limb a mainly spastic movement disorder.

Upper limb

Typical upper limb posturing includes adduction and internal rotation at the shoulder, pronation and flexion at the elbow/forearm and flexion and ulnar deviation at the wrist with flexed digits, and "thumb in palm." The muscles typically involved in each pattern are indicated in Table 14.1, along with guidelines for injection of BoNT-A as Botox® (Allergan Ltd., Irvine, CA).

Without intervention, spastic posturing in the hemiplegic upper limb can progress to painful fixed contracture and deformities that further impair function and cosmesis.

It is tempting to think that the spasticity or dystonia is the main functional limitation in the hemiplegic upper limb, and that relaxing the overactive muscles will necessarily restore function. On the contrary, the main barriers to function are impaired selective motor control and sensation. Muscle relaxation may set the stage for functional gains, but may not be adequate by itself. Therefore, focal treatment with BoNT alone is rarely indicated and should usually be combined with a program of splinting and occupational therapy or upper limb training.

Lower limb

The involved lower limb is usually slightly shorter than that on the uninvolved side, with muscle atrophy especially affecting the calf muscle. Typically, involvement is more pronounced distally than proximally (see Box 14.2).

> **Box 14.2** Grading of lower limb involvement in spastic hemiplegia
>
> (Modified after Winters *et al.* [1987])
>
>   Type I: a drop foot in the swing phase of gait but no calf contracture.
>
>   Type II: spastic or contracted gastrocsoleus resulting in equinus gait.
>
>   Type III: involvement extends to the knee with spasticity and co-contraction of the hamstrings and rectus femoris.
>
>   Type IV: involvement extends to the hip, which is typically flexed, adducted, and internally rotated.

In younger children, the hemiplegic lower limb can be managed quite effectively using a combination of focal injections of BoNT, the use of an ankle-foot orthosis (AFO), and a physical therapy program. An AFO is useful in all four types because it controls drop foot in swing. In type II, injection of BoNT once calf spasticity is noted can be very effective in improving gait and function. We usually start injection of the gastrocsoleus from the age of 18 months to 2 years and continue until age 6 years. By this time either the spasticity is well controlled or a contracture has developed, which is more effectively treated by an orthopedic, muscle tendon lengthening procedure. Types III and IV hemiplegia may be treated with multilevel injections of BoNT in the younger child, and multilevel surgery in the older child. Multilevel injections typically are directed to the spastic gastrocsoleus, sometimes the tibialis posterior if the posturing is equinovarus, the hamstrings, the hip adductors and hip flexors, and occasionally the rectus femoris when there is a stiff knee gait.

Bilateral cerebral palsy: spastic diplegia

Children with spastic diplegia have usually been born prematurely and have generalized lower limb spasticity but normal cognition and few medical co-morbidities. Walking is typically delayed until aged 2–5 years in children with spastic diplegia

and when they first walk, it is typically with a "tip toe" gait pattern. Spastic equinus is very common and may impair stability in stance and the ability to progress in standing and walking (Figure 14.3a, 3b). In the younger child, spastic equinus is safely and effectively managed by injection of BoNT into the gastrocsoleus muscles and the provision of AFOs in the context of a physical therapy program. This allows many children to achieve flat foot and to progress in standing and walking at a faster rate than would be otherwise the case.

Older children with spastic diplegia frequently develop fixed contractures of the flexor muscles including the iliopsoas at the hip, the hamstrings at the knee, and the plantarflexors of the ankle. There are also frequently torsional abnormalities of the long bones including medial femoral torsion and lateral tibial torsion. There may be instability of the hip joint and breakdown of the mid foot. These more advanced musculoskeletal problems are best dealt with by multilevel orthopedic surgery typically between the ages of 6 and 10 years. However, the use of spasticity management in the younger child is still an excellent option for these children. It avoids the need for early surgery, eliminates the need for repeated surgery, and allows the orthopedic procedures to be performed at an age when an outcome is much more predictable. The sequence of early management by focal injections of BoNT followed by multilevel orthopedic surgery yields superior functional outcomes than have been achieved in the past by serial orthopedic procedures. A small number of children with spastic diplegia have such severe lower limb spasticity that it is not amenable to multilevel injections of BoNT. Such children are more effectively managed by selective dorsal rhizotomy.

Bilateral cerebral palsy: spastic quadriplegia

Children with spastic quadriplegia have spasticity and/or dystonia in all four limbs and have much greater functional impairment than children with

(a)

(b)

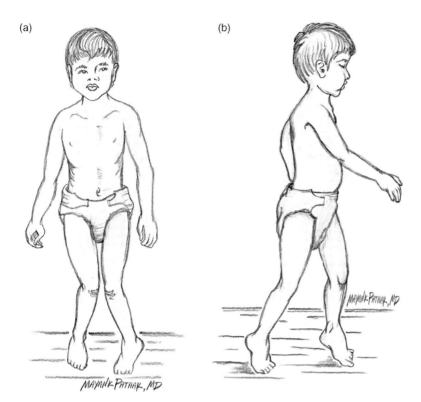

Figure 14.3 Spastic diplegia frontal (a) and lateral (b) views. Muscles that are commonly overactive in spastic diplegia are hamstrings, gastrocnemius, and soleus.

spastic diplegia. Some children can stand for transfers and walk short distances (GMFCS level IV). However some children lack head control and sitting balance, and are unable to stand or transfer. These children are transported in a wheelchair and are dependent for all aspects of their care (Figure 14.4a and 4b).

Functional walking is not a goal for these children, but spasticity management can still be very useful to prevent postural deformities becoming fixed and to make care and comfort easier for these children and adolescents. Focal injections of BoNT are sometimes useful in the upper limb to permit easier use of wheelchair controls for children at GMFCS level IV. Injections of the hip adductors (Chapter 13, Figure 13.13) and hamstrings (Chapter 13, Figure 13.15) may aid sitting position when standing and walking are not functional goals. Injections of the calf muscles may permit more comfortable sitting; allow the orthoses, shoes, and

socks to be worn; and keep the feet on a wheelchair foot plate.

Progression of spastic posturing to fixed contractures and joint instability is very common in these children. The majority will develop hip instability which can be detected by serial radiographic examination of the hips. Injection of BoNT into the hip adductors may slow the progression of hip displacement but the majority will eventually require preventative or reconstructive orthopedic surgery. If spastic dystonia is severe and causing discomfort or difficulties with care, the use of an intrathecal baclofen pump can be very effective.

Treatment techniques

Following definition of treatment goals and a discussion of the risks and benefits of the medication, the patient is prepared for the procedure. Patients

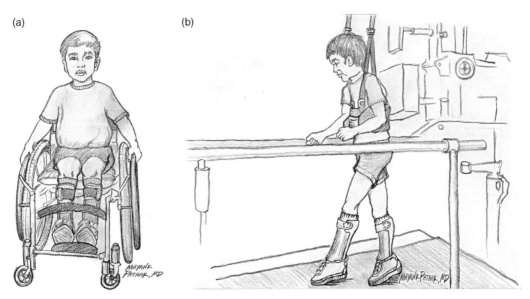

Figure 14.4 (a and b) Spastic quadriplegia. Almost any muscle group may be affected by spasticity or dystonia or more frequently a mixture of both. The target muscles which benefit most from BoNT injection are the hip adductors and hamstrings. In the upper limbs, injection of the elbow flexors and finger flexors may improve reach, grasp and release.

often prefer some measure of local anesthesia. Topical lidocaine cream or ethyl chloride as a local coolant is helpful at the time of injection. Additionally, oral midazolam can be utilized as an anxiolytic. While most children and adults can tolerate the procedure well, combative patients, such as those with autism or extreme anxiety, may benefit from general anesthesia. Parents traditionally prefer to stay for the injections and provide reassurance (Russman *et al.*, 2002).

Assistance from technicians or medical personnel is important to stabilize and appropriately position the child. The patient is placed in a position to activate the muscle of interest, e.g., frog-legged for injection of the adductors. The skin is prepared with alcohol or povidone-iodine and universal precautions are utilized. While palpation is the most commonly and easily utilized method, electromyographic or electrical stimulation guidance may be very helpful when surface landmarks are not easily localized or when precise targeting of smaller muscles in the upper extremities is required. Ultrasonography is useful, especially to accurately

localize muscles and confirm the presence of the needle in muscles that are deeper and hard to reach.

Treatment guidelines

Dosing guidelines for Botox (BoNT-A) have been developed by experienced injectors, which reflect concern for avoidance of antibody-based resistance while delivering a clinically effective dose to the target muscles (Box 14.3) (Russman *et al.*, 2002). Because of the maximum dose limitation, not all muscles may be injected in one treatment session. For up-to-date information on dosing schedules see WE MOVE website (www.wemove.org/).

Adverse effects

When used according to published guidelines, BoNT is safe for use in most children with cerebral palsy. The most common side effects are at the site

---

Box 14.3 Guidelines for dosing of Botox
for children

1. Maximum dosing per session: the lesser of 15 U/kg
   or 400 U
   Experienced injectors may use more
2. Dose range:
   Upper extremity: 0.5–2 U/kg
   Lower extremity smaller muscles: 1–3 U/kg and larger
     muscles 3–6 U/kg
   No more than 50 U per injection site
3. Reinjection interval 3 months or greater
4. Dilution 1–2 cc of non-bacteriostatic saline
   per 100 U vial
5. Spread of the toxin is 4–5 cm in the muscle. Thus
   muscles may need more than one injection site based
   on size, fascial planes, and dose

---

of the injection and include muscle soreness and bruising. These complications are minor and self-limiting. There are no reports of deep infection after intramuscular injection or permanent neurovascular injury. Remote side effects, including incontinence and dysphagia, have occasionally been reported. Incontinence is of great concern to parents but usually resolves quickly. Dysphagia, which may lead to aspiration and chest infection, is the most serious complication. Children with spastic quadriplegia with pseudobulbar palsy seem to be much more sensitive to systemic spread after focal injection of BoNT, and treatment may be relatively contraindicated in this group for this reason.

Treatment planning and considerations

Botox is approved for use in cerebral palsy in some countries (including Canada) but not others (including the United States), and the age threshold

varies by country as well. Off-label use is common but ideally should be in the context of approved clinical trials. There is reasonable clinical evidence to suggest that younger children respond more fully and for longer periods of time than do older children. This may simply be because of the progression from dynamic posturing to fixed contracture in the older child.

Children with spastic hemiplegia and spastic diplegia can be safely injected from age 18–24 months. Treatment seems to be most effective between the ages of 2 and 6 years, and should be in the context of a global tone management program including the use of orthoses, serial casting, and physical therapy. By age 6–10 years, children will have plateaued in terms of physical functioning, and many no longer require injection therapy. Some will have developed fixed contractures and are more effectively managed by orthopedic surgical procedures.

REFERENCES

Koman, L. A., Smith, B. P. & Shilt, J. S. (2004). Cerebral palsy. *Lancet*, **363**(9421), 1619–31.

Palisano, R. J., Rosenbaum, P., Walter, S., *et al.* (1997). Development and reliability of a system to classify gross motor function in children with cerebral palsy. *Dev Med Child Neurol*, **45**, 113–20.

Russman, B. S., Tilton, A. H. & Gormley, M. E. Jr. (2002). Cerebral palsy: a rational approach to a treatment protocol, and the role of botulinum toxin in treatment. In N. H. Mayer & D. M. Simpson, eds., *Spasticity: Etiology, Evaluation, Management, and the Role of Botulinum Toxin*. New York: WE MOVE, pp. 134–43.

Winters, T. F. Jr., Gage, J. R. & Hicks, R. (1987). Gait patterns in spastic hemiplegia in children and young adults. *J Bone Joint Surg Am*, **69**, 437–41.

15

Hyperhidrosis

Henning Hamm and Markus K. Naumann

Definition, prevalence, and diagnosis

Hyperhidrosis may generally be defined as excessive sweating or sweating beyond physiological needs. It may be divided into generalized, regional, and localized/focal types and, according to whether the cause is known or not, into primary or idiopathic forms. Secondary hyperhidrosis can be induced by a wealth of infectious, endocrine, metabolic, cardio-vascular, neurological, psychiatric, and malignant conditions, and can also be caused by certain drugs and poisoning. The prevalence of hyperhidrosis in the US population has been calculated at 2.8% (Strutton et al., 2004). Of those, primary axillary hyperhidrosis appears to be the most frequent type, severely affecting 0.5%.

According to a consensus statement, primary focal hyperhidrosis (PFH) can be diagnosed as explained in Table 15.1 (Hornberger et al., 2004). It usually starts in childhood or adolescence and mainly involves the armpits, palms, soles, and cra-niofacial region, either alone or in various combin-ations. There are well-known, emotional triggers of sweating episodes, but the exact pathogenesis of the overstimulation of eccrine sweat glands is still poorly understood apart from a clear genetic background.

As measured by standardized questionnaires, PFH negatively affects many aspects of daily life to a significant extent, including emotional status, personal hygiene, work and productivity, leisure activities and self-esteem (Hamm et al., 2006). The so-called hyperhidrosis disease severity scale (HDSS) (Table 15.2), a single-item question allowing four gradations of the tolerability of sweating and its interference with daily activities, offers a simple and useful way to estimate the impairment of quality of life (Lowe et al., 2007).

History taking is the most important tool to diag-nose PFH and to exclude secondary types. Physical examination should focus on visible evidence of excessive sweating in the characteristic locations and on detection of signs that suggest a secondary cause. Laboratory tests are not needed if the pre-sentation is characteristic and if evidence of sec-ondary causes is lacking. In contrast, generalized forms of sweating and asymmetric patterns have to be evaluated for underlying disorders (Hornberger et al., 2004). Gravimetric quantification of sweat production in predominantly involved sites is not routinely performed but may be helpful to support the diagnosis, to rate the severity, and in clinical research. Minor's iodine-starch test is used to out-line the sweating area prior to botulinum toxin treatment or local surgery.

Conventional treatment options

There is quite a large number of treatment options for PFH, the utility of which partly depend on the site involved (Haider & Solish, 2005).

Manual of Botulinum Toxin Therapy, ed. Daniel Truong, Dirk Dressler and Mark Hallett. Published by Cambridge University Press.
© Cambridge University Press 2009.

Table 15.1. Diagnostic criteria of primary focal hyperhidrosis

Focal, visible, excessive sweating of at least 6 months duration without apparent cause with at least two of the following characteristics:
- bilateral and relatively symmetric sweating
- impairment of daily activities
- frequency of at least one episode per week
- age of onset less than 25 years
- positive family history
- cessation of focal sweating during sleep

Table 15.2. Hyperhidrosis disease severity scale

Question: How would you rate the severity of your sweating?
1: Sweating is never noticeable and never interferes with daily activities.
2: Sweating is tolerable and sometimes interferes with daily activities.
3: Sweating is barely tolerable and frequently interferes with daily activities.
4: Sweating is intolerable and always interferes with daily activities.

Note:
Only severity scores of 3 and 4 should be assigned to true hyperhidrosis.

When seeking medical advice, most patients with primary axillary hyperhidrosis have already tried over-the-counter antiperspirants without success. The majority of them, particularly those with mild to moderate hyperhidrosis, can be treated effectively with topical aluminum chloride salts mechanically obstructing the sweat gland ducts. We prefer aluminum chloride hexahydrate 15% in aqueous solution thickened with methylcellulose (aluminum chloride hexahydrate 15.0, methylcellulose 1.5, distilled water ad 100.0 cc); others recommend absolute alcohol or salicylic acid gel as the base for the preparation. To minimize skin irritation, the solution should be applied to dry, clean armpits at bedtime and washed off after getting up in the morning. Initially, it is used every other evening until euhidrosis is achieved. The frequency of application can often be tapered to once every 1–3 weeks to maintain the effect. Continued treatment may lead to atrophy of the secretory cells. If ineffective, every evening application or higher concentrations may be tried, but will often not be tolerated by the patient. In contrast, the irritative potential of aluminum chloride salts is less severe on palms and soles so that concentrations may possibly be increased to 25–35%. Nevertheless, this treatment has proved less potent and less feasible in sites other than the axillary region.

Tap water iontophoresis using direct current (DC) or DC plus alternating current (AC) is regarded as the most effective non-invasive therapy for palmar and plantar hyperhidrosis. Iontophoresis is thought to work by blockage of the sweat gland at the stratum corneum level, but its exact mode of action is unclear. Hands or feet are placed in a shallow basin filled with tap water through which an electric current at 15–20 mA is passed for 15–30 minutes. Initially, patients undergo three to seven treatments per week, and six to ten treatments are usually required to achieve euhidrosis. Side effects include burning, tingling ("pins and needles"), irritation, erythema, skin dryness, transient paresthesias, and rarely vesicles; wounds have to be protected by petrolatum. To maintain the effect, regular sessions about once or twice a week are necessary, which is why many patients refrain from continuation of the time-consuming procedure. The method is less practical for axillary hyperhidrosis, and it is contraindicated in pregnancy and in patients with a pacemaker or metal implant.

Oral anticholinergic drugs are able to suppress sweating for a short time, but their effect is almost invariably accompanied by side effects such as dry mouth, blurred vision, dizziness, urinary retention, and constipation. Glycopyrrolate, diazepam, amitryptiline, beta-blockers, diltiazem, clonidine, gabapentin, indomethacin, and oxybutynin are further oral agents that have been tried in a limited number of hyperhidrosis patients with variable success.

Surgery can be used as a last choice in severe cases. Various techniques of local elimination or destruction of sweat glands have been proposed to treat axillary hyperhidrosis (Naumann & Hamm, 2002). En bloc excision of the entire sweating area as the simplest and most effective method has largely been abandoned since it inevitably leads to large unsightly scars. Nowadays, curettage and liposuction techniques that may be performed under local or tumescent local anesthesia are favored in respect of far better cosmetic results (Proebstle *et al.*, 2002). However, bleeding, hematomas, seromas, wound infection, skin necrosis, prolonged wound healing, paresthesias, prominent scars, and wound contractures interfering with arm mobility are possible complications, and only about 70% of patients benefit from these local procedures in the long run.

Endoscopic thoracic sympathectomy (ETS) interrupting the transmission of sympathetic nerve impulses from ganglia to nerve endings is the most efficient but also most invasive method to treat focal hyperhidrosis. Usually, thoracic sympathetic ganglia T3 and T4 are destroyed or cut through by electrocautery for treatment of palmar hyperhidrosis, and, in addition, T2 in craniofacial hyperhidrosis. In about 98% of patients with palmar hyperhidrosis, immediate and complete anhidrosis occurs, with only low rates of recurrence, whereas results in axillary hyperhidrosis are less convincing. Acute and early complications including bleeding, hemo-, pneumo- and chylothorax, pleural adhesion or effusion, neuralgia, and complete or incomplete Horner's syndrome are rare. However, compensatory sweating mainly of the back, abdomen, and legs develops regularly some months after surgery, as well as gustatory sweating in up to half of the patients. Incapacitating compensatory sweating is claimed by about 5–10% of patients (Dumont *et al.*, 2004). Therefore, ETS should be reserved for patients with severe palmar hyperhidrosis who have not responded to any other treatments available.

Treatment algorithms for primary axillary and primary palmar hyperhidrosis worked out in an international consensus conference are presented in Tables 15.3 and 15.4 (Hornberger *et al.*, 2004).

Table 15.3. Treatment algorithm for primary axillary hyperhidrosis

Topical over-the-counter antiperspirants
⇩
Topical aluminum chloride hexahydrate 10–35%
⇩
Intradermal injections of botulinum toxin type A
⇩
Topical sweat gland resection by curettage or liposuction techniques

Source: Adapted from Hornberger *et al.* (2004) with permission.

Table 15.4. Treatment algorithm for primary palmar hyperhidrosis

Topical aluminum chloride 10–35%
or
Tap water iontophoresis
⇩
Intradermal injections of botulinum toxin type A
⇩
Endoscopic thoracic sympathectomy

Source: Adapted from Hornberger *et al.* (2004) with permission.

Botulinum toxin therapy

A decade ago, botulinum toxin type A (BoNT-A) was introduced as a novel, minimally invasive therapeutic modality for focal hyperhidrosis. When injected intradermally it blocks the release of acetylcholine from sympathetic nerve fibers that stimulate eccrine sweat glands and causes a localized, long-lasting but reversible abolishment of sweating (Glaser, 2006).

Botulinum toxin type A has been evaluated most extensively in primary axillary hyperhidrosis. Three large randomized, placebo-controlled, double-blind studies and several open-label studies clearly document its effectiveness and safety in this indication.

In a European study enrolling 320 patients, 94% of patients treated with 50 mouse units (U) Botox® per axilla were treatment responders at week 4 (> 50% reduction in sweat production from baseline gravimetric measurement) with an average reduction in sweat production of 83.5% (Naumann & Lowe, 2001). In a 12-month follow-up study, 207 of these patients received up to 3 further BoNT-A injections. Response rates and satisfaction with treatment remained consistently high with no diminution of effect and no confirmed positive results for neutralizing antibodies to BoNT-A with repeated treatments (Naumann *et al.*, 2003). Mean duration of benefit was about 7 months after a single treatment. Twenty-eight percent of patients did not require more than one injection, indicating a long-lasting benefit of at least 16 months. No major side effects occurred, with subjective increase in non-axillary sweating perceived by 4% of the patients being the most frequent complaint. Botulinum toxin type A treatment also markedly improved the quality of life of patients (Naumann *et al.*, 2002).

In a multicenter North American trial in 322 patients comparing 50 U Botox per axilla to 75 U Botox per axilla and placebo, responders were defined as having at least a 2-grade reduction in their HDSS score. There was a 75% response rate in the verum groups compared to a 25% response rate in the placebo-treated patients, but without significant difference between the groups treated with different Botox doses (Lowe *et al.*, 2007). Eighty to 84% of the treatment groups had at least a 75% reduction in sweat production, compared to only 21% in the placebo group. Median duration of the BoNT-A effect was again approximately 7 months. These studies brought about the license of Botox for axillary hyperhidrosis in many countries worldwide. Currently, it is the only botulinum toxin formulation licensed for use in hyperhidrosis.

A randomized, placebo-controlled, double-blind study in 145 German patients with one axilla being treated with either 100 or 200 U Dysport® and the contralateral one with placebo obtained similar results with regard to efficacy and safety (Heckmann *et al.*, 2001). A significant decrease in sweat production compared to placebo was observed after 2 weeks and maintained 24 weeks after injection. The two doses proved equally effective in reducing axillary sweating.

There are a number of smaller controlled and observational studies showing that BoNT-A is also a valuable treatment option in palmar hyperhidrosis. However, treatment is more complex, injections are more painful, higher doses are needed, and the effect is less pronounced and less long-lasting than in axillary hyperhidrosis.

Reduction or elimination of pain during palmar injections can best be achieved by median and ulnar nerve blocks performed a few centimeters proximal to the wrist. However, transient paresthesias and the potential risk of permanent nerve damage particularly with regard to repeated treatments have to be considered. Cryoanesthesia with ice cubes, cold packs, liquid nitrogen spray, liquid ethylchloride or dichlorotetrafluoroethane (Frigiderm®) may be a reasonable alternative in many patients. Moreover, vibratory anesthesia, regional intravenous anesthesia (Bier block), and general sedation have been advocated. The usual dose is 100 U Botox per palm but 150 U or more may be required depending on its size. Sweating is reduced to about half the pretreatment amount, and the effect lasts about 4 months on average (Lowe *et al.*, 2002). Mild weakness of intrinsic hand muscles may occur in a minority of patients for up to 4–6 weeks and is usually insignificant. This most frequent side effect should be particularly pointed out to manual workers.

In axillary hyperhidrosis, BoNT-A treatment is now the treatment of choice if topical treatments prove ineffective. In palmar hyperhidrosis, it should be considered if topical treatments and iontophoresis have failed. Another excellent indication for BoNT-A treatment is gustatory sweating which is discussed more detailed in Chapter 12.

According to a few smaller studies injections of botulinum toxin type B (BoNT-B) seem to be similarly effective as BoNT-A in axillary and palmar hyperhidrosis. Doses used were 2000–5000 U NeuroBloc® per axilla and 5000 U per palm. Compared to BoNT-A, side effects occur considerably more often with BoNT-B, especially systemic adverse events including dryness of the mouth and throat, dryness of eyes, indigestion, and heartburn (Dressler *et al.*, 2002; Baumann *et al.*, 2005).

Botulinum toxin type A has also been used for primary hyperhidrosis of other sites, such as scalp (Figure 15.1), forehead (Kinkelin *et al.*, 2000), and soles, and in certain types of regional secondary hyperhidrosis, such as Ross syndrome (Figure 15.2) and compensatory sweating. Experience in these indications is much more limited than in axillary and palmar hyperhidrosis and no general recommendations can be given.

Technique of botulinum toxin treatment in primary axillary hyperhidrosis

Preparation of axillary BoNT-A treatment includes the following:
- avoid shaving and use of antiperspirants 48 hours prior to treatment
- exclude contraindications (pregnancy, lactation, severe coagulopathies, certain neuromuscular diseases, intake of aminoglycoside antibiotics and cumarins)
- obtain informed consent

As shown in Figure 15.3 the sequence of axillary BoNT-A treatment is as follows:

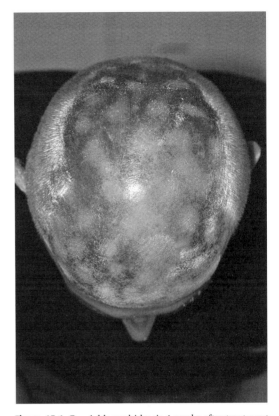

Figure 15.1 Cranial hyperhidrosis 4 weeks after treatment with botulinum toxin type A injections. Areas in which sweating is abolished are visualized by iodine-starch test.

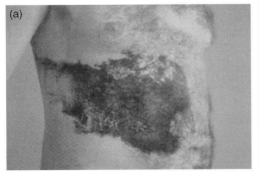
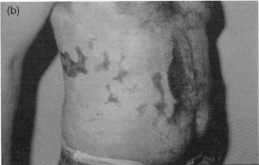

Figure 15.2 Segmental hyperhidrosis in Ross syndrome (a) before and (b) 4 weeks after treatment with botulinum toxin type A injections. Sweating areas are visualized by iodine-starch test.

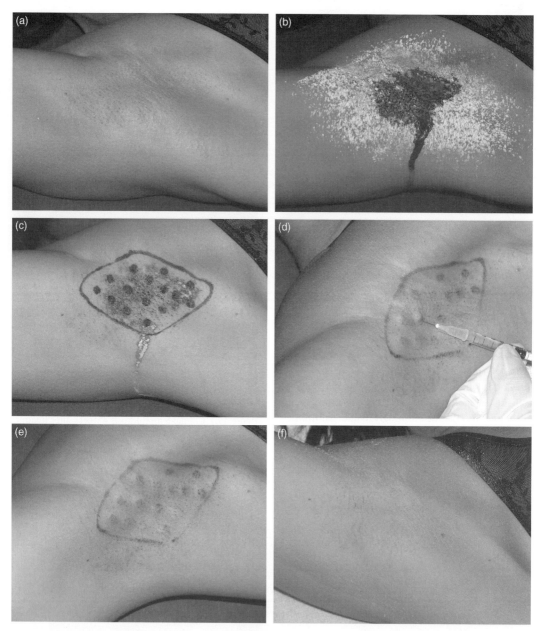

Figure 15.3 Treatment of primary axillary hyperhidrosis with botulinum toxin type A injections. (a) Right axilla and surrounding area covered with 2% iodine solution; (b) blue-black demarcation of sweating area after application of corn starch; (c) marking of sweating area and 15 injection points; (d) intradermal injection of botulinum toxin type A by the use of 1 cc syringe and 30 gauge needle; (e) state immediately after termination of treatment procedure; (f) iodine-starch test 4 weeks after treatment demonstrating abolishment of sweating.

- clean and dry the axilla
- wipe 2% iodine solution (iodine doubly sublimated 5.0, ricinus oil 25.0, pure ethyl alcohol 80% ad 250.0) onto axillary and surrounding skin (Figure 15.3a)
- sprinkle corn starch onto the dry iodine by dint of a caster
- wait for delineation of the sweating area by blue-black discoloration (Figure 15.3b) and outline the sweating area with a pen
- take a picture for documentation
- clean, disinfect, and wipe the axilla dry
- mark 10–15 injection points evenly distributed about 2 cm apart from each other on the outlined area (Figure 15.3c)
- dilute 100 U Botox (alternatively 500 U Dysport) with 4 or 5 cc of sterile normal saline
- use 1 cc syringe with 0.05 division and a 30 gauge needle
- inject 3–4 U Botox intradermally into each injection point totaling 50 U per axilla (alternatively 6–16 U Dysport per injection point totaling 100–200 U per axilla) (Figures 15.3d, 15.3e)
- clean the axilla

Patients should be re-treated when the sweating returns at a level of concern but not within 16 weeks of the last treatment. The time interval between injections can be extended by using aluminum chloride hexahydrate.

Technique of botulinum toxin treatment in primary palmar hyperhidrosis

Before treatment, the following should be considered:
- exclude contraindications (see above)
- obtain informed consent (off-label use!)

Nerve block for anesthesia of the palm is performed as shown in Figures 15.4a and b:
- patient in lying position
- fill up 5 cc syringe with lidocaine or mepivacaine 1% without epinephrine and use a 27 gauge needle
- inject 3 cc of local anesthetic a few centimeters proximal of the wrist radial of the tendon of the palmaris longus muscle in distal direction and 2 cc of local anesthetic ulnar of the ulnar artery in direction to the pisiform bone

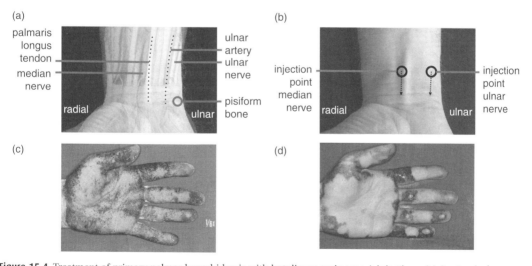

Figure 15.4 Treatment of primary palmar hyperhidrosis with botulinum toxin type A injections. (a) Anatomical structures of orientation for median and ulnar nerve block. (b) Points and direction of injection for median and ulnar nerve block. (c) Iodine-starch test before and (d) 4 weeks after treatment demonstrating virtual abolishment of sweating in treated areas.

- exclude intravasal injection by repeated aspiration
- stop injection if patient feels pain or sensation in distribution of the nerve
- wait 30 minutes after anesthesia before starting treatment

Alternatively, cryoanesthesia with ice cubes, cold packs, or liquid nitrogen spray immediately before injections may be used.

The sequence of the treatment procedure of palmar hyperhidrosis is as follows:

- clean and dry the palm
- iodine-starch test usually not needed as the entire palm and volar aspects of all fingers have to be treated (Figure 15.4c)
- mark about 20–25 injection points evenly distributed about 2 cm apart from each other on the palm including the ulnar side of the hand by use of a grid or stamp
- mark five evenly distributed injection points on each finger including the finger tip
- dilute 100 U Botox with 4 or 5 cc of sterile normal saline
- use 1 cc syringe with 0.05 division and a 30 gauge needle
- inject 2–3 U Botox intradermally into each injection point totaling 100 (–150) U per palm
- use a 30 gauge needle and hold it obliquely to reduce back flow
- clean the palm
- advise the patient not to drive a car or perform dangerous manual work on the day of treatment

Patients should be re-evaluated about 4 weeks after treatment (Figure 15.4d) and re-treated when the sweating returns at a level of concern, but not within 16 weeks of the last treatment. The time interval between injections can be extended by using tap water iontophoresis or aluminum chloride hexahydrate.

ACKNOWLEDGMENTS

We thank Dr. Diana Anders and Dr. Stephanie Moosbauer for photodocumentation of the axillary BoNT-A treatment.

REFERENCES

Baumann, L., Slezinger, A., Halem, M., *et al.* (2005). Double-blind, randomized, placebo-controlled pilot study of the safety and efficacy of Myobloc (botulinum toxin type B) for the treatment of palmar hyperhidrosis. *Dermatol Surg*, **31**, 263–70.

Dressler, D., Adib Saberi, F. & Benecke, R. (2002). Botulinum toxin type B for treatment of axillar hyperhidrosis. *J Neurol*, **249**, 1729–32.

Dumont, P., Denoyer, A. & Robin, P. (2004). Long-term results of thoracoscopic sympathectomy for hyperhidrosis. *Ann Thorac Surg*, **78**, 1801–7.

Glaser, D. A. (2006). The use of botulinum toxins to treat hyperhidrosis and gustatory sweating syndrome. *Neurotox Res*, **9**, 173–7.

Haider, A. & Solish, N. (2005). Focal hyperhidrosis: diagnosis and management. *CMAJ*, **172**, 69–75.

Hamm, H., Naumann, M. K., Kowalski, J. W., *et al.* (2006). Primary focal hyperhidrosis: disease characteristics and functional impairment. *Dermatology*, **212**, 343–53.

Heckmann, M., Ceballos-Baumann, A. O. & Plewig, G. (2001). Botulinum toxin A for axillary hyperhidrosis (excessive sweating). *N Engl J Med*, **344**, 488–93.

Hornberger, J., Grimes, K., Naumann, M., *et al.* (2004). Recognition, diagnosis, and treatment of primary focal hyperhidrosis. *J Am Acad Dermatol*, **51**, 274–86.

Kinkelin, I., Hund, M., Naumann, M. & Hamm, H. (2000). Effective treatment of frontal hyperhidrosis with botulinum toxin A. *Br J Dermatol*, **143**, 824–7.

Lowe, N. J., Yamauchi, P. S., Lask, G. P., Patnaik, R. & Iyer, S. (2002). Efficacy and safety of botulinum toxin type a in the treatment of palmar hyperhidrosis: a double-blind, randomized, placebo-controlled study. *Dermatol Surg*, **28**, 822–7.

Lowe, N. J., Glaser, D. A., Eadie, N., *et al.* (2007). Botulinum toxin type A in the treatment of primary axillary hyperhidrosis: a 52-week multicenter double-blind, randomized, placebo-controlled study of efficacy and safety. *J Am Acad Dermatol*, **56**, 604–11.

Naumann, M. & Hamm, H. (2002). Treatment of axillary hyperhidrosis. *Br J Surg*, **89**, 259–61.

Naumann, M. & Lowe, N. J. (2001). Botulinum toxin type A in treatment of bilateral primary axillary hyperhidrosis: randomised, parallel group, double blind, placebo controlled trial. *BMJ*, **323**, 596–9.

Naumann, M. K., Hamm, H. & Lowe, N. J. (2002). Effect of botulinum toxin type A on quality of life measures in patients with excessive axillary sweating: a randomized controlled trial. *Br J Dermatol*, **147**, 1218–26.

Naumann, M., Lowe, N. J., Kumar, C. R. & Hamm, H. (2003). Botulinum toxin type a is a safe and effective treatment for axillary hyperhidrosis over 16 months: a prospective study. *Arch Dermatol*, **139**, 731–6.

Proebstle, T. M., Schneiders, V. & Knop, J. (2002). Gravimetrically controlled efficacy of subcorial curettage: a prospective study for treatment of axillary hyperhidrosis. *Dermatol Surg*, **28**, 1022–6.

Strutton, D. R., Kowalski, J. W., Glaser, D. A. & Stang, P. E. (2004). US prevalence of hyperhidrosis and impact on individuals with axillary hyperhidrosis: results from a national survey. *J Am Acad Dermatol*, **51**, 241–8.

16

Cosmetic uses of botulinum toxins

Dee Anna Glaser

Clinical aspects and pathophysiology

The twenty-first century has seen an explosion in the numbers of individuals seeking out ways to look younger and more beautiful. As the demand for procedures increases, so does the desire for less invasive therapy with shortened downtimes. Botulinum toxin (BoNT) has become the most common aesthetic procedure performed in the USA with more than three million such procedures performed in 2005 (The American Society for Aesthetic Plastic Surgery, 2007).

For cosmetic uses, the target of BoNT is primarily the muscles of facial expression. These muscles generally have soft tissue attachments and when contracted, move the overlying skin. With age, there is atrophy of the underlying facial support, including the muscles (Spencer, 2006). The skin thins and with repeated muscle contraction there is folding and pleating of the skin, which becomes permanent creases over time. Botulinum toxin will temporarily weaken hyperfunctional muscles, thereby improving or eliminating the overlying skin creases. The position and interplay of opposing muscle actions contribute to the appearance of facial aging, and, again, BoNT can be used to alter such relationships. In fact, patients report a change in appearance within 2 weeks of receiving botulinum toxin type A (BoNT-A) and by 4 weeks after therapy to the upper face, report looking 3 years younger than baseline (Carruthers & Carruthers, 2007).

At the time of this writing, Botox® (Allergan Inc., Irvine, CA) is the only BoNT-A that is available in the USA, and the only BoNT-A with a cosmetic indication (treatment of glabellar lines) and it is Food and Drug Administration (FDA)-approved for the treatment of hyperhidrosis. Dysport®, (Ipsen Ltd., Slough, UK) is registered in over 70 countries and has been studied for both aesthetic and hyperhidrosis indications. There is no agreed upon conversion ratio although 2.5:1 to 5:1 (Dysport units: Botox units) has been suggested (Rzany *et al.*, 2007; Talarico-Filho *et al.*, 2007) Xeomin® (Merz, Frankfurt/M, Germany), also a BoNT-A is available in Europe but not yet in the USA. It is reported to have a conversion ratio of 1:1 with Botox (Jost *et al.*, 2005, 2007). Doses in this chapter are for the Botox brand of BoNT-A unless otherwise specified.

Review of the anatomy

When used for cosmetic purposes, BoNT-A is primarily used to target the muscles of facial expression (Figure 16.1). These are unique in that most have soft tissue attachments and move the skin and related structures to help communicate and express emotional states (on the body, muscles typically have bony attachments via ligaments and result in skeletal body movement). With muscle contracture, the overlying skin can develop creases,

Manual of Botulinum Toxin Therapy, ed. Daniel Truong, Dirk Dressler and Mark Hallett. Published by Cambridge University Press.
© Cambridge University Press 2009.

Figure 16.1 Muscular anatomy of the face.

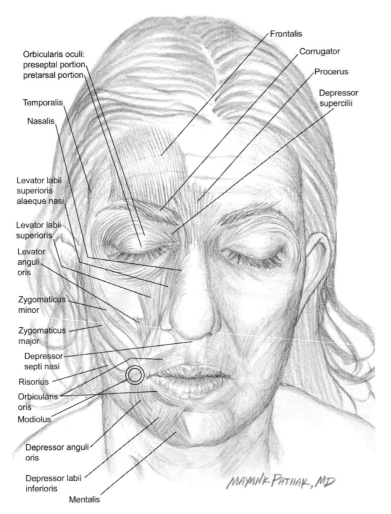

Frontalis

Orbicularis oculi:
preseptal portion
pretarsal portion

Corrugator

Procerus

Depressor
supercilii

Temporalis

Nasalis

Levator labii
superioris
alaeque nasi

Levator labii
superioris

Levator
anguli
oris

Zygomaticus
minor

Zygomaticus
major

Depressor
septi nasi

Risorius

Orbicularis
oris

Modiolus

Depressor anguli
oris

Depressor labii
inferioris

Mentalis

MAYANK PATHAK, MD

wrinkles, or folds that are perpendicular to the axis of the muscle contraction. The seventh cranial nerve, facial nerve, provides motor function of the face. Injection points are determined by the muscles and not the course of the nerve.

Treatment techniques and guidelines

Reconstitution of Botox can be performed using preserved normal saline despite the manufacturer's recommendations of the use of non-preserved saline. The benzyl alcohol preservative in the former decreases patient discomfort without altering efficacy (Alam *et al.*, 2002). The amount of diluent used varies among physicians with typical ranges of 1–5 cc but can be as high as 10 cc per 100 unit vial. Syringe selection also varies with most physicians using insulin syringes or 1 cc tuberculin syringes. The latter will result in wastage of the product in the needle hub and special syringes (Figure 16.2) with a bullet-shaped plunger are

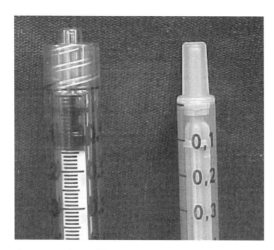

Figure 16.2 One cubic centimeter syringes. A tuberculin syringe on the left vs. the syringe on the right which is designed to reduce wastage due to the shape of the plunger.

available to reduce any wastage. Small gauge needles should be used for facial injections; most commonly 30–32 gauge needles are used.

To reduce the risk of bruising, patients should stop the use of anticoagulants, aspirin, non-steroidal anti-inflammatory agents, and supplements such as vitamin E, gingko, and garlic 7 days prior to their injection appointment. Although ideal, it is not necessary to postpone injection should the patient fail to stop such agents.

Patients should be placed in a comfortable position, ideally with their head supported. An upright or slightly reclined position is ideal for cosmetic injections. Pain is usually minimal but some patients will prefer the use of a topical anesthetic prior to injections. This can be especially valuable around the mouth. The application of ice prior to injections may also help reduce discomfort and may reduce the risk of bruising, especially in high-risk areas such as the lateral orbital rim and lower eyelid.

Although there are no controlled studies to support the need for special postoperative recommendations, many physicians recommend the following:

- Contract the treated muscles immediately after injection, ranging from 10 minutes to several hours
- Do NOT bend over for 2–3 hours, such as to pick up objects from floor, put on shoes
- Do NOT massage the treated areas for 2–4 hours
- Do NOT lay down for 2–4 hours
- Limit heavy physical activity for 2–4 hours

Cosmetic uses of botulinum toxin

Treatment should always begin with an accurate assessment of the patient. In particular, the patient's needs and their desires or goals should be addressed. Adjuvant therapy with fillers, lasers, resurfacing, or surgery may need to be combined with BoNT to achieve maximum improvement.

The following text serves as a guideline for the treatment of the aging face. It is always best to customize therapy based on the individual's needs and desires as discussed with close attention to the anatomy and muscle size and function. Ideally muscles should be visualized and/or palpated prior to injection. The use of the non-dominant thumb and finger can help localize and stabilize the muscle during injection (Figure 16.3).

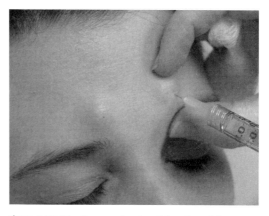

Figure 16.3 Use the non-dominant thumb and finger to stabilize the treated muscle while the dominant hand injects. Note the erythema and the distention of the skin is commonly seen and is transient. Botox was reconstituted with 2.0 cc/100 units and 5 units (0.1 cc) injected into each corragutor muscle.

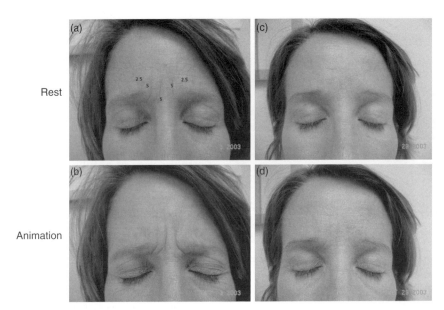

Rest

Animation

Figure 16.4 Treatment of the glabella. The glabellar lines at rest (a) are accentuated with frowning (b). After treatment with 20 units (a) the lines are diminished and the eyebrows are elevated at rest (c) and with frowning (d). The numbers represent the units of Botox used and the approximate location of injection.

Glabella

The glabellar frown lines represent one of the most commonly performed cosmetic units treated. Four muscles pull the brows down and in: corrugator superciliaris, orbicularis oculi, procerus, and depressor supercilii. Most commonly five injection sites are used to treat the glabella, but can range from three to seven sites. Botox doses of 20–30 units are a good starting point but may need to be altered depending on the muscle mass and desires of the patient.

Having the patient frown or animate is the best way to visualize the muscles but landmarks are available to guide the injections (Figure 16.4). The procerus can be injected at the center of an "X" that intersects the medial brows and the contralateral medial canthi if it is not clearly visualized (Figure 16.5). It is important that the brow be used and not the eyebrow since the eyebrows can be reshaped and distorted in terms of their anatomical landmarks. Five to ten units of Botox are injected

into the procerus muscle and can be massaged to help diffusion into the depressor supercilii muscles. Some injectors grab the procerus with the non-dominant thumb and index finger to improve accuracy. The corrugator muscles are identified with animation and can best be visualized superior to the medial canthus. The belly of the muscle is supported up by the non-dominant thumb and ~5 units are injected (Figure 16.3). The tail of the corrugator muscle frequently will need to be treated as well and is usually located ~1 cm above the supraorbital notch near the midpupillary line. A typical dose is 2.5–5 units into each tail of the corrugator.

Forehead

Horizontal forehead lines are easily treated by targeting the frontalis muscle. In many individuals frontalis fibers are not present in the superior midline section of the forehead which is replaced with membranous galea. If this is the case, injection into this area is unnecessary. The frontalis muscle is the

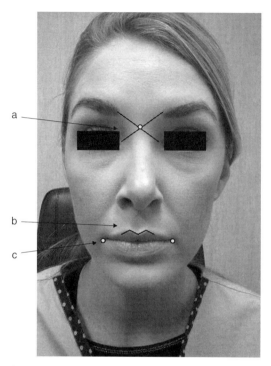

Figure 16.5 Cosmetic landmarks.
a. The procerus muscle can be injected at the cross-point between the medial eyebrow and medial canthus.
b. The cupid's bow of the mouth is usually not injected when treating radial lip lines.
c. The oral commisure can be used as a landmark when injecting the depressor anguli oris muscle in the lower face.

only levator muscle of the upper face, which elevates the brow, eyebrows, and the skin of the forehead. High doses or incorrect placement of BoNT-A can result in a real or perceived brow or eyebrow ptosis.

To avoid a lowering of the eyebrows or brow, injections should start 2–3 cm superior to the orbital rim and doses should be low. Doses of 10–20 units for women or 15–30 units for men should be considered (Figure 16.6). The pattern of injection and doses needed will vary depending on the height of the forehead, the volume of muscle, and the placement of the eyebrows at rest.

Frontalis muscle fibers can extend laterally and if not treated adequately, a "Mr. Spock" appearance

can develop unilaterally or bilaterally. An additional 2–4 units should be used to bring the peaked brow down (Figure 16.7).

Eyes

The "crow's feet" or wrinkles at the lateral canthus are caused by contraction of the lateral portion of the orbicularis oculi muscle and, to a lesser degree, the zygomaticus and risorius muscles of the mouth. At the lateral canthus, the vertically oriented fibers of the orbicularis oculi muscle can easily be treated but injections should stay above the zygomatic notch to avoid lip ptosis. The subcutaneous fat can be injected through the thin skin with good diffusion of Botox into the muscle. Typically two to four injection points are required with a starting dose of 10–15 units per canthus (Figure 16.8).

A prominent bulge of the lower eyelid with smiling or animation is caused by the pretarsal portion of the orbicularis oculi muscle. One injection at the midpupillary line approximately 2 mm inferior to the lid margin with 1–2 units is usually sufficient to reduce this bulge (Figures 16.9 and 16.10). In addition a more open and almond-shape of the eye can be produced. Bruising is common in this area (Figure 16.11) and lid ectropion can occur. Injections medial to the midpupillary line can weaken the blink reflex and result in dry eyes. Injections lateral to the midpupillary line increases the risk for lower lid ectropion.

Brow lift

Brow ptosis is common and, like the frown, has a negative connotation, giving the individual a tired, run-down appearance. When treating eyebrow ptosis, it is important to assess for asymmetry of the eyebrow, a very common finding in middle-aged women (Carruthers & Carruthers, 2003). It is important to review the defect with the patient prior to injection and to adjust the dosing appropriately if better symmetry is required (Figures 16.9 and 16.10). The depressor muscles should be treated while maintaining elevator muscle (frontalis)

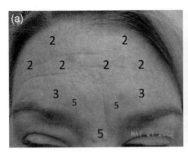
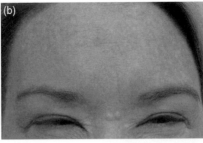

Figure 16.6 Glabella and forehead injections before (a) and after (b) injection of 21 units into the glabella and 12 units into the frontalis muscle. The numbers represent the units of Botox used and the approximate location of injection.

function. Treatment of the glabellar complex as described can be combined with treatment of the superolateral portions of the orbicularis oculi (usually at the lateral brow at its junction with the temporal fusion line) using 2–6 units. Injections of the lateral canthus (crow's feet) can also be helpful.

Nose

Nasal scrunch or "bunny lines" are produced by the transverse nasalis muscle and are accentuated with speech, smiling, and frowning. These vertical lines may develop in some patients after treatment with BoNT in the glabella or may naturally occur. Very small doses of Botox are needed, typically 1–3 units per side, which can be injected subcutaneously due

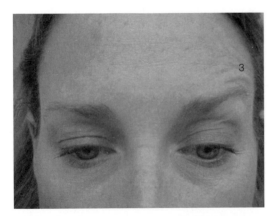

Figure 16.7 Asymmetric raised lateral eyebrow following forehead injections. An additional 3 units of Botox in the lateral frontalis will effectively return the brow to the desired position.

to the thin skin at the lateral wall of the nasal bridge (Figure 16.12). Placement is particularly important on the nose as the levator labii superioris alaeque nasi and the levator labii superioris both originate along the medial aspect of the malar prominence.

Mouth

Rejuvenation of the mouth can be achieved using small doses of BoNT-A. Outcomes are usually maximized when combined with other techniques such as fillers or resurfacing.

"Smoker's" lines or vertical lip lines are common, especially in women. Repetitive pursing or movement of the orbicularis oris muscle contribute to the development of these lines which interfere with lipstick use as it may run into the wrinkles (Figure 16.13). Four to ten units can be used for the upper lip while 3–8 units are needed for the lower lip. Injections do not need to be placed into the lines and should be placed 1–2 mm away from the pink border of the lip to decrease discomfort. I avoid the lateral quarter of each lip and usually do not inject the cupid's bow (Figures 16.14, 16.15, and 16.5). Prepare patients for a possible (sometimes not perceived by others) change in speech and word pronunciation which typically resolves in ~ 2 weeks if it occurs at all.

The corners of the mouth represent another very important point of cosmetic enhancement. As the corners of the mouth turn downwards with age, it portrays sadness or anger. The depressor anguli oris (DAO) muscle can be injected with 3–5 units as a starting dose and increased as needed to achieve a

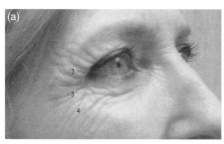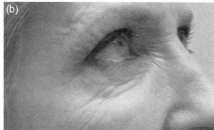

Figure 16.8 Treatment of the crow's feet with 10 units of Botox before (a) and (b) after. The numbers represent the units of Botox used.

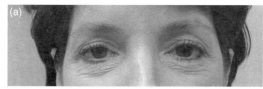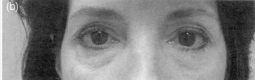

Figure 16.9 Eyebrow asymmetry before Botox (a) and after injection to lift the brows (b).

reduction in the marionette lines and a more neutral or upturned corner of the mouth (Figure 16.16).

The depressor labii inferioris (DLI) muscle which lies beneath and slightly medial to the DAO must be avoided. An inferior and lateral approach to the DAO is best. Have the patient make a "sad or disappointed" face or make an exaggerated pronunciation of the letter "e" to palpate or visualize the DAO. If not easily identified, injections should be made ~ 8–10 mm lateral to the oral commissure and 10–15 mm inferior to this point (Figure 16.5).

Chin

A deep mental crease, chin puckering or a prominent chin can be improved with BoNT-A. A total of 4–8 units can be injected into the mentalis muscle, ideally at the inferior and near midline to avoid the DLI muscle (Figure 16.17).

Neck

Vertical neck bands and cords may be prominent in some individuals at rest and with animation (Figure 16.18). The superficial platysma muscle is

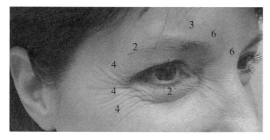

Figure 16.10 Injection pattern for the brow lift and reduction of a lower lid bulge. The left side was treated as well. The numbers represent the units of Botox used.

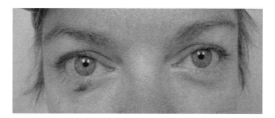

Figure 16.11 Lower lid ecchymosis 14 days after injection of 1 unit Botox in the pretarsal orbicularis oculi.

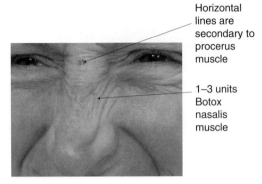

Horizontal lines are secondary to procerus muscle

1–3 units Botox nasalis muscle

Figure 16.12 Nasal scrunch or "bunny lines" are produced by the nasalis muscle whereas the horizontal lines at the root of the nose are secondary to the procerus muscle.

injected into the bands using 2–4 units every 1–2 cm. It may be helpful to have the patient exaggerate the bands for the physician to grab and then have the patient relax the muscle contraction for the actual injection, which is very superficial. A bleb should be seen with each injection (Figure 16.19). Doses of 50 units or more may be required to treat an entire neck, but high doses can be associated with neck weakness and even trouble swallowing.

Horizontal neck lines can be treated but are much less responsive than the vertical neck bands and patients need to be adequately counseled on expected outcomes.

Mandibular contouring

A square-appearing jawline can widen the lower face and for women, give a more masculine appearance. In some patients, this is secondary to masseter muscle hypertrophy, which with treatment can return the face to a more oval shape. Reductions of up to 30% in masseter muscle volume or a mean decrease in thickness of 2.9 mm have been reported (Ahuja *et al.*, 2001; Park *et al.*, 2003). To accentuate the contours of the masseter at the angle of the jaw, ask the patient to strongly clench the teeth. Approximately six to eight injections will be required with doses in the 25–30 units per side. A one-inch needle is used and the deeper portions of the muscle should be injected. Localized aching and swelling can develop and post-injection ice for 24–48 hours can be helpful.

Side effects

Adverse events are relatively uncommon when BoNT is injected by an experienced physician. Side effects will vary depending on the part of the face that is being treated. Some patients may not achieve the desired cosmetic effect and should be counseled preoperatively.

Adverse events of short duration
- Mild stinging or discomfort with injection
- Erythema and edema at injection site
- Headache, transient, usually lasting 4–8 hours
- Bruising
- Asymmetry
- Localized numbness or paresthesias at the injection site, transient

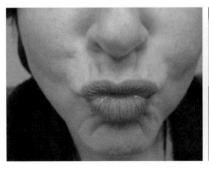

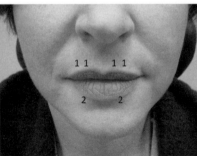

Figure 16.13 Small doses of Botox to treat perioral lines which can be accentuated with puckering. Initially start with low doses, avoiding the lateral portions.

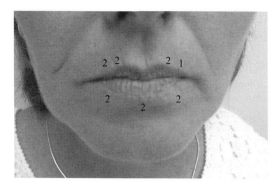

Figure 16.14 Woman with vertical lip lines treated with a total of 13 units Botox.

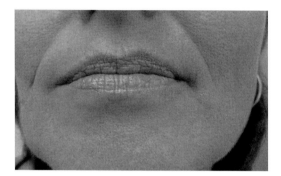

Figure 16.15 Excellent reduction in vertical lines in the same patient shown in Figure 16.14 without the use of fillers.

- Focal twitching
- Mild nausea
- Malaise and myalgias

Adverse events of longer duration, often technique dependent
- Blepharoptosis

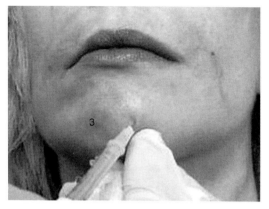

Figure 16.17 Injection of a total of 6 units Botox into the mentalis muscle to reduce chin puckering. Injections should be inferior and medial to avoid the depressor labii inferioris muscle.

- Brow ptosis
- Diplopia
- Decreased tearing and xerophthalmia
- Ectropion
- Lagophthalmus
- Oral incompetence
- Decreased neck strength
- Dysphagia
- Dysarthria

Adverse events, of immediate hypersensitivity type reactions
- Urticaria
- Dyspnea
- Angioedema
- Anaphylaxis

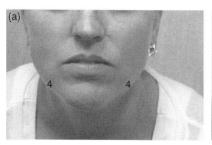

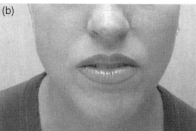

Figure 16.16 Injection of 4 units Botox into depressor anguli oris (a) results in elevation of the corners of mouth (b).

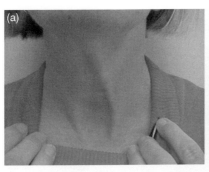
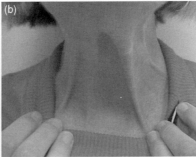

Figure 16.18 Vertical neck bands at rest (a) and with animation (b).

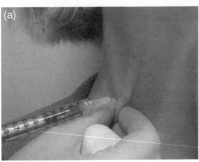
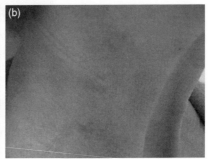

Figure 16.19 Grab the superficial platysma muscle band with the non-dominant hand (a) and inject 2–4 units of Botox every 1–2 cm (b).

REFERENCES

Alam, M., Dover, J. & Arndt, K. (2002). Pain associate with injection of botulinum A exotoxin reconstituted using isotonic sodium chloride with and without preservative. *Arch Dermatol*, **138**, 510–14.

Carruthers, J. & Carruthers, A. (2003). *Using Botulinum Toxins Cosmetically*. London: Martin Dunitz, pp. 17–32.

Carruthers, J. & Carruthers, A. (2007). Botulinum toxin type A treatment of multiple upper facial sites: patient-reported outcomes. *Dermatol Surg*, **33**(S1), S10–17.

Jost, W., Brinkmann, S. & Comes, G. (2005). Efficacy and tolerability of a botulinum toxin type A free of complexing proteins (NT 201) compared with commercially available botulinum toxin type A (BOTOX) in healthy volunteers. *J Neural Transm*, **112**(7), 905–13.

Jost, W., Blumel, J. & Grafe, S. (2007). Botulinum neurotoxin type A free of complexing proteins (XEOMIN) in focal dystonia. *Drugs*, **67**(5), 669–83.

Park, M. Y., Ahn, K. Y. & Jung, D. S. (2003). Botulinum toxin type A treatment for contouring the lower face. *Dermatol Surg*, **29**, 477–83.

Rzany, B. D., Dill-Muller, D., Grablowitz, D., Heckmann, M. & Daird, D. (2007). Repeated botulinum toxin A injections for the treatment of lines in the upper face: a retrospective study of 4,103 treatments in 945 patients. *Dermatol Surg*, **33**(S1), S18–25.

Spencer, J. M. (2006). Facial anatomy and use of botulinum toxin. In A. Benedetto, ed., *Botulinum Toxin in Clinical Dermatology*. Abingdon, Oxfordshire: Taylor & Francis, pp. 33–44.

Talarico-Filho, S., Nascimento, M. M., De Macedo, F. S. & De Sanctis Pecora, C. (2007). A double-blind, randomized, comparative study of two type A botulinum toxins in the treatment of primary axillary hyperhidrosis. *Dermatol Surg*, **33**(S1), S44–50.

The American Society for Aesthetic Plastic Surgery. (2007) Cosmetic Surgery National Data Bank. 2005 Statistics, multi specialty expanded data for 2005. www.surgery.org.

To, E. W., Ahuja, A. T., Ho, W. S., *et al.* (2001). A prospective study of the effect of botulinum toxin A on masseteric muscle hypertrophy with ultrasonographic and electromyographic measurement. *Br J Plast Surg*, **54**, 197–200.

17

Botulinum toxin in the gastrointestinal tract

Vito Annese and Daniele Gui

Cricopharyngeal dysphagia

The cricopharyngeal muscle, or upper esophageal sphincter (UES), corresponds to the most inferior portion of the inferior constrictor muscle. It constitutes a sphincter separating the hypopharynx from the esophagus, preventing the inlet of air into the esophagus during inspiration and the esophageal reflux into the pharynx. It is myoelectrically silent at rest and active during swallowing.

Cricopharyngeal dysphagia arises from its dysfunction which can be primary or secondary to a number of pathological conditions including cerebrovascular accidents, amyotrophic lateral sclerosis, oculopharyngeal muscular dystrophy, skull basal lesion, etc. Oropharyngeal dysphagia is the clinical presentation, and possibly correlates with aspiration or penetration of liquid or food in the upper airways. During manometry an incomplete relaxation of the UES or an increased intrabolus pressure may be demonstrated (Figure 17.1a).

Cricopharyngeal muscle dysfunction has been traditionally treated with surgical myotomy, mechanical dilation, or plexus neurectomy. Localized injections of botulinum toxin (BoNT) into the dorsomedial or ventrolateral parts of the muscle have also been successfully performed endoscopically by means of electromyographic (EMG) guidance, or percutaneously with EMG guidance (Figure 17.1b) and eventual computerized tomography or fluoroscopic

control (Moerman, 2006). Unfortunately, there are no standards or guidelines and the administered dose ranges widely between 10 and 120 (mouse) units of Botox® per patient, usually selected on the basis of symptom severity. Local injections are relatively simple, safe (complication rate about 7%) and effective, although the effect wanes after 4–6 months (Moerman, 2006). Injection in the horizontal part of the muscle and an adequate (i.e., high enough) starting dose are predictors of greater efficacy. The toxin can be used as part of the diagnostic evaluation to ascertain the role of cricopharyngeal spasm in the explanation of patient's symptoms; moreover, it may help to identify those patients who are more likely to benefit from surgical myotomy.

Paradoxically, BoNT can cause transient oropharyngeal dysphagia as a complication of local injections for cervical and oromandibular dystonia.

Achalasia

Achalasia is a rare neuromuscular disorder of the esophagus characterized by loss of peristalsis and failure of the lower esophageal sphincter (LES) to relax normally. This results in functional obstruction with retention of food and saliva in the lumen, and subsequent risk of aspiration, malnutrition, and weight loss. The etiology is unknown but the early pathological changes consist of a myenteric

Manual of Botulinum Toxin Therapy, ed. Daniel Truong, Dirk Dressler and Mark Hallett. Published by Cambridge University Press.
© Cambridge University Press 2009.

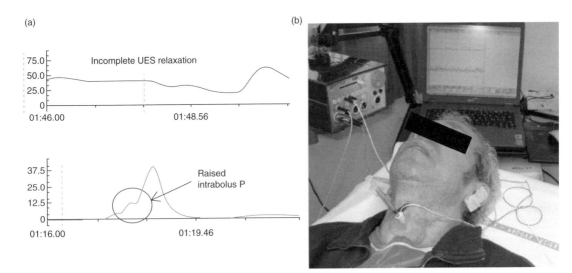

Figure 17.1 (a) Example of manometry of the upper esophageal sphincter (UES) demonstrating incomplete relaxation and raised intrabolus pressure (P) at the pharyngeal level. Manometry should be combined to videofluoroscopy in the careful evaluation of UES dysfunction (*courtesy of Professor A. Zaninotto, J Gastr Surg*). (b) Electromyography of the UES could be recorded by means of a portable computer-assisted equipment. A 50 mm long (26 gauge) concentric needle electrode is inserted at the infero-lateral aspect of the cricoid cartilage and rotated medially after insertion to record the cricopharyngeal muscle electrical activity. Subsequently, the electrode is connected to a insulin syringe and 4–10 units of Botox (Allergan Inc., Irvine, CA, USA) are injected (*courtesy of Professor G. Zaninotto, J Gastr Surg*). © 2004, The Society for Surgery of the Alimentary Tract.

plexus inflammation with subsequent loss of ganglion cells and fibrosis. Degenerative (retrograde?) changes of the vagal nerves and dorsal vagal nuclei have also been described. The impairment of LES relaxation and peristaltic propagation of contractions is due to selective loss of inhibitory nerve endings whose neurotransmitters are nitric oxide and vasoactive intestinal polypeptide. Conversely, the excitatory cholinergic pathway is preserved and may lead to increased resting LES pressure.

Current therapies are aimed to mechanically reduce the LES tone through pneumatic dilation or surgical myotomy. Both procedures, although effective in the large majority of patients (65–90%), carry a significant risk of complications; a 2% rate of perforation and reduced efficacy over time (about 50%) for dilation, and a 10–30% risk of gastroesophageal reflux after myotomy (Pehlivanov & Pasricha, 2006). Moreover, especially for myotomy, functional results are largely influenced by the surgeon's experience.

These limitations prompted PJ Pasricha in 1994 to assess, for the first time, the usefulness of intrasphincteric injection of BoNT (Pehlivanov & Pasricha, 2006). The rationale behind this was that the selective loss of the inhibitory nerves in achalasia upset the excitatory (cholinergic) influences on the LES. By blocking the acetylcholine release, locally injected toxin might reduce the LES pressure and improve the esophageal emptying. The efficacy of this treatment modality has been evaluated in a number of uncontrolled and controlled trials, also comparing its cost/effectiveness with dilation and surgical myotomy (Annese & Bassotti, 2006; Leyden *et al.*, 2006). The toxin is injected through a standard sclerotherapy needle during an upper gastrointestinal endoscopy under conscious sedation. Eighty to 100 units of toxin (Botox or the equivalent dose of Dysport®) are injected in each quadrant of the LES at four or eight sites (preferred) in 1 or 0.5 cc aliquots (Figure 17.2a and b). Injections of toxin

(a)   (b)

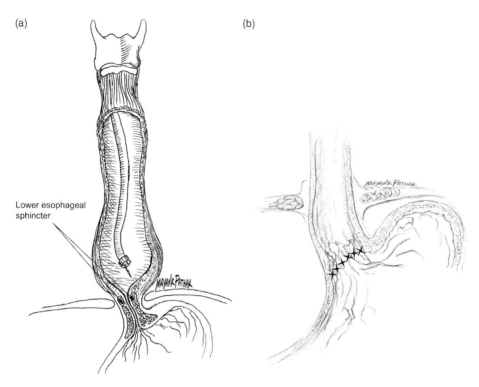

Lower esophageal
sphincter

Figure 17.2 (a) Botulinum toxin is injected into the lower esophageal sphincter (LES) in patients with esophageal achalasia during a standard endoscopy with conscious sedation, through a sclerotherapy needle (23 gauge) is used. 100 units of Botox or 250 units of Dysport (Ipsen) diluted in 4 cc, are delivered in four or (preferably) eight radial sites starting at the Z-line and 1 cm above. (b) Following the botulinum toxin injection the pressure of LES is reduced and the esophagus empties by gravity. This allows in the early stage of disease also the reduction of esophageal diameter.

by means of endoscopic fundic retroversion or endoscopic ultrasonography do not enhance the efficacy. Although BoNT injection is remarkably safe (about 10% of patients report a mild chest pain) and effective in the short term (70–90%) (Annese & Bassotti, 2006; Leyden *et al.*, 2006), there are a number of limitations: (1) the mean duration of efficacy is one year or less, although single cases with prolonged (3–4 years) benefit have been reported; (2) after repeated injections a decline of efficacy (antibodies?) has been reported; and (3) repeated toxin injections may increase the difficulty of a subsequent surgical myotomy, although functional results seem similar (Annese & Bassotti, 2006). The use of BoNT is currently recommended

in poor candidates for surgery, old and very old patients, or as a temporizing measure (Pehlivanov & Pasricha, 2006). A potential benefit of BoNT prior to pneumatic dilation has been suggested but not adequately proven.

Spastic esophageal disorders

Diffuse esophageal spasm (DES) is a rare esophageal motility disorder characterized by a severe reduction of esophageal peristalsis, often accompanied by prolonged and high-amplitude esophageal contractions and impaired LES relaxation. Isolated LES hypertension is another infrequent motility disorder, usually characterized by a normal esophageal peristalsis and LES relaxation. The etiology for both disorders is unknown but a deranged function of the myenteric plexus is suspected. The major symptom for both disorders is chest pain, with or without concurrent dysphagia. No satisfactory pharmacological therapy is available, and rarely a surgical myotomy is required. Moreover, pneumatic dilation is usually poorly effective on chest pain. A therapeutic role of BoNT has been reported in the literature, although in limited case series and uncontrolled observations (Storr *et al.*, 2001). For LES hypertension the same treatment technique used for achalasia has been employed, while in patients with DES, multiple injections along the esophageal wall are suggested, beginning at the LES region and moving proximally at 1–2 cm intervals, into endoscopically visible contraction rings (Figure 17.3) (Storr *et al.*, 2001).

Sphincter of Oddi dysfunction

Recurrent upper abdominal pain is a common clinical problem affecting 10% or more patients undergoing cholecystectomy. Sphincter of Oddi dysfunction (SOD) has been implicated in the etiology of 10–20% of these cases. Although rare, SOD can cause recurrent pancreatitis. Unfortunately, this disorder is difficult to diagnose with non-invasive techniques; sphincter of Oddi (SO) manometry is useful in diagnosis, but carries a potential risk of pancreatitis and cholangitis. Moreover, it shows a great technical complexity with a considerable rate of false-positives and -negatives. High pressure of the sphincter is relieved by endoscopic sphincterotomy, which is considered as the treatment of choice for SOD; however, in many patients this procedure does not relieve symptoms and might determine risk of pancreatitis, bleeding, and perforation.

Preliminary studies on animals demonstrated that locally injected BoNT significantly reduces the sphincter wave amplitudes and phasic contractile activity, probably through a selective inhibition of cholinergic influences. In this setting, two potential

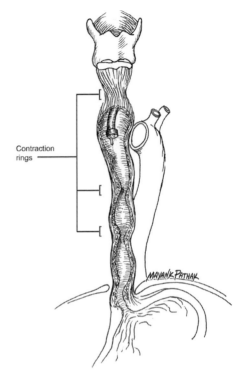

Contraction rings

Figure 17.3 In patients with diffuse esophageal spasm multiple injections of toxin are given, beginning at the LES region and moving proximally at 1–2 cm intervals to reduce the strength of esophageal contractions.

uses of toxin could be hypothesized: firstly, intrasphincteric injection may serve as a simple test to identify patients whose pain is really caused by SOD. Secondly, once efficacy is established, BoNT may prove to be an effective and safer therapeutic modality than sphincterotomy (Whermann *et al.*, 2000). The technique is rather simple, consisting of a single injection into the major papilla of 100 units of Botox with a sclerotherapy needle (Figure 17.4a and b). However, controlled and prospective studies are lacking.

Obesity

Genetic, social, psychological, and behavioral factors make it difficult both to prevent and to treat

(a)   (b)

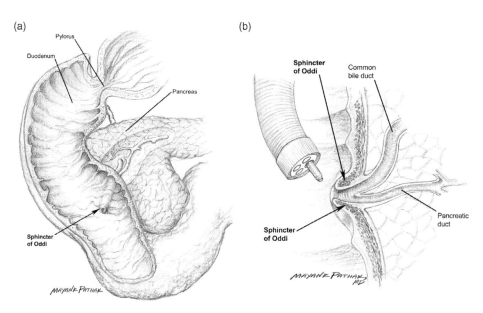

Figure 17.4 (a and b) In patients with sphincter of Oddi dysfunction (demonstrated by biliary manometry and/or colangio-magnetic nuclear resonance plus secretin stimulation), the toxin is delivered with a side-view endoscope through a sclerotherapy needle at the papilla. The arrows indicate sphincter of Oddi sites.

obesity. High caloric intake in obese patients is difficult to control and the achievement of early satiety is an important goal. In the stomach, rings of contraction originate in the antrum and sweep distally; the strongest ones occlude the gastric lumen entirely, propelling chyme through the pylorus, into the duodenum (Figures 17.5a–d). Even though several neuromediators are present in the gastrointestinal tract and the complex gastric activity is influenced by endocrine and paracrine mediators, motility is mostly dependent on acetylcholine. This suggests a possible effect of BoNT injections into the antral muscles, weakening the propulsive contractions and interfering with gastric emptying.

We treated rats with BoNT gastric injections, reporting a parallel reduction of body weight and food intake (Gui *et al.*, 2000). Another study showed that this effect was related to a significant reduction of gastric emptying (Coskun *et al.*, 2005).

Currently, BoNT intraparietogastric injections in obese patients are still experimental. In the six studies reported in the literature, a total of 55 patients were treated (Rollnik *et al.*, 2003; Albani *et al.*, 2005; Garcia-Compean *et al.*, 2005; Gui *et al.*, 2006; Junior *et al.*, 2006; Foschi *et al.*, 2007). Botox (100–500 units) was injected under endoscopic control, using a sclerotherapy injector needle, in 8, 16, 20 or 24 sites around the gastric antral circumferences, starting at a distance of 3 cm from the pyloric ring. In one study the fundus was also injected; in our hands, the toxin was injected at the angular level (Figure 17.6) (Gui *et al.*, 2006). The procedure was safe and no side effects of the treatment were observed; however, results are still uncertain. Studies were not conducted consistently, so, given the small size of the series, it is difficult to draw conclusions about gastric emptying times, alimentary diary, and caloric intake after BoNT treatment. Early satiety sensation was consistently reported as the most frequent subjective effect of the treatment. Body weight variations differed greatly and in only one of the studies did the difference between treated and control patients reach

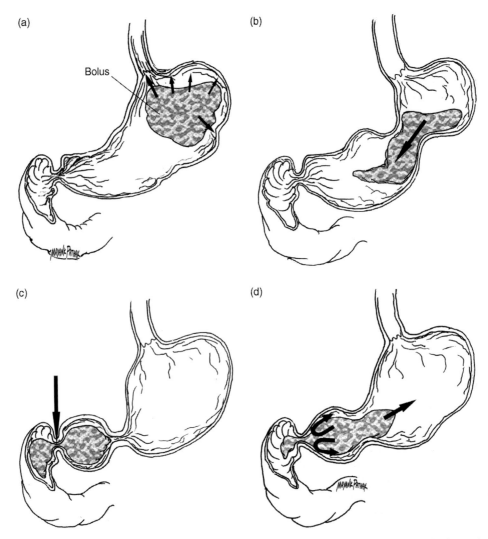

(a)

Bolus

(b)

(c)

(d)

Figure 17.5 Phases of the peristaltic activity in the stomach. Receptive relaxation of the fundus upon food ingestion (a), followed by the peristaltic movements, causing the food to advance towards the antrum and pylorus (b and c). On the basis of the antral pump strength and of the pylorus contraction, the food may partly go through the duodenum or be totally repelled towards the gastric body and remixed (d).

statistical significance $(11 \pm 1.09$ vs. $5.7 \pm 1.1\,$kg, $P < 0.001)$ (Foschi *et al.*, 2006).

In conclusion, BoNT intraparietogastric injections seem to play a role in the manipulation of appetite, but further studies are required to explore optimal modalities and possibilities of this new application.

Gastroparesis

Gastroparesis is an uncommon gastric motility disorder, mostly idiopathic or related to diabetes, which results in delayed gastric emptying, early satiety, postprandial fullness, bloating, epigastric pain, nausea, vomiting, and weight loss. Pro-motility

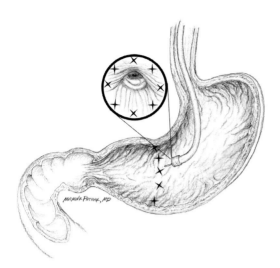

Figure 17.6 Endoscopic injection of the stomach. A gastroscope is inserted into the stomach. A sclerotherapy needle advances inside the endoscope and is inserted in the gastric wall to inject the toxin (not shown in the picture). The signs (X) indicate, both frontally and laterally, the eight sites where the toxin was injected during the study conducted by the authors on obese patients in order to relent the antral propulsive peristalsis.

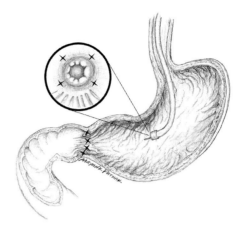

Figure 17.7 Endoscopic injection of the stomach. The signs (X) indicate, both frontally and laterally, the sites on the pylorus quadrants where the toxin is injected in gastroparetic affections.

drugs such as metoclopramide, erythromycin, domperidone (and the recently introduced tegaserod), have been extensively used, unfortunately, with poor results and prominent side effects.

Botulinum toxin injection into the pyloric ring, aimed at relaxing the sphincter, can reduce pyloric resistance and accelerate gastric emptying as shown in several small series, where 80–200 units of Botox were administered in four to five sites circumferentially, using an endoscope (Figure 17.7). The reported reduction in symptoms lasted for 1–3 months in the majority of cases (Bromer *et al.*, 2005). In a recent large study involving 63 patients, mostly with idiopathic gastroparesis, a more limited response rate (43%) to Botox treatment was reported. Male gender was associated with a greater probability of success. As a major pre-existing symptom, vomiting was an indicator of poor response. Moreover, Botox was administered to resolve the pyloric spasm after the Whipple

procedure (duodeno-cephalo-pancreatectomy) with pylorus preservation, although results were inconsistent (Gui *et al.*, 2003). The toxin has been occasionally used in cases of pyloric obstruction syndrome (after pyloroplasty for ulcer, pancreas transplantation, total esophagectomy) and in infants with hypertrophic pyloric stenosis, but results were unsatisfactory (Gui *et al.*, 2003).

Chronic anal fissure

Anal fissure is a frequent, highly painful condition, affecting both genders in the young, otherwise healthy, population. The principal symptom is intense, long-lasting, post-defecatory pain. The first lesion is a mucosal tear, usually in the posterior anal commissure (Figure 17.8a). Even though constipation is frequently associated, the pathogenesis has not been completely elucidated and the internal anal sphincter (IAS) hypertonus is deemed to play a critical role. The mucosal lesion causes intense pain and the reflex action of pain seems to cause spastic contraction of the IAS, leading to compression of the small arterial vessels running

(a)   (b)

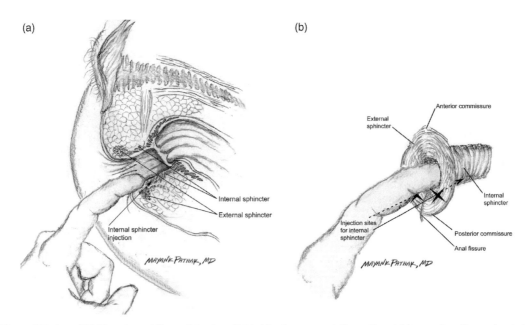

Figure 17.8 (a and b) Chronic anal fissure injection. Guided by the surgeon's finger tip, which perceives the contracted internal anal sphincter, the needle is inserted into the sphincter and the toxin is injected. The arrows indicate the injection sites.

through the muscular fibers of the sphincter. The blood shortage of the mucosa impairs the healing of the lesion, resulting in a vicious circle. The lesion lasting over 3 months is considered "chronic" (CAF) as it doesn't tend to spontaneously heal.

Current therapies of CAF aim to reduce the IAS tone, interrupting the sequence of pain and spasm. Surgical treatment (lateral internal sphincterotomy, anal dilation) achieves this scope mechanically, reducing the strength of the muscle. Anal dilation techniques have been progressively abandoned because of poor results and frequent side effects; lateral sphincterotomy is the most frequent surgical technique applied today, with a high success rate (97%), although incontinence of flatus or feces, up to 35% and 5.3% respectively, has been reported (Khubchandani & Reed, 1989).

Medical spasmolitic therapies (i.e. topically applied nitroglycerin, isosorbide dinitrate or nifedipine) are effective to a limited extent, but are often unpractical and may be associated with tedious general side effects such as headache.

"Chemical sphincterotomy" with a single Botox injection into the IAS was introduced in 1994 (Gui *et al.*, 1994). It has the advantage of a long-term effect (up to 4 months), reversibility of action, minimal invasiveness, and a healing rate slightly short of results offered by surgery. The very rare side effects include short-term incontinence of flatus or feces, anal hematomas, acute inflammation of hemorrhoids, and hemorrhoidal prolapse. Botulinum toxin treatment is performed in the outpatient setting. No sedation or local analgesia are required.

In most cases, the IAS is easily identified by the surgeon's finger and the toxin is injected in the muscle using a syringe with a 27 gauge needle (Figure 17.8b). Although the optimal dose of Botox has not yet been established, usually a total of 10–50 units is administered, preferentially in both sides of the anterior commissure (Gui *et al.*, 2003).

Within this range, greater doses are said to give higher success rates, with a minimal increase in side effects. Many authors consider BoNT the front-line therapy of CAF, but often it is regarded as an expensive alternative.

Puborectalis syndrome

Outlet obstruction related to pelvic floor dyssynergia is not an infrequent cause of constipation in the elderly and middle-aged woman. It is characterized by a failure of the puborectalis muscle to relax during evacuation efforts or by its paradoxical contraction with reduction of the ano-rectal angle, thus impeding the expulsion of feces from the rectum. Biofeedback training and relaxation exercises are beneficial in many patients, however, they are time consuming and lose effectiveness over time. Surgical division of the puborectalis muscle has been proposed, but it is associated with a high rate of incontinence.

Botulinum toxin injected into the muscle is a reversible and less invasive approach that can relax the spasm and increase the ano-rectal angle during straining, thus allowing for evacuation. A few studies have been reported in the literature (Gui *et al.*, 2003). Injections are administered without sedation, in the outpatient setting, under ultrasonographic or EMG control or otherwise guided by the surgeon's finger. With the patient in the litotomy position, the needle is inserted into the perianal skin, 2–2.5 cm laterally of the anal orifice (Figure 17.9) (Maria *et al.*, 2006).

Although the treatment remains an experimental procedure and optimal dose or standard technique have yet to be determined, BoNT injections seem to be an effective approach in the outlet obstruction syndrome related to pelvic floor dyssynergia, particularly in parkinsonian patients (Cadeddu *et al.*, 2005).

Proctalgia fugax

This rare affliction is defined as a sudden and severe pain in the anal region, mostly occurring at

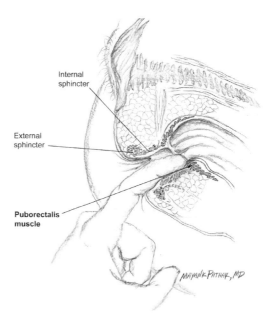

Figure 17.9 Puborectal muscle injection. To infiltrate the puborectal muscle, the procedure is substantially the one described for the internal anal sphincter. The surgeon inserts his finger more deeply into the anal canal in order to perceive the bulging muscle which encompasses the rectum in a semicircular way. This procedure may also be performed under transanal ultrasonographic guidance. The arrows indicate the injection sites.

night and lasting for several seconds or minutes, then completely disappearing. The pathophysiology remains unclear, but it has been suggested that IAS spasm might be the cause. Data concerning the treatment of this disorder is very scarce. Diltiazem, clonidine, salbutamol, and nitroglycerin ointments have been applied with some beneficial results (Bharucha *et al.*, 2006).

A few cases of BoNT IAS injections have been reported in literature. The injection technique is quite similar to the one used in anal fissure (Figure 17.8), but in proctalgia the four quadrants of the sphincter (IAS) are injected. Results are described as promising and further studies are needed to establish indications, doses, and effectiveness of this therapy (Katsinelos *et al.*, 2001).

REFERENCES

Albani, G., Petroni, M. L., Mauro, A., *et al.* (2005). Safety and efficacy of therapy with botulinum toxin in obesity: a pilot study. *J Gastroenterol*, **40**, 833–5.

Annese, V. & Bassotti, G. (2006). Non-surgical treatment of esophageal achalasia. *World J Gastroenterol*, **12**, 5763–6.

Bharucha, A. E., Wald, A., Enck, P. & Rao, S. (2006). Functional anorectal disorders. *Gastroenterology*, **130**, 1510–18.

Bromer, M. Q., Friedenberg, F., Miller, L. S., *et al.* (2005). Endoscopic pyloric injection of botulinum toxin A for the treatment of refractory gastroparesis. *Gastrointest Endosc*, **61**, 833–9.

Cadeddu, F., Bentivoglio, A. R., Brandara, F., *et al.* (2005). Outlet type constipation in Parkinson's disease: results of botulinum toxin treatment. *Aliment Pharmacol Ther*, **22**, 997–1003.

Coskun, H., Duran, Y., Dilege, E., *et al.* (2005). Effect on gastric emptying and weight reduction of botulinum toxin-A injection into the gastric antral layer: an experimental study in the obese rat model. *Obes Surg*, **15**, 1137–43.

Foschi, D., Corsi, F., Lazzaroni, M., *et al.* (2007). Treatment of morbid obesity by intraparietogastric administration of botulinum toxin: a randomized, double-blind, controlled study. *Int J Obes (Lond)*, **31**, 707–12. [Epub 2006 Sep 26]

Garcia-Compean, D., Mendoza-Fuerte, E., Martinez, J. A., Villarreal, I. & Maldonado, H. (2005). Endoscopic injection of botulinum toxin in the gastric antrum for the treatment of obesity. Results of a pilot study. *Gastroenterol Clin Biol*, **29**, 789–91.

Gui, D., Cassetta, E., Anastasio, G., *et al.* (1994). Botulinum toxin for chronic anal fissure. *Lancet*, **344**, 1127–8.

Gui, D., De Gaetano, A., Spada, P. L., *et al.* (2000). Botulinum toxin injected in the gastric wall reduces body weight and food intake in rats. *Aliment Pharmacol Ther*, **14**, 829–34.

Gui, D., Rossi, S., Runfola, M. & Magalini, S. C. (2003). Review article: botulinum toxin in the therapy of gastrointestinal motility disorders. *Aliment Pharmacol Ther*, **18**, 1–16.

Gui, D., Mingrone, G., Valenza, V., *et al.* (2006). Effect of botulinum toxin antral injection on gastric emptying and weight reduction in obese patients: a pilot study. *Aliment Pharmacol Ther*, **23**, 675–80.

Junior, A. C., Savassi-Rocha, P. R., Coelho, L. G., *et al.* (2006). Botulinum A toxin injected into the gastric wall for the treatment of class III obesity: a pilot study. *Obes Surg*, **16**, 335–43.

Katsinelos, P., Kalomenopoulou, M., Christodoulou, K., *et al.* (2001). Treatment of proctalgia fugax with botulinum A toxin. *Eur J Gastroenterol Hepatol*, **13**, 1371–3.

Khubchandani, I. T. & Reed, J. F. (1989). Sequelae of internal sphincterotomy for chronic fissure in ano. *Br J Surg*, **76**, 431–4.

Leyden, J. E., Moss, A. C. & MacMathuna, P. (2006). Endoscopic pneumatic dilation versus botulinum toxin injection in the management of primary achalasia. *Cochrane Database Syst Rev*, **18**(4), CD005046.

Maria, G., Cadeddu, F., Brandara, F., Marniga, G. & Brisinda, G. (2006). Experience with type A botulinum toxin for treatment of outlet-type constipation. *Am J Gastroenterol*, **101**, 2570–5.

Moerman, M. B. (2006). Cricopharyngeal Botox injection: indications and technique. *Curr Opin Otolaryngol Head Neck Surg*, **14**, 431–6.

Pehlivanov, N. & Pasricha, P. J. (2006). Achalasia: botox, dilatation or laparoscopic surgery in 2006. *Neurogastroenterol Motil*, **18**, 799–804.

Rollnik, J. D., Meier, P. N., Manns, M. P. & Goke, M. (2003). Antral injections of botulinum a toxin for the treatment of obesity. *Ann Intern Med*, **138**, 359–60.

Storr, M., Allescher, H. D., Rosch, T., *et al.* (2001). Treatment of symptomatic diffuse esophageal spasm by endoscopic injections of botulinum toxin: a prospective study with long-term follow-up. *Gastrointest Endosc*, **54**, 754–9.

Whermann, T., Schmitt, T. H., Arndt, A., *et al.* (2000). Endoscopic injection of botulinum toxin in patients with recurrent acute pancreatitis due to sphincter of Oddi dysfunction. *Aliment Pharmacol Ther*, **14**, 1469–77.

Zaninotto, G., Ragona, R. M., Briani, C., *et al.* (2004). The role of botulinum toxin injection and upper esophageal sphincter myotomy in treating oropharyngeal dysphagia. *J. Gastr. Surg.*, **8**, 997–1006.

18

Botulinum toxin in urological disorders

Brigitte Schurch and Dennis D. Dykstra

Introduction

Botulinum toxins (BoNTs) are licensed for the treatment of a number of conditions characterized by striated muscle spasticity. However, in recent years, their unlicensed use in the treatment of lower urinary tract conditions has been described (Smith *et al.*, 2004). Chief amongst these are conditions characterized by detrusor overactivity. Treatment of vulvodynia and chronic pelvic pain, benign prostate hyperplasia, and detrusor sphincter dyssynergia are other emerging indications with promising positive results.

Overactive bladder

The International Continence Society (ICS) report of 2002 defined the overactive bladder syndrome as urgency, with or without urge incontinence, usually with frequency and nocturia, in the absence of local pathological or hormonal factors (Abrams *et al.*, 2002). The prevalence in Europe and USA was estimated to be 3% among men 40–44 years of age, 9% among women 40–44 years of age, 42% among men 75 years of age or older, and 31% among women 75 years of age or older (Tubaro, 2004). The symptoms of overactive bladder have many potential causes and contributing factors. Urination involves the higher cortex of the brain, the pons, the spinal cord, the peripheral autonomic, somatic, and sensory afferent innervation of the lower urinary tract, and the anatomical components of the lower urinary tract itself. Disorders of any of these structures may contribute to the symptoms of overactive bladder (Figure 18.1).

A variety of efferent and afferent neural pathways, reflexes, and central and peripheral neurotransmitters are involved in urine storage and bladder emptying. Acetylcholine, which interacts with muscarinic receptors on the detrusor muscle, is the predominant peripheral neurotransmitter responsible for bladder contraction. The muscarinic receptor subtype M3 appears to be the most clinically relevant in the human bladder. Acetylcholine interacts with the M3 receptor, initiating a cascade of events that result in contraction of the detrusor muscle. The M2 receptor may also facilitate bladder contraction by reducing intracellular levels of cyclic adenosine monophosphate. Pathological states can alter sensitivity to muscarinic stimulation. For example, bladder-outflow obstruction appears to enhance responsiveness to acetylcholine, a phenomenon similar to denervation supersensitivity.

Many classes of drugs, especially anticholinergics, have been studied or proposed for the treatment of symptoms of overactive bladder. All anticholinergic drugs can have bothersome side effects. Although dry mouth is the most common, constipation,

Manual of Botulinum Toxin Therapy, ed. Daniel Truong, Dirk Dressler and Mark Hallett. Published by Cambridge University Press.
© Cambridge University Press 2009.

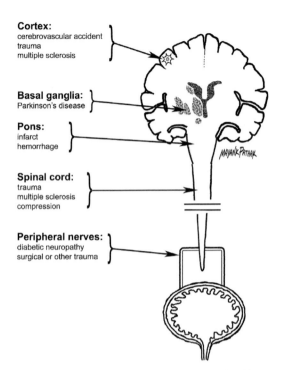

Figure 18.1 Anatomical lesions and neurogenic bladder.

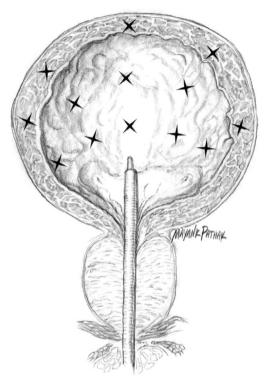

Figure 18.2 BoNT-A injection into the bladder: detrusor mapping.

gastroesophageal reflux, blurry vision, urinary retention, and cognitive side effects can also occur. Since various forms of dementia are routinely treated with cholinesterase inhibitors, the potential for adverse cognitive effects and delirium due to antimuscarinic drugs is a particular concern in the older population. Direct injection of BoNT into the detrusor muscle (which inhibits acetylcholine at the presynaptic cholinergic junction but may also have an important role on the afferent pathways of the lower urinary tract) (Apostolidis *et al.*, 2006) appears to ameliorate detrusor hyperreflexia in patients with spinal cord injury (Schurch *et al.*, 2000, 2005; Giannantoni *et al.*, 2004). It also has therapeutic value in selected patients with severe refractory symptoms of overactive bladder (Kessler *et al.*, 2005; Popat *et al.*, 2005; Schmid *et al.*, 2006; Sahai *et al.*, 2007). Injection technique consists of injecting mainly the detrusor and sparing the trigone (Figure 18.2) using a rigid or a flexible cystoscope.

Patients have either no, mild conscious sedation or general anesthesia. Injection doses reported in the literature have varied between 100 and 300 (mouse) units of BoNT-A (Botox®) and 500 and 1000 units of BoNT-A (Dysport®) for neurogenic detrusor overactivity (NDO).

Injection doses have varied between 100 and 300 units of Botox and 300 units of Dysport for idiopathic detrusor overactivity (IDO). Injection sites have varied between 20 and 30 for NDO and 10 to 30 for IDO.

Mean duration of improvement has varied between 3 and 9 months with Botox and between 5 and 10 months with Dysport. The continence improvement rate is 86.5% with Botox and 86% with Dysport.

No side effects related to the injection itself have been reported. There are occasional reports of general weakness using Botox (2 of the 340 treated patients [0.6%]), whereas general weakness has been described in 2.5–5% with Dysport (255 treated patients). Botulinum toxin type B (NeuroBloc®/ Myobloc®) is efficient in treating IDO (Dykstra *et al.*, 2003; Ghei *et al.*, 2005), but due to its short duration of action, it is better used as secondary treatment in patients who become resistant to BoNT-A (Ghei *et al.*, 2005).

Conclusion: BoNT for overactive bladder appears to be a treatment with high efficacy that meets evidence-based medicine level 1 criteria (i.e. a prospective, randomized, controlled clinical trial with masked outcome assessment, in a representative population), with a good safety profile. Repeated injections appear as effective as the first one (Karsenty *et al.*, 2006). Additional controlled, double-blind studies and dose finding studies especially in IDO are needed to further explore this treatment option.

Vulvodynia and chronic pelvic pain

Vulvodynia

Vulvodynia is a chronic disorder in women characterized by provoked or constant vulvar pain of varying intensity without obvious concomitant clinical pathology. Two subtypes of vulvodynia are recognized: generalized and localized. The latter is currently referred to as vestibulodynia or vestibulitis (Bachmann *et al.*, 2006).

In addition to vulvar pain, there is typically burning and, less often, itching. Onset is usually abrupt and the typical patient is between 20 and 45 years of age. Vulvodynia has been shown to affect 15–20% of the female population in the United States (Bachmann *et al.*, 2006).

There is a limited number of studies on the use of BoNT for the treatment of vulvodynia (Brin & Vapnek, 1997; Shafik & El-Sibai, 2000; Gunter & Brewer, 2002; Ghazizadeh & Nikzad, 2004; Gunter *et al.*, 2004, 2005; Dykstra *et al.*, 2006). Initial studies targeted overactive muscle sites in the vagina and pelvic floor with the intention of decreasing muscle spasm and therefore pain. Because recent research suggests BoNT may affect peripheral and central sensitization, researchers have targeted overactive muscles and painful tissue areas with the intent of relaxing muscle and inhibiting the release of neurotransmitters that can cause pain and inflammation (substance P and calcitonin gene-related peptide) (Dykstra & Presthus, 2006).

Injection techniques with BoNT for vulvodynia range from 10 units to 50 units (Botox) and 150 units to 400 units (Dysport). Dilutions of toxin have ranged from 0.5 cc to 1.0 cc. Injection sites have included the anterior vaginal wall muscles, the puborectalis, pubococcygeus, perineal body, bulbocavernosus, and bulbospongiosus muscles (Figure 18.3). The number of injections into each muscle has varied from one to three sites. Needle size has been between 23 and 30 gauge. Patients had either no sedation or mild conscious sedation. Electromyography (EMG) has been used in a few studies to better localize the muscles being injected. Studies have been mainly single or multiple case series with single or multiple follow-up injections. One study was controlled (Shafik & El-Sibai, 2000). All studies showed improvement in most patients regarding pain, muscle spasm, quality of life, and sexual activity. Duration of effects lasted from 4 weeks to 2 years. A small number of patients were cured. No significant adverse effects were noted in any study.

Chronic pelvic pain

Chronic pelvic pain is a non-cyclic pain for a duration of six or more months localized to the anatomic pelvis, anterior abdominal wall at or below the umbilicus, the lumbosacral back or the buttocks and is of sufficient severity to cause functional disability or lead to medical care (Howard, 2003).

Approximately 15–20% of women aged 18–50 years have chronic pelvic pain of greater than 1 year duration (an estimated number greater than migraine, asthma, and back pain) (Howard, 2003).

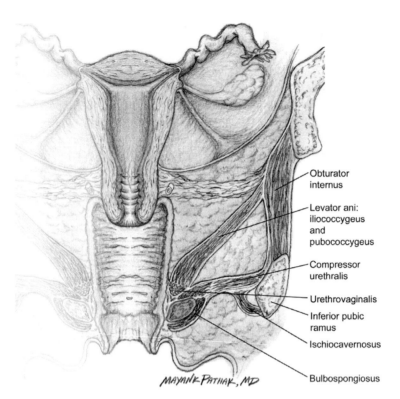

Figure 18.3 Vaginal and pelvic floor muscles.

Obturator internus

Levator ani: iliococcygeus and pubococcygeus

Compressor urethralis

Urethrovaginalis

Inferior pubic ramus

Ischiocavernosus

Bulbospongiosus

MAYANK PATHAK, MD

Chronic pelvic pain may result from psychological disorders or neurological diseases both central and peripheral. Sufficient evidence strongly suggests that several of the most common disorders in women such as endometriosis, interstitial cystitis, irritable bowel syndrome, and pelvic inflammatory disease are causes of chronic pelvic pain (Howard, 2003).

Patients with chronic pelvic pain may have generalized or localized pelvic pain, pain with intercourse, pain exacerbation after sexual intercourse, pain exacerbated both premenstrually and menstrually, and complain of voiding symptoms of frequency, urgency, and nocturia (Howard, 2003).

There is a limited number of studies on the use of BoNT for the treatment of chronic pelvic pain (Zermann *et al.*, 2000, 2001; Jarvis *et al.*, 2004; Thompson *et al.*, 2005; Meredith *et al.*, 2006). These studies have included both male and female patients. Injection techniques with BoNT for

chronic pelvic pain have ranged from 40 to 200 units of Botox. Dilutions have ranged from 2 to 4 cc. Injection sites have included the puborectalis, pubococcygeus, and external urethral sphincter muscles (Figure 18.4). The number of injections into each muscle has ranged from three to five sites, and a 22 gauge needle is usually used. Patients have had either no sedation or only mild conscious sedation. Electromyography was used in one study to improve muscle localization. The studies were multiple case series and all studies showed improvement in most patients regarding pain, spasm, quality of life, and sexual activity. Duration of effect was 12 weeks to 1.5 years. No adverse effects were noted.

Conclusion: the use of BoNT for the treatment of vulvodynia and chronic pelvic pain may be a viable option for patients. Controlled, double-blind studies are needed to further explore this treatment option.

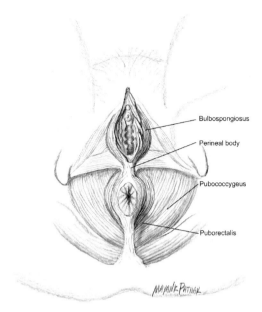

Figure 18.4 Pelvic floor muscles.

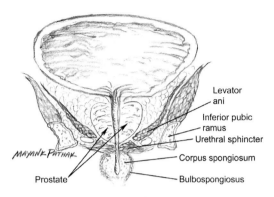

Figure 18.5 Male genitalia and prostate.

Benign prostatic hyperplasia

Benign prostatic hyperplasia (BPH) is a non-malignant enlargement of the prostate and is regarded as a major cause of bladder outlet obstruction (Chuang *et al.*, 2005).

Because surgical denervation was known to produce profound atrophy in the rat prostate, BoNT-A was used to show selective chemical denervation and subsequent atrophy of the rat prostate (Doggweiler *et al.*, 1998).

The pathophysiology of BPH may involve a dynamic component that reflects the smooth muscle tone within the gland and a static component that is related to the mass effect of the enlarged prostate. Botulinum may have an effect on both components by relaxing smooth muscle and causing atrophy of glandular tissue (Chuang, 2005).

There have been a few studies on the use of BoNT in humans (Maria *et al.*, 2003; Chuang *et al.*, 2005; Kuo, 2005; Park *et al.*, 2005). One hundred to 200 units of BoNT-A (Botox) were injected at two to ten sites with 4–20 cc dilution factor. Botulinum toxin was injected into the transition zone at the lateral lobes and median lobes of the prostate or both lateral lobes of the prostate (Figure 18.5). Needle size was 21, 22 or 23 gauge. Injections were done via rectal ultrasound, transrectal ultrasound or via a cystoscope. Injections were done without sedation or anesthesia or under light intravenous sedation or general anesthesia. All studies except one were case series. One study was randomized, placebo-controlled.

In all studies patients showed improvement in mean prostate volumes, symptom scores, quality-of-life measurements, post-void residual urine volumes, peak flow rates, and serum prostate-specific antigen concentration. Onset of effects was within 1 week of injection and duration was from 3 to 9 months.

Conclusion: the use of BoNT-A for the treatment of BPH may be a viable option for selected BPH patients. Controlled, double-blind studies are needed to further explore this treatment option.

Detrusor sphincter dyssynergia

Detrusor sphincter dyssynergia (DSD) is an involuntary contraction of the external urethral sphincter (Figures 18.6 and 18.7) during detrusor contraction. Patients with spinal cord injuries are particularly vulnerable to this problem. Detrusor sphincter dyssynergia causes voiding dysfunction

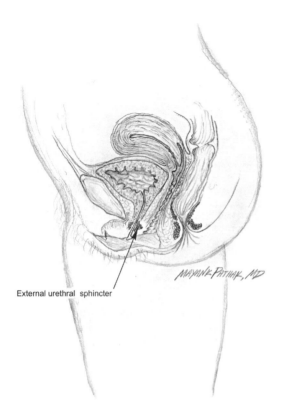

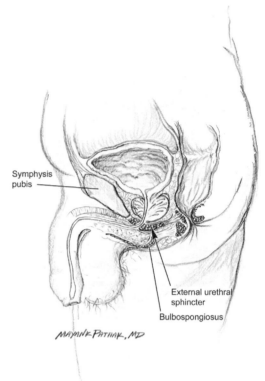

Figure 18.6 External urethral sphincter injection using EMG in female. The arrowhead indicates approximate injection site.

Figure 18.7 External urethral sphincter injection using EMG in male. The arrowhead indicates approximate injection site.

and can lead to high intravesical pressure, autonomic hyperreflexia, hydroureteronephrosis, infection, and renal failure (Gallien *et al.*, 1998).

There is a limited number of studies available on the use of BoNT for the treatment of DSD (Dykstra *et al.*, 1988; Dykstra & Sidi, 1990; Schurch *et al.*, 1996, 1997, 1999; Gallien *et al.*, 1998, 2005; Petit *et al.*, 1998; Wheeler *et al.*, 1998; Mall *et al.*, 2001; Phelan *et al.*, 2001; de Seze *et al.*, 2002). Botulinum toxin dose ranges from 40 to 100 units (Botox) and 150 to 250 units (Dysport). Injections have been performed either transperineally or endoscopically with 21–23 gauge needles using both EMG (Figures 18.6 and 18.7) and non-EMG techniques. Early techniques used frequent injections (weekly or monthly), because initial findings suggested that more frequent injections lasted longer. Due to

immunogenic concerns, however, injections are now limited to at least 3-month intervals. Currently, injections into the external sphincter are performed using one to four injection sites with a volume of 1–4 cc (Figures 18.6 and 18.7). Autonomic dysreflexia is monitored during the injections.

Results in patients with spinal cord injury and DSD show improvement in urodynamic parameters such as post-void residual volume, detrusor pressure on voiding and urethral pressure profiles. Duration of effects lasts from 2 to 9 months. However, patients with multiple sclerosis (MS) and DSD who were injected with a single dose of 100 units of BoNT-A (Botox) did not show similar favorable results (Gallien *et al.*, 2005).

Conclusion: the use of BoNT for patients with spinal cord injury and DSD appears to be a viable treatment option. Its use in MS patients with DSD does not appear helpful. Further controlled trials are needed to clarify dose, technique, response, and ideal patient population.

REFERENCES

Abrams, P., Cardozo, L., Fall, M., *et al.* (2002). The standardisation of terminology of lower urinary tract function: report from the Standardisation Sub-committee of the International Continence Society. *Neurourol Urodyn*, **21**(2), 167–78.

Apostolidis, A., Dasgupta, P. & Fowler, C. J. (2006). Proposed mechanism for the efficacy of injected botulinum toxin in the treatment of human detrusor overactivity. *Eur Urol*, **49**(4), 644–50.

Bachmann, G. A., Rosen, R., Pinn, V. W., *et al.* (2006). Vulvodynia: a state-of-the-art consensus on definitions, diagnosis and management. *J Reprod Med*, **51**(6), 447–56.

Brin, M. F. & Vapnek, J. M. (1997). Treatment of vaginismus with botulinum toxin injections. *Lancet*, **349** (9047), 252–3.

Chuang, Y. C., Chiang, P. H., Huang, C. C., Yoshimura, N. & Chancellor, M. B. (2005). Botulinum toxin type A improves benign prostatic hyperplasia symptoms in patients with small prostates. *Urology*, **66**(4), 775–9.

de Seze, M., Petit H., Gallien, P., *et al.* (2002). Botulinum a toxin and detrusor sphincter dyssynergia: a double-blind lidocaine-controlled study in 13 patients with spinal cord disease. *Eur Urol*, **42**(1), 56–62.

Doggweiler, R., Zermann, D. H., Ishigooka, M. & Schmidt, R. A. (1998). Botox-induced prostatic involution. *Prostate*, **37**(1), 44–50.

Dykstra, D., Enriquez, A. & Valley, M. (2003). Treatment of overactive bladder with botulinum toxin type B: a pilot study. *Int Urogynecol J Pelvic Floor Dysfunct*, **14**(6), 424–6.

Dykstra, D. D. & Presthus, J. (2006). Botulinum toxin type A for the treatment of provoked vestibulodynia: an open-label, pilot study. *J Reprod Med*, **51**(6), 467–70.

Dykstra, D. D. & Sidi, A. A. (1990). Treatment of detrusor-sphincter dyssynergia with botulinum A toxin: a double-blind study. *Arch Phys Med Rehabil*, **71**(1), 24–6.

Dykstra, D. D., Sidi, A. A., Scott, A. B., Pagel, J. M. & Goldish, G. D. (1988). Effects of botulinum A toxin on detrusor-sphincter dyssynergia in spinal cord injury patients. *J Urol*, **139**(5), 919–22.

Gallien, P., Robineau, S., Verin, M., *et al.* (1998). Treatment of detrusor sphincter dyssynergia by transperineal injection of botulinum toxin. *Arch Phys Med Rehabil*, **79**(6), 715–17.

Gallien, P., Reymann, J. M., Amarenco, G., *et al.* (2005). Placebo controlled, randomised, double blind study of the effects of botulinum A toxin on detrusor sphincter dyssynergia in multiple sclerosis patients. *J Neurol Neurosurg Psychiatry*, **76**(12), 1670–6.

Ghazizadeh, S. & Nikzad, M. (2004). Botulinum toxin in the treatment of refractory vaginismus. *Obstet Gynecol*, **104** (5 Pt 1), 922–5.

Ghei, M., Maraj, B. H., Miller, R., *et al.* (2005). Effects of botulinum toxin B on refractory detrusor overactivity: a randomized, double-blind, placebo controlled, crossover trial. *J Urol*, **174**(5), 1873–7; discussion 1877.

Giannantoni, A., Di Stasi, S. M., Stephen, R. L., *et al.* (2004). Intravesical resiniferatoxin versus botulinum-A toxin injections for neurogenic detrusor overactivity: a prospective randomized study. *J Urol*, **172**(1), 240–3.

Gunter, J. & Brewer, A. (2002). Botulinum toxin A for generalized vulvar dysaesthesia. *J Pain*, **21**(April 3 (2Suppl 1)), Abstract 681.

Gunter, J., Brewer, A. & Tawfik, O. (2004). Botulinum toxin a for vulvodynia: a case report. *J Pain*, **5**(4), 238–40.

Gunter, J., Quan, D., Martel, R. & Teal, S. (2005). A prospective study of botulinum toxin for vestibulodynia. Toxin Meetings Denver Co June 23.25, 2005. Abstract 39A.

Howard, F. M. (2003). Chronic pelvic pain. *Obstet Gynecol*, **101**(3), 594–611.

Jarvis, S. K., Abbott, J. A., Lenart, M. B., Steensma, A. & Vancaillie, T. G. (2004). Pilot study of botulinum toxin type A in the treatment of chronic pelvic pain associated with spasm of the levator ani muscles. *Aust N Z J Obstet Gynaecol*, **44**(1), 46–50.

Karsenty, G., Reitz, A., Lindemann, G., Boy, S. & Schurch, B. (2006). Persistence of therapeutic effect after repeated injections of botulinum toxin type A to treat incontinence due to neurogenic detrusor overactivity. *Urology*, **68**(6), 1193–7.

Kessler, T. M., Danuser, H., Schumacher, M., *et al.* (2005). Botulinum A toxin injections into the detrusor: an effective treatment in idiopathic and neurogenic detrusor overactivity? *Neurourol Urodyn*, **24**(3), 231–6.

Kuo, H. C. (2005). Prostate botulinum A toxin injection–an alternative treatment for benign prostatic obstruction in poor surgical candidates. *Urology*, **65**(4), 670–4.

Mall, V., Glocker, F. X., Frankenschmidt, A., *et al.* (2001). Treatment of neuropathic bladder using botulinum toxin A in a 1-year-old child with myelomeningocele. *Pediatr Nephrol*, **16**(12), 1161–2.

Maria, G., Brisinda, G., Civello, I. M., *et al.* (2003). Relief by botulinum toxin of voiding dysfunction due to benign prostatic hyperplasia: results of a randomized, placebo-controlled study. *Urology*, **62**(2), 259–64; discussion 264–5.

Meredeth, M., Karp, B., Bartrum, D., Zimmer, C. & Stratton, P. (2006). Botulinum toxin in the treatment of chronic pain and endometriosis. *J Soc for Gynecol Investig*, **13**(2(Suppl)), 276A.

Park, D. S., Lee, Y. K., Jeong, H. S., *et al.* (2005). The initial experience of intraprostatic injection of botulinum toxin type A for benign prostatic hyperplasia: a comparative study of short-term effect with transurethral resection of prostate. *Koran J Urol*, **46**(11), 1173–9.

Petit, H., Wiart, L., Gaujard, E., *et al.* (1998). Botulinum A toxin treatment for detrusor-sphincter dyssynergia in spinal cord disease. *Spinal Cord*, **36**(2), 91–4.

Phelan, M. W., Franks, M., Somogyi, G. T., *et al.* (2001). Botulinum toxin urethral sphincter injection to restore bladder emptying in men and women with voiding dysfunction. *J Urol*, **165**(4), 1107–10.

Popat, R., Apostolidis, A., Kalsi, V., *et al.* (2005). A comparison between the response of patients with idiopathic detrusor overactivity and neurogenic detrusor overactivity to the first intradetrusor injection of botulinum-A toxin. *J Urol*, **174**(3), 984–9.

Sahai, A. (2007). Efficacy of botulinum toxin-A for treating idiopathic detrusor overactivity: results from a single center, randomized, double-blind placebo controlled trial. *J Urol*, **177**(6), 2231–6.

Schmid, D. M., Sauermann, P., Werner, M., *et al.* (2006). Experience with 100 cases treated with botulinum-A toxin injections in the detrusor muscle for idiopathic overactive bladder syndrome refractory to anticholinergics. *J Urol*, **176**(1), 177–85.

Schurch, B., Hauri, D., Rodic, B., *et al.* (1996). Botulinum-A toxin as a treatment of detrusor-sphincter dyssynergia: a prospective study in 24 spinal cord injury patients. *J Urol*, **155**(3), 1023–9.

Schurch, B., Hodler, J. & Rodic, B. (1997). Botulinum A toxin as a treatment of detrusor-sphincter dyssynergia

in patients with spinal cord injury: MRI controlled transperineal injections. *J Neurol Neurosurg Psychiatry*, **63**(4), 474–6.

Schurch, B., Schmid, D. M. & Knapp, P. A. (1999). An update on the treatment of detrusor-sphincter dyssynergia with botulinum toxin type A. *Eur J Neurol*, **6**(Suppl 4), S83–9.

Schurch, B., Stöhrer, M., Kramer, G., *et al.* (2000). Botulinum-A toxin for treating detrusor hyperreflexia in spinal cord injured patients: a new alternative to anticholinergic drugs? Preliminary results. *J Urol*, **164**(3 Pt 1), 692–7.

Schurch, B., de Sèze, M., Denys, P., *et al.* (2005). Botulinum toxin type a is a safe and effective treatment for neurogenic urinary incontinence: results of a single treatment, randomized, placebo controlled 6-month study. *J Urol*, **174**(1), 196–200.

Shafik, A. & El-Sibai, O. (2000). Vaginismus: results of treatment with botulinum toxin. *J Obstet Gynaecol*, **20**(3), 300–2.

Smith, C. P., Somogyi, G. T. & Boone, T. B. (2004). Botulinum toxin in urology: evaluation using an evidence-based medicine approach. *Nat Clin Pract Urol*, **1**(1), 31–7.

Thompson, A. J., Jarvis, S. K., Lenart, M., Abbott, J. A. & Vancaillie, T. G. (2005). The use of botulinum toxin type A (Botox) as treatment for intractable chronic pain associated with spasms of the levator ani muscles. *BJOG*, **112**(2), 247–9.

Tubaro, A. (2004). Defining overactive bladder: epidemiology and burden of disease. *Urology*, **64**(6 Suppl 1), 2–6.

Wheeler, J. S., Jr., Walter, J. S., Chintam, R. S. & Rao, S. (1998). Botulinum toxin injections for voiding dysfunction following SCI. *J Spinal Cord Med*, **21**(3), 227–9.

Zermann, D., Ishigooka, M., Schubert, J. & Schmidt, R. A. (2000). Perisphincteric injection of botulinum toxin type A. A treatment option for patients with chronic prostatic pain? *Eur Urol*, **38**(4), 393–9.

Zermann, D. H., Ishigooka, M., Doggweiler-Wiygul, R., Schubert, J. & Schmidt, R. A. (2001). The male chronic pelvic pain syndrome. *World J Urol*, **19**(3), 173–9.

19

Use of botulinum toxin in musculoskeletal pain and arthritis

Amy M. Lang

Introduction

Since the mid 1990s, botulinum toxins (BoNTs) have been proposed in the treatment of over 100 musculoskeletal conditions. Although initial reports from open-label studies, retrospective reviews, and case series have been encouraging, clinical evidence from large controlled trials is largely lacking, mixed, or negative in regard to the efficacy of botulinum toxins for neck and back pain (Cheshire *et al.*, 1994; Brashear *et al.*, 1999; Brin *et al.*, 1999; Foster *et al.*, 2001; Benzon *et al.*, 2003; De Andres *et al.*, 2003; Lang, 2003, 2004; Gobel *et al.*, 2006; Jabbari *et al.*, 2006; Jabbari, 2007). These differences reflect the complexities of pain syndromes, variations in dosing regimens and injection methodologies, and importance of individual muscles to regional kinematics and function.

The use of BoNT for treatment of myofascial pain (MP), arthritis, and other conditions that are beyond the Food and Drug Administration (FDA)-approved labeling should be considered investigational. Numerous studies have found BoNT type A (BoNT-A) and BoNT type B (BoNT-B) to be safe and well tolerated at doses used for the treatment of cervical dystonia, but side effects can be seen at the higher doses used for cervicothoracic and lumbosacral pain.

Precautions should be taken around breast implants, pacemakers, and other implanted devices. Care should be exercised in regard to the depth of any injection over the trunk so as to avoid pneumothorax. The scalenes should not be injected in patients with chronic obstructive pulmonary disease (COPD), sleep apnea, or other respiratory condition in which these muscles may be crucial as accessory muscles of inspiration. If there is a question of underlying radiculopathy, electromyography (EMG) should be performed prior to treatment with BoNT. Fluoroscopic, EMG, and/or ultrasound guidance is required for infiltration of deep compartment muscles. Cervicothoracic muscles should not be targeted with BoNT in patients with hypermobility syndrome.

The pain-relieving effects of BoNT are not fully explained by focal muscle relaxation alone. In addition to blocking acetylcholine release, inactivation of the SNARE (soluble N-ethylmaleimide-sensitive factor attachment protein receptor) complex by BoNT may also interrupt exocytosis of nociceptive peptides and transmitters such as glutamate, substance-P, and calcitonin gene-related peptide. Numerous in-vitro and in-vivo studies of BoNT have demonstrated inhibitory effects on neuropeptides and inflammatory mediators, and support a role for BoNT as a neuromodulator in prevention of central sensitization (Gilio *et al.*, 2000; Welch *et al.*, 2000; Durham *et al.*, 2004; Aoki, 2005).

Botulinum toxin therapy should not be considered a stand-alone treatment for refractory pain

Manual of Botulinum Toxin Therapy, ed. Daniel Truong, Dirk Dressler and Mark Hallett. Published by Cambridge University Press. © Cambridge University Press 2009.

syndromes. Patients should be guided to make ergonomic and lifestyle changes, and perform stabilization exercises to help prevent recurrent pain. Some patients may require instruction with regard to sleep hygiene and relaxation techniques, or formal psychological counseling to address maladaptive responses to chronic pain. Patients unwilling to adopt lifestyle changes may not be optimal candidates for BoNT therapy.

Myofascial pain

Myofascial pain (MP) is a regional pain syndrome defined by the presence of a localized, hyperirritable trigger point (TrP), a palpable knot or mass (usually 3–6 mm in diameter), in a taut band of muscle associated with tenderness and referred pain into well-defined areas remote from the Trp area (Borg-Stein & Simons, 2002). Trigger points have a high degree of correlation with acupuncture meridians (Dorsher, 2006). Myofascial pain is characterized by chronic, focal muscle pain, associated with stiffness, tenderness, and fatigue (Simons *et al.*, 1999). Palpation of an active TrP is often associated with a local twitch response or jump sign, a palpable or visible contraction of the taut muscle band with digital palpation. A latent TrP is clinically silent until activated, typically by trauma, but may cause pain on palpation. There is the potential for rather significant variability among examiners rating TrPs, unlike the situation for fibromyalgia tender points, where the examination is simple with good reliability and validity (Gerwin *et al.*, 1997). Laboratory testing, radiographic studies, diagnostic ultrasound and other standard tests are not helpful in making a diagnosis of MP, but they may be useful for excluding other diagnoses.

A neuroplastic mechanism may be involved in the development of myofascial TrPs (Hong & Simons, 1998; Calandre *et al.*, 2006). In response to trauma or stress, excessive amounts of intracellular calcium are liberated, initiating a cascade of uncontrolled shortening of the involved muscle fibers. Dysfunctional motor end plates of neurons

release excessive amounts of acetylcholine to sustain contraction, thereby impeding muscle perfusion, increasing metabolic demand, and causing accumulation of toxic metabolites. This exacerbates the energy crisis to perpetuate the cycle within the taut band. This hypothesis is supported by studies demonstrating abnormal firing of motor end plates, low oxygen tension, and decreased high-energy phosphates in TrPs. Trigger points are also associated with localized autonomic signs, such as vasoconstriction and pilomotor reactions.

In addition to peripheral sensitization, a form of central sensitization in the spinal cord has also been implicated as the neural mechanism for pain associated with TrPs. The receptive field of the neuron at the dorsal horn of the spinal cord expands in response to chronic nociceptive stimuli, accounting for the zone of referred pain associated with TrPs. Due to the more pervasive central sensitization that occurs in patients with fibromyalgia, TrPs may be more irritable and less responsive to treatment than those in individuals with regional MP alone. Trigger points can also become recalcitrant due to mechanical factors of chronic muscle shortening and development of contracture or adhesions that inhibit sliding of muscle fibers. These perpetually shortened bands cause dysfunction of reciprocal activation–inhibition relationships in surrounding muscles.

Although it is seen as a primary regional soft tissue pain syndrome, refractory MP may indicate that pain is multifactorial (Mennell, 1992; McPartland, 2004). Myofascial pain can be precipitated or perpetuated by trauma, mechanical factors such as muscle overload and poor postural habits, nutritional deficiencies, endocrinopathy or other metabolic dysfunction, and stress. It is a regional disorder commonly affecting cervicothoracic (Table 19.1), lumbosacral, and/or pelvofemoral muscles (Darlow *et al.*, 1987; Simons *et al.*, 1999, Simons, 2004).

Myofascial pain should be distinguished from fibromyalgia syndrome (FM), a generalized condition of which the hallmark is the tender point. Trigger points should be distinguished from FM tender points (Durette *et al.*, 1991). By criteria

Table 19.1. Differential diagnoses of cervicothoracic pain

Cervical dystonia	Medication effects
Disc pathology	Metabolic disease
Endocrinopathy	Neoplastic syndrome
Facet syndrome	Neurological disorders
Fibromyalgia	Nutritional conditions
Infectious disease	Psychological disorders
Inflammatory conditions	Radiculopathy
Joint disorders	Regional soft tissue disorders
Mechanical stresses	Visceral referred pain

according to the American College of Rheumatology, FM is a more widespread pain condition (three or more body regions above and below the waist) lasting for three or months associated with pain in at least 11 or 18 tender point sites on digital palpation with a force of approximately 4 kg. Tender points are not associated with a "twitch" on palpation and are usually clinically silent unless stimulated by palpation. Tender points typically do not cause a referred pain pattern on palpation. Patients with FM tend to have more constitutional symptoms than those with MP. Some investigators consider MP and FM to be the same disease process at opposite ends of the localized to generalized spectrum.

Approaches to treating MP are numerous and include soft tissue modalities such as electrical stimulation and ultrasound, massage, manipulation, vapocoolant spray and passive stretch, active stretching and exercise programs, dry needling, injections of anesthetic with or without corticosteroids, acupressure, acupuncture, and pharmacotherapy. Virtually any intervention that improves perfusion of the affected muscle improves MP (Lang, 2002). Oral medications have been used with variable success alone or in combination: corticosteroids and non-steroidal anti-inflammatory drugs, skeletal muscle relaxants, vasodilators, opioids, and adjuvant analgesics such as antidepressants and anti-epileptic drugs (Porta, 2000; Lang, 2002). The problem with many of these medications is their systemic side effects and long-term risks in patients having other medical problems; cognitive changes or sedating qualities that are particularly limiting in

certain occupations and in the elderly; the dependency or abuse potential of opioids and some skeletal muscle relaxants; and the medicolegal risks and regulatory issues relevant to prescribing these medications.

Travell and Simons popularized the spray and stretch technique as a treatment for MP (Simons *et al.*, 1999). The purpose is to desensitize the TrP and stretch and relax the taut band of muscle. Ice may be used instead of vapocoolant sprays. Whether or not this technique is as efficacious as TrP injections is arguable, but it is useful as a non-invasive technique and adjunct to other therapies including independent stretching and exercise.

Along with spray and stretch techniques, physical therapy (PT) and PT modalities are probably the most commonly used approaches in early MP (Calillet, 1977; Carter, 1998; Borg-Stein & Simons, 2002; Graff-Radford, 2004). Therapeutic heat, cold therapy, transcutaneous nerve stimulation, electrical muscle stimulation, ultrasound, iontophoresis, myofascial release, massage, hydrotherapy, stretching and strengthening exercises (passive and active) can be helpful. In chronic MP, PT modalities are often combined with Trp injections to maximize response to the injections during the beneficial response phase.

Borg-Stein and Simons (2002) reviewed the medical literature on Trp injections and concluded that, although such injections have widespread clinical acceptance, evaluation of their efficacy is hindered by difficulties in definitions as well as variations in technique. The authors noted that, although inter-rater reliability is somewhat suspect, it improves with training (Borg-Stein & Simons, 2002). In clinical practice, a 25–27 gauge, 1.5 inch needle is most often used with volumes of 2–10 cc depending on the size of the muscle. Efficacy has been demonstrated with dry needling, sterile water, lidocaine (plain 1% and 2%), bupivacaine, diclofenac, and prednisone (Frost *et al.*, 1980; Borg-Stein & Simons, 2002). It appears that the nature of the injected substance is not a critical factor and reports conflict as to whether any therapeutic substance injected provides more benefit than dry needling alone.

Local anesthetics reduce post-injection soreness and for that reason are most commonly used. Most authors do not feel that steroids are needed unless there is an associated inflammatory process such as bursitis, tendonitis, or scar neuroma. Skin depigmentation, tendon atrophy, and depression of plasma cortisol levels have been associated with local corticosteroid injections. Tissue necrosis is sometimes observed following repeated injections with local anesthetics. Trigger point injections should be limited to a series of three to four in patients who derive only temporary benefit from the procedure, and offered in conjunction with a comprehensive treatment program rather than as sole therapy.

When MP becomes refractory to treatment, consideration should be given to treatment with BoNT. Reduction of MP by neurolysis has been attributed to the ability of BoNT to block acetylcholine release from motor end plates at the neuromuscular junction, the core of the TrP. Results may be enhanced by injecting the neurotoxin evenly throughout the mid-belly of muscles rather than by administering it with conventional TrP injection techniques (Lang, 2000; Ferrante *et al.*, 2005).

In general, results of clinical trials of BoNT in MP have been mixed. Preliminary studies found that BoNT-A may be beneficial in the treatment of MP (Cheshire *et al.*, 1994; Wheeler *et al.*, 1998; Lang, 2000). Ferrante *et al.* (2005) conducted a randomized, double-blind, placebo-controlled trial of BoNT-A in the treatment of 132 patients with cervicothoracic MP, and concluded that injections of BoNT-A directly into TrP do not improve this condition. Such varied results reflect differences in protocols, dosing regimens, and injection methodologies for treatment of cervicothoracic pain with BoNT. Collectively, these studies illustrate the need to consider several factors with regard to BoNT treatment of cervicothoracic and lumbosacral pain syndromes: patient selection, muscle selection, serotype, concentration, and injection technique, dose per muscle, dose per treatment session, aftercare, and dosing on re-treatment. Postural kinematics and regional effects of BoNT

as a focally acting skeletal muscle relaxant are more important determinants of efficacy than simply targeting TrP in the treatment of MP.

Key point: the goal with BoNT is to make a biomechanical change, taking advantage of the focally acting skeletal muscle relaxation effects of BoNT to achieve a neutral spine position and restore normal kinematics. Botulinum toxin is NOT used to target TrPs.

Myofascial pain involving the gluteus and piriformis muscles can mimic sciatica. Before considering treatment of lumbosacral pain with BoNT, a careful assessment should be undertaken to assure that target muscles are not simply overworked or weakened muscles compensating for hip flexion contractures, arthritis, sacroiliac joint dysfunction, or disc pathology.

Unfortunately, due to the lack of consensus on diagnosis and treatment of MP as well as variability in examination findings, there is no clear consensus on appropriate treatment. Good controlled outcome studies are uniformly lacking. As with all chronic pain conditions, a multidisciplinary approach is prudent since it is the rare patient in which a single modality is curative.

Forward head posture

In general, the degree to which a patient is in forward head posture (mild, moderate, severe, or profound) determines the range of BoNT dose selected; specifically, lower doses are indicated in suboccipital and upper back muscles with progressive forward head posture. It may at first seem paradoxical to use lower dose ranges in patients demonstrating greater deviation in head forward posture. However, it is important to realize that suboccipital paraspinals and upper back muscles shorten in forward head posture (Fernandez-de-Las-Penas *et al.*, 2006). These muscles sustain greater static workloads to hold up the head which is extended forward as if on a lever arm. Larger dose ranges create a sense of head heaviness and shoulder girdle weakness in such patients.

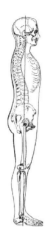

Neutral spine is defined by a plumb line:
⇩ *tragus of the ear*
⇩ *anteromedial upper trapezius ridge*
⇩ *lumbar vertebral bodies*
⇩ *posterior to the mid-center of the hip joint*
⇩ *anterior to the knee joint axis*
⇩ *through the calcaneo-cuboid joint*

Neutral pelvis is defined by a parallel line:
⇩ *ASIS and pubic ramus along the same plane*

Figure 19.1 Neutral spine. Neutral spine position is defined by a plumb line falling from the tragus of the ear through the anterior upper trapezius ridge, continuing through the lower lumbar vertebral bodies, and then passing posterior to the hip, anterior to the knee, and through the mid-foot; with the anterior superior iliac spine (ASIS) and pubic ramus in line along a parallel plane.

Pectoral muscles may have to be injected for the relief of mid-back pain and to improve postural mechanics in patients with moderate to severe forward head posture. Treatment of interscapular muscles should be avoided, since further weakening of these compensatory over-lengthened muscles may only worsen shoulder mechanics and pain. Doses of BoNT-A higher than those for the pectoral muscles can cause secondary compensatory pain in the subclavius.

As head forward posture progresses to severe level, anterior and middle scalenes shorten, narrowing the outlet for the brachial plexus. This can result in a cervicobrachial syndrome with pain and sensory symptoms radiating into the upper extremities. Anterior and middle scalenes can be treated to alleviate the upper extremity symptoms, but BoNT-A (Botox®) doses higher than 25 mouse units (U) per scalene can result in swallowing difficulties, particularly if bilateral treatments are administered.

Patients should be informed that they will most likely observe clinical benefits within 8–12 weeks post-injection. Patients should continue their home exercise programs, with particular emphasis on pectoral stretching, mid-back strengthening/scapular stabilization, and maintaining a neutral spine position (Figure 19.1). For patients with moderate to severe head forward posture, cervical stretching exercises are best performed in supine lying without a pillow. Chiropractic interventions utilizing rapid thrust techniques should be avoided, as a new range of motion end points emerge following treatment with BoNT.

Forward head posture, with either anterior or posterior pelvic tilt, promotes changes in the length of cervicothoracic muscles and secondary effects on shoulder kinematics. Muscles acting on the shoulder girdle work synergistically to counterbalance and stabilize the scapula in all planes for maintenance of normal glenohumeral joint position. Over-lengthened or fixed shortened muscles are unable to produce the same amount of force as they would from an optimal length. Muscles that are fixed at a position other than their optimal length are less efficient at shoulder stabilization, fatigue faster, and are prone to injury, especially with repetitive reaching and lifting tasks. Eccentric contractions by over-lengthened muscles are at the highest risk for strain or sprain injury due to a decrease in the number of overlapping sarcomeres in the stretched position. This explains the increased incidence of mid-back strain or sprain in the presence of a fixed forward head posture (Figure 19.2) (Griegel-Morris *et al.*, 1992; Greenfield *et al.*, 1995; Haughie *et al.*, 1995).

Forward head posture can be described in terms of fingerbreadths of anterior translation of the tragus of the ear anterior to the upper medial trapezius ridge. Primary and secondary pain patterns that

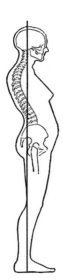

Fixed forward head posture

Shortened muscles:
➢ suboccipital paraspinals
➢ splenius capitis
➢ scalenes
➢ sternocleidomastoid
➢ levator scapulae
➢ upper trapezius
➢ pectoralis major/minor

Over-lengthened muscles:
➢ rhomboids
➢ middle/lower trapezius
➢ thoracic paraspinals

Figure 19.2 Forward head posture. In forward head posture the center of gravity is shifted by varying degrees to cause secondary changes in muscle length and function.

Primary pain:
➢ upper trapezius

Secondary pain:
➢ levator scapulae

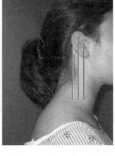

Figure 19.3 Fixed forward head posture: 2 fingerbreadths.

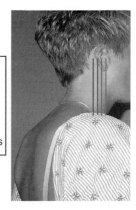

Primary pain:
➢ interscapular muscles

Secondary pain:
➢ lower thoracic paraspinals

Figure 19.4 Fixed forward head posture: 3 fingerbreadths.

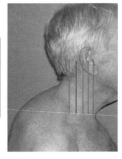

Primary pain:
➢ cervicobrachial symptoms

Secondary pain:
➢ mid-back region

Figure 19.5 Fixed forward head posture: 4 fingerbreadths.

emerge in fixed forward head posture can be predicted by the muscles involved at each position of fixed anterior translation of 1, 2, 3, or 4 fingerbreadths. Primary pain often progresses over the course of usual daily activities, and secondary pain emerges with forward reaching or lifting tasks that place a greater lever arm of gravity against the neutral plumb line to pull the body forward.

The most common presentation of fixed forward head posture is 2 fingerbreadths of anterior translation in which primary pain focuses along the upper medial trapezius ridge (Figure 19.3). With

forward reaching or lifting tasks secondary pain emerges at the levator scapulae, close to its insertion at the upper medial border of the scapula.

A "follow the pain" paradigm for muscle selection in BoNT therapy only works for milder fixed postural deviations of 1 or 2 fingerbreadths of forward head posture. With more advanced fixed postural deviations of 3 or 4 fingerbreadths (Figure 19.4), a "follow the pain" paradigm will aggravate symptoms by targeting over-lengthened and compensatory muscles. Resolution of pain in such cases demands a "postural paradigm" that considers the effects of BoNT on kinematics of the shoulder girdle.

The thoracic outlet narrows with progressive fixed forward head posture such that by 4 fingerbreadths (Figure 19.5) of anterior translation symptoms begin radiating into the upper limb, especially with reaching or lifting tasks. Cervicobrachial symptoms

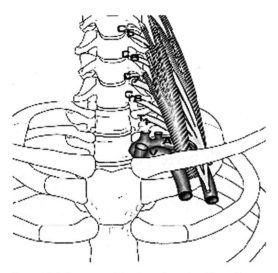

Figure 19.6 Anatomy of the thoracic outlet. (From Simons *et al.*, 1999).

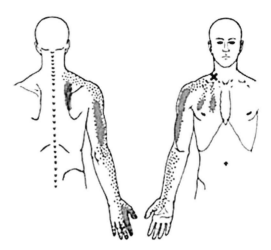

Figure 19.7 Scalene MP referral pattern. (From Simons *et al.*, 1999).

mimic those of classic thoracic outlet syndrome (Figure 19.6), but classic features of thoracic outlet syndrome are lacking on diagnostic screens.

Cervicobrachial syndrome (Fig. 19.7)

Cervicobrachial syndrome, International Classification of Diseases [ICD-9 723.3], is characterized as follows:
- Symptoms mimic thoracic outlet syndrome
- Develops as a result of narrowing of the thoracic outlet, hypertrophy of the scalenes, and/or compression of neurovascular structures beneath the pectoralis minor tendon
- May emerge due to forward head posture, buxom habitus, cervical dystonia, COPD, or sleep apnea
- Provocative maneuvers of shoulder abduction/ external rotation cause sensory complaints WITHOUT a pulse deficit
- Physical exam is normal
- EMG/nerve conduction studies (NCS) are normal
  Regional MPs must also be distinguished from other conditions with similar pain referral patterns. Cervicothoracic MPs frequently occur in association with cervical facet syndrome, pain referring

from the spinal zygapophyseal (facet) joints. Pain referral patterns from cervical facet joints coincide with classic myofascial TrP at the suboccipital paraspinals, upper trapezius, and scapular regions. The diagnosis of cervical facet syndrome should be suspected in patients with degenerative changes in spine radiographs or other imaging studies, and in post-trauma cases, particularly if pain has been recurrent or refractory to treatment. Pain referral patterns associated with cervical nerve root irritation, impingement, or radiculopathy radiate into shoulder girdle muscles and into upper extremities depending upon the level and severity of involvement. Neck and shoulder girdle muscles may initially contract reflexively to splint or protect the region. The regional MP evolves secondary to sustained contraction. Pain in the cervicothoracic region can also occur with visceral disorders such as cardiac disease, gastric ulcer, gallstones, tumors, and metastatic lesions. Diagnostic evaluation should be considered in any patient with atypical or refractory pain.

Although challenges still exist with regard to muscle selection and optimal dose per injection site, successful outcomes hinge upon restoration of neutral biomechanics (Table 19.2). Myofascial

Table 19.2. Muscle selection guide for botulinum toxin therapy – based on a postural paradigm and forward head posture

Fingerbreadths	Primary pain	Secondary pain	Muscle selection
1	Suboccipital region	Upper trapezius	Semispinalis capitis Splenius capitis Upper trapezius
2	Upper trapezius	Levator scapulae	Upper trapezius Levator scapula ±Sp. capitis and Semi capitis
3	Inter-scapular muscles	Lower thoracic paraspinals	Pectoralis major Pectoralis minor Sternocleidomastoid
4	Cervicobrachial symptoms	Mid-back region	Anterior scalene Middle scalene Pectoralis major Pectoralis minor

pain can result from a failure of biomechanical balance, and disruption of the normal interactions of many tissues and structures. Restoring biomechanical balance and improving function by relieving associated pain may improve the effectiveness of rehabilitative efforts. As part of an overall long-term pain management strategy, BoNT can be combined with physical therapy to be more effective in minimizing pain over the long term as opposed to the sole use of analgesics. The rationale for combining BoNT therapy with physical treatments is based on evidence that muscle shortening increases spindle sensitivity and spasticity (Maier *et al.*, 1972; Williams, 1980; Gioux and Petit, 1993). Applying treatment to relax the muscle along with physical treatment should maximize the potential for muscle lengthening (Figure 19.8). Additionally, in contrast to pharmacotherapy, the lack of systemic effects associated with BoNT is especially important in patients actively participating in stretching and exercise programs.

Key issue: preservative-free normal saline should be used for reconstitution of BoNT-A (Botox). Bacterostatic saline can bind albumin and lead to decreased efficacy of BoNT therapy.

The injections are administered either unilaterally or bilaterally, distributing BoNT (varying

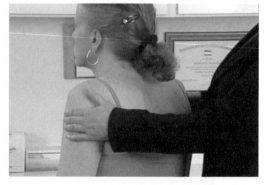

Figure 19.8 Botulinum toxin alone is inadequate for reduction of forward head posture. Patients should be instructed in regard to neutral spine positioning and scapulothoracic stabilization exercises.

doses) evenly throughout the mid-belly of surface muscles (Table 19.3).

A grid-like pattern is utilized for the upper trapezius (Figure 19.9), consisting of incremental injections at 1- to 2-cm intervals perpendicular to muscle fibers, and one or two sites longitudinally between the above to complete a grid. The injections should be confined to the medial half of the upper trapezius ridge, as more lateral injections can lead to weakness of shoulder elevation due to

Table 19.3. DOSING GUIDELINES FOR CERVICOTHORACIC MUSCLES: Unilateral dosing for BoNT-A (Botox) (25 U/cc Normal Saline)

Muscle	Dose* (U)	Comments
Semispinalis capitis	12.5 F; 25 M	Single injection site perpendicular to the muscle at the suboccipital region
Splenius capitis	12.5 F; 25 M	Single injection site perpendicular to the muscle at the apex of the posterior triangle
Upper trapezius	75 F; 100 M	Grid pattern: infiltrate 1 cc increments in two sites perpendicular and one to two sites longitudinal through muscle mid-belly
Levator scapulae	50	At the upper medial scapular border: infiltrate 1 cc perpendicular then angle cephalid to infiltrate 1 cc longitudinal to muscle fibers
Pectoralis major	25	Single injection site 3 fingerbreadths below the axillary fold, angled superomedially through the muscle
Pectoralis minor	25	Single injection site 3 fingerbreadths inferomedial to the midpoint of the deltopectoral groove, perpendicular to the muscle
Sternocleidomastoid	12.5 F; 25 M	Single injection site in the superior aspect of the muscle perpendicular to the muscle fibers
Anterior scalene	25	Anterior to posterior approach for anterior scalene; single injection site per muscle under EMG
Middle scalene	25	Lateral to medial approach for middle scalene; single injection site per muscle under EMG

Note:
*F = female; M = male; Note: Botox should be injected unilaterally or bilaterally (as warranted) based on whether or not chronic tension type headaches are unilateral or bilateral.

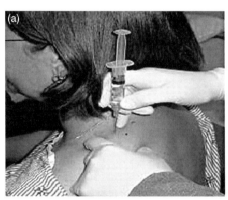 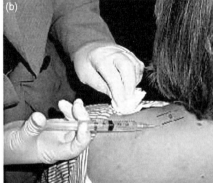

Figure 19.9 (a and b) Upper trapezius grid pattern injection technique (BoNT-A [Botox] 25 U/cc normal saline per injection site): the upper trapezius is injected using a grid pattern technique that has been previously described. This technique requires anatomical localization of the mid-belly of the upper trapezius along the medial half of the upper trapezius ridge. The mid-belly is infiltrated in a grid pattern at two sites perpendicular and one or two sites longitudinal to the muscle, using a 25 gauge 1.5 inch needle.

regional spread into the supraspinatus. The levator scapulae is infiltrated from one site, first perpendicular then longitudinal to muscle fibers. The splenius capitis and semispinalis capitis are each injected at a single site perpendicular to the muscle fibers. The splenius capitis is injected at the apex of the posterior cervical triangle where it is readily accessible as a surface muscle. The semispinalis

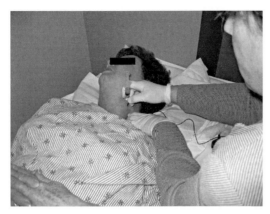

Figure 19.10 The anterior scalene is identified and infiltrated using EMG guidance. The muscle is approached in an anterior to posterior direction 3 cm above the clavicle, through the lateral border of the sternocleidomastoid, and activated by deep inspiration.

capitis lies beneath the upper trapezius at the base of the occiput. The injection site is located approximately 2 fingerbreadths below the occipital protuberance. Injection of the muscles in the interscapular region – rhomboids, middle and lower trapezius – should be avoided due to risk of destabilizing the scapulae. Target muscles in the cervicothoracic region may be identified and infiltrated using anatomical localization or EMG (Figure 19.10). Electromyographic localization of cervical muscles requires a disposable injectable insulated monopolar EMG needle electrode, commercially available in 26 gauge by 37 mm (1.5 inch), or other sufficient length to achieve the required depth for target muscles (Table 19.4; Figure 19.11).

Piriformis syndrome

Both BoNT-A and BoNT-B have been shown to improve pain associated with piriformis syndrome. The piriformis muscle can be identified in most cases under EMG guidance and infiltrated using a 100–120 mm injectable monopolar electrode needle (Figure 19.12). The piriformis is infiltrated close to the sacrum in the superomedial aspect

Table 19.4. Dosing adjustments

Clinical situation	Dosing adjustment
Small muscle bulk	Use lower end of dose ranges
Thoracic kyphosis	Avoid thoracic paraspinals
Hypermobility syndrome	Limit treatment to craniofacial regions if needed, and avoid cervical injections
COPD, asthma, apnea	Avoid scalenes injections
Upper and lower back treated simultaneously	Use lower doses in both regions
Repetitive reaching and lifting required	Use lower doses for cervicothoracic muscles
Repeat treatments	Re-evaluate target muscles and reduce doses if needed to avoid atrophy

Note:
Clinical considerations such as those above require special consideration and/or decrease in the BoNT dose by as much as 25–50%.

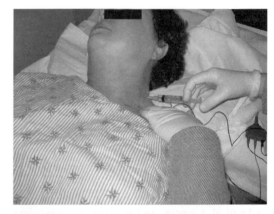

Figure 19.11 The middle scalene is identified and infiltrated using EMG guidance. The muscle is approached in a lateral to medial direction 3 cm above the clavicle, posterior to the lateral border of the sternocleidomastoid, and activated by deep inspiration.

of the muscle for maximal efficacy. Typical dosing for the piriformis muscle is 100 U BoNT-A (Botox) in 1–2 cc preservative-free normal saline; or 5000 U (1 cc) BoNT-B (NeuroBloc®/Myobloc®) injected without additional dilution.

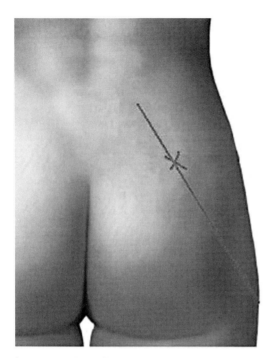

Figure 19.12 The piriformis muscle can be identified and infiltrated under EMG guidance using a 100–120 mm injectable monopolar electrode needle. The needle is infiltrated perpendicular to the muscle at a point marking the proximal third of a line drawn from the posterior superior iliac spine notch to the greater trochanter. The muscle is activated by external rotation of the ipsilateral foot.

Wong *et al.* (2005) evaluated BoNT-A in a randomized, double-blind, placebo-controlled trial of 60 patients with lateral epicondylitis. Following injection of 60 U of Botox, mean visual analog scale (VAS) scores decreased from 65.5 mm at baseline to 25.3 mm at 4 weeks, and at week 12, mean VAS scores were 23.5 mm for the Botox treated group compared to 43.5 mm for the placebo group (Wong *et al.*, 2005). A follow-up double-blind, randomized, controlled pilot study in 40 patients with chronic tennis elbow failed to show a net benefit in pain, quality of life or grip strength at 3 months post-injection (Hayton *et al.*, 2005). Twenty patients had been randomized to receive intramuscular injections of 50 U of Botox, administered 5 cm distal to the maximum point of tenderness at the

lateral epicondyle in line with the middle of the wrist (Hayton *et al.*, 2005). The differences in the outcomes between these two trials may be due to the smaller number of patients, lower doses of Botox used in the latter treatment protocol, and injection methodology. Patients should be informed that injections of BoNT for tennis elbow can result in transient weakness of finger extension.

Intra-articular pain

Anti-nociceptive effects of BoNT-A have been reported in non-muscle treatment models such as intra-articular injections for arthritis (Singh *et al.*, 2004a, b; Mahowald *et al.*, 2006). Singh *et al.* reported that injection of 50–100 U of BoNT-A decreased refractory shoulder pain in 6 frail elderly patients by $\geq 50\%$ in 7/9 injected joints, and improved active shoulder abduction and flexion without causing any regional weakness or other deleterious effects (Singh *et al.*, 2004a). Pain relief lasted 6–11 weeks. These authors also conducted a retrospective review of five patients injected with BoNT-A for refractory knee and/or ankle pain associated with moderate to severe rheumatoid arthritis (two patients), osteoarthritis (two patients), and psoriatic arthritis (one patient). Pain was reduced by 50% in 3/6 joints injected, and by 30% in 5/6 joints. Lower extremity function improved in four of the five patients. Double-blind studies for shoulder and knee injections are currently underway.

Phantom limb pain

Preliminary reports demonstrate efficacy of BoNT-A and BoNT-B in phantom limb pain of upper and lower extremity amputees (Kern *et al.*, 2004a, b, c). Improvements in pain resulted even from differing approaches to the injection of either regional muscles or painful soft tissues. Dosing ranges reported for phantom limb pain are 100 U for Botox or 2500–5000 U for BoNT-B (NeuroBloc/Myobloc) (Kern *et al.*, 2004a, b).

Conclusions

Botulinum toxin is emerging as an important addition to the pain treatment algorithms for neck and back pain due to its ability to sustain muscle relaxation. The patient whose evaluation rules out other non-muscular pain sources, and whose pain has failed other conservative treatments, may be an appropriate candidate for BoNT therapy.

Preclinical data supporting possible antinociceptive effects of BoNT are promising, and may open new pathways to the treatment of chronic pain that obviate the systemic risks inherent to traditional pharmacotherapies.

Successful treatment of neck and back pain with BoNT requires consideration of postural mechanics to guide muscle selection, adherence to recommended dosing guidelines and injection techniques, and patient education to incorporate neutral spine positioning into activities of daily living.

REFERENCES

Aoki, K. R. (2005). Review of a proposed mechanism for the antinociceptive action of botulinum toxin type A. *Neurotoxicology*, **26**, 785–93.

Benzon, H. T., Katz, J. A., Benzon, H. A. & Iqbal, M. S. (2003). Piriformis syndrome: anatomic considerations, a new injection technique, and a review of the literature. *Anesthesiology*, **98**, 1442–8.

Borg-Stein, J. & Simons, D. G. (2002). Focused review: myofascial pain. *Arch Phys Med Rehabil*, **83**, S40–7, S48–9.

Brashear, A., Lew, M. F., Dykstra, D. D., *et al.* (1999). Safety and efficacy of NeuroBloc (botulinum toxin type B) in type A-responsive cervical dystonia. *Neurology*, **53**, 1439–46.

Brin, M. F., Lew, M. F., Adler, C. H., *et al.* (1999). Safety and efficacy of NeuroBloc (botulinum toxin type B) in type A-resistant cervical dystonia. *Neurology*, **53**, 1431–8.

Calandre, E. P., Hidalgo, J., Garcia-Leiva, J. M. & Rico-Villademoros, F. (2006). Trigger point evaluation in migraine patients: an indication of peripheral sensitization linked to migraine predisposition? *Eur J Neurol*, **13**, 244–9.

Calillet, R. (1977). *Soft Tissue Pain and Disability*. Philadelphia: FA Davis Co.

Carter, J. E. (1998). Surgical treatment for chronic pelvic pain. *JSLS*, **2**, 129–39.

Cheshire, W. P., Abashian, S. W. & Mann, J. D. (1994). Botulinum toxin in the treatment of myofascial pain syndrome. *Pain*, **59**, 65–9.

Darlow, L. A., Pesco, J. & Greenberg, M. S. (1987). The relationship of posture to myofascial pain dysfunction syndrome. *J Am Dent Assoc*, **114**, 73–5.

De Andres, J., Cerda-Olmedo, G., Valia, J. C., *et al.* (2003). Use of botulinum toxin in the treatment of chronic myofascial pain. *Clin J Pain*, **19**, 269–75.

Dorsher, P. (2006). Trigger points and acupuncture points. *Acupunct Med*, **17**, 21–5.

Durette, M. R., Rodriquez, A. A., Agre, J. C. & Silverman, J. L. (1991). Needle electromyographic evaluation of patients with myofascial or fibromyalgic pain. *Am J Phys Med Rehabil*, **70**, 154–6.

Durham, P. L., Cady, R. & Cady, R. (2004). Regulation of calcitonin gene-related peptide secretion from trigeminal nerve cells by botulinum toxin type A: implications for migraine therapy. *Headache*, **44**, 35–42; discussion 42–3.

Fernandez-de-las-Penas, C., Alonso-Blanco, C., Cuadrado, M. L. & Pareja, J. A. (2006). Forward head posture and neck mobility in chronic tension-type headache: a blinded, controlled study. *Cephalalgia*, **26**, 314–19.

Ferrante, F. M., Bearn, L., Rothrock, R. & King, L. (2005). Evidence against trigger point injection technique for the treatment of cervicothoracic myofascial pain with botulinum toxin type A. *Anesthesiology*, **103**, 377–83.

Foster, L., Clapp, L., Erickson, M. & Jabbari, B. (2001). Botulinum toxin A and chronic low back pain: a randomized, double-blind study. *Neurology*, **56**, 1290–3.

Frost, F. A., Jessen, B. & Siggaard-Andersen, J. (1980). A control, double-blind comparison of mepivacaine injection versus saline injection for myofascial pain. *Lancet*, **1**, 499–500.

Gerwin, R. D., Shannon, S., Hong, C. Z., Hubbard, D. & Gevirtz, R. (1997). Interrater reliability in myofascial trigger point examination. *Pain*, **69**, 65–73.

Gilio, F., Curra, A., Lorenzano, C., *et al.* (2000). Effects of botulinum toxin type A on intracortical inhibition in patients with dystonia. *Ann Neurol*, **48**, 20–6.

Gioux, M. & Petit, J. (1993). Effects of immobilizing the cat peroneus longus muscle on the activity of its own spindles. *J Appl Physiol*, **75**, 2629–35.

Gobel, H., Heinze, A., Reichel, G., Hefter, H. & Benecke, R. (2006). Efficacy and safety of a single botulinum type A toxin complex treatment (Dysport) for the relief of upper back myofascial pain syndrome: results from a randomized double-blind placebo-controlled multicentre study. *Pain*, **125**, 82–8.

Graff-Radford, S. B. (2004). Myofascial pain: diagnosis and management. *Curr Pain Headache Rep*, **8**, 463–7.

Greenfield, B., Catlin, P. A., Coats, P. W., *et al.* (1995). Posture in patients with shoulder overuse injuries and healthy individuals. *J Orthop Sports Phys Ther*, **21**, 287–95.

Griegel-Morris, P., Larson, K., Mueller-Klaus, K. & Oatis, C. A. (1992). Incidence of common postural abnormalities in the cervical, shoulder, and thoracic regions and their association with pain in two age groups of healthy subjects. *Phys Ther*, **72**, 425–31.

Haughie, L. J., Liebert, I. M. & Roach, K. E. (1995). Relationship of forward head posture and cervical backward bending to neck pain. *J Man Manip Ther*, **3**, 91–7.

Hayton, M. J., Santini, A. J., Hughes, P. J., *et al.* (2005). Botulinum toxin injection in the treatment of tennis elbow. A double-blind, randomized, controlled, pilot study. *J Bone Joint Surg Am*, **87**, 503–7.

Hong, C. Z. & Simons, D. G. (1998). Pathophysiologic and electrophysiologic mechanisms of myofascial trigger points. *Arch Phys Med Rehabil*, **79**, 863–72.

Jabbari, B. (2007). Treatment of chronic low back pain with botulinum neurotoxins. *Curr Pain Headache Rep*, **11**, 352–8.

Jabbari, B., Ney, J., Sichani, A., *et al.* (2006). Treatment of refractory, chronic low back pain with botulinum neurotoxin A: an open-label, pilot study. *Pain Med*, **7**, 260–4.

Kern, U., Martin, C., Scheicher, S. & Muller, H. (2004a). Does botulinum toxin A make prosthesis use easier for amputees? *J Rehabil Med*, **36**, 238–9.

Kern, U., Martin, C., Scheicher, S. & Muller, H. (2004b). Effects of botulinum toxin type B on stump pain and involuntary movements of the stump. *Am J Phys Med Rehabil*, **83**, 396–9.

Kern, U., Martin, C., Scheicher, S. & Muller, H. (2004c). [Long-term treatment of phantom- and stump pain with Botulinum toxin type A over 12 months. A first clinical observation]. *Nervenarzt*, **75**, 336–40.

Lang, A. M. (2000). A pilot study of botulinum toxin type A (BOTOX), administered using a novel injection technique, for the treatment of myofascial pain. *Am J Pain Manage*, **10**, 108–12.

Lang, A. M. (2002). Botulinum toxin therapy for myofascial pain disorders. *Curr Pain Headache Rep*, **6**, 355–60.

Lang, A. M. (2003). Botulinum toxin type A therapy in chronic pain disorders. *Arch Phys Med Rehabil*, **84**, S69–73; quiz S74–5.

Lang, A. M. (2004). Botulinum toxin type B in piriformis syndrome. *Am J Phys Med Rehabil*, **83**, 198–202.

Mahowald, M. L., Singh, J. A. & Dykstra, D. (2006). Long term effects of intra-articular botulinum toxin A for refractory joint pain. *Neurotox Res*, **9**, 179–88.

Maier, A., Eldred, E. & Edgerton, V. R. (1972). The effects on spindles of muscle atrophy and hypertrophy. *Exp Neurol*, **37**, 100–23.

McPartland, J. M. (2004). Travell trigger points–molecular and osteopathic perspectives. *J Am Osteopath Assoc*, **104**, 244–9.

Mennell, J. M. (1992). *The Musculoskeletal System: Differential Diagnosis from Symptoms and Physical Signs*. Gaithersburg, Maryland: Aspen Publishers, Inc.

Porta, M. (2000). A comparative trial of botulinum toxin type A and methylprednisolone for the treatment of myofascial pain syndrome and pain from chronic muscle spasm. *Pain*, **85**, 101–5.

Simons, D. G. (2004). Review of enigmatic MTrPs as a common cause of enigmatic musculoskeletal pain and dysfunction. *J Electromyogr Kinesiol*, **14**, 95–107.

Simons, D. G., Travell, J. G. & Simons, L. (1999). *Travell and Simons' Myofascial Pain and Dysfunction: The Trigger Point Manual, Vol. 1. Upper Half of Body 2nd edn.*, Baltimore: Lippincott Williams & Wilkins.

Singh, J., Mahowald, M. & Dykstra, D. (2004a). Intra-articular botulinum A toxin for chronic shoulder pain in the elderly. *J Invest Med*, **52**, S380.

Singh, J., Mahowald, M. & Dykstra, D. (2004b). Report on intraarticular botulinum toxin type A for refractory joint pain. *J Pain*, **5**, S60.

Welch, M. J., Purkiss, J. R. & Foster, K. A. (2000). Sensitivity of embryonic rat dorsal root ganglia neurons to Clostridium botulinum neurotoxins. *Toxicon*, **38**, 245–58.

Wheeler, A. H., Goolkasian, P. & Gretz, S. S. (1998). A randomized, double-blind, prospective pilot study of botulinum toxin injection for refractory, unilateral, cervicothoracic, paraspinal, myofascial pain syndrome. *Spine*, **23**, 1662–6; discussion 1667.

Williams, R. (1980). Sensitivity changes shown by spindle receptors in chronically immobilized skeletal muscle. *J Physiol*, **306**, 26P–7P.

Wong, S. M., Hui, A. C., Tong, P. Y., *et al.* (2005). Treatment of lateral epicondylitis with botulinum toxin: a randomized, double-blind, placebo-controlled trial. *Ann Intern Med*, **143**, 793–7.

20

The use of botulinum toxin in the management of headache disorders

Stephen D. Silberstein

Summary of clinical aspects of headache disorders

Headache affects over 45 million individuals in the United States, which makes it one of the most common nervous system disorders (NINDS, 2002). The International Headache Society (IHS) classifies primary headache disorders as those in which headache itself is the illness, with no other etiology diagnosed. Examples include migraine and tension-type headache (TTH) (IHS, 2004). Headache disorders can be further classified as episodic (< 15 headache days per month) or chronic (≥ 15 headache days per month for more than 3 months) (IHS, 2004).

Migraine is a progressive debilitating disorder characterized by enhanced sensitivity of the nervous system (Silberstein, 2000); it is associated with a combination of neurological, gastrointestinal, and autonomic disturbances (Silberstein, 2004). The IHS diagnostic criteria for this condition includes headache associated with at least two of the following: unilateral location, pulsating quality, moderate or severe pain intensity, and aggravation by or causing avoidance of routine physical activities; at least one of the following during headache: nausea and/or vomiting, photophobia, and phonophobia; and headache not attributable to another disorder (IHS, 2004). It is estimated that 28 million Americans, including 18% of women and 7% of men, are afflicted with severe, disabling migraines

(Lipton et al., 2001). The World Health Organization (WHO) ranks migraine as one of the world's most disabling illnesses, profoundly impacting quality of life, causing functional impairment, and disruption of household or social activities (WHO, 2004).

Chronic daily headache (CDH) is a heterogeneous group of headache disorders that can include chronic migraine, chronic TTH (CTTH), and other headache types that occur 15 days or more per month in the absence of structural or systemic disease (Silberstein et al., 2005) and affects 4% to 5% of the general population worldwide (Scher et al., 1998; Castillo et al., 1999; Wang et al., 2000). Patients with CDH often overuse acute headache medications (Silberstein et al., 2005) and have greater disability and lower quality of life than patients with episodic headache (Meletiche et al., 2001; Bigal et al., 2003).

Tension-type headache is the most common of the primary headache disorders, with an annual prevalence as high as 38% (Schwartz et al., 1998). It is associated with bilateral pain that is pressing or tightening in quality and mild to moderate in intensity. It is not associated with nausea/vomiting or routine physical activity but may be associated with photophobia or phonophobia (IHS, 2004). Frequent episodic (at least ten episodes occurring on ≥ 1 but < 15 days per month) or chronic (≥ 15 days per month) TTH is associated with greatly decreased quality of life and high disability (Schwartz et al., 1998; IHS, 2004).

Manual of Botulinum Toxin Therapy, ed. Daniel Truong, Dirk Dressler and Mark Hallett. Published by Cambridge University Press. © Cambridge University Press 2009.

Pathophysiology of headache disorders

Migraine is believed to arise from activation of blood vessel nociceptors, along with a change in central pain modulation mediated by the trigeminal system (Silberstein, 2004). In response to stimulation of the trigeminal sensory neurons, perivascular nerve fibers that innervate blood vessels release peptide mediators, neurokinin A, substance P, and calcitonin gene-related peptide (CGRP), which transmit nociceptive activity to the brain stem autonomic nuclei via glutamate-mediated transduction (see Figure 20.1). The trigeminovascular system can be activated by cortical spreading depression, a process characterized by shifts in cortical steady state potential; transient increases in potassium, nitric oxide, and glutamate; and transient increases followed by sustained decreases in cortical blood flow (see Figure 20.2) (Silberstein, 2004). Trigeminal activation results in release of vasoactive peptide-producing neurogenic inflammation, vasodilation, and sensitization of nerve fibers, and, ultimately, pain and associated symptoms (Silberstein, 2004). Migraine pain is likely a result of the combination of activation of pain-producing intracranial structures and reduction in endogenous pain control pathways (Silberstein *et al.*, 2001; Silberstein, 2004).

The pathophysiology underlying TTH is not well understood (WHO, 2004). The relative contributions of peripheral and central pain mechanisms to TTH remain unclear (Silberstein *et al.*, 2006).

Treatment of headache

Acute (abortive) migraine treatments, which patients take at the time of occurrence, in an attempt to relieve pain and disability and prevent progression, include migraine-specific medications, such as ergots or triptans, and non-specific agents, such as analgesics or opioids (Silberstein, 2004). Patients with acute TTH typically self-medicate with over-the-counter analgesics, such as aspirin, acetaminophen, or non-steroidal anti-inflammatory drugs (NSAIDs), which could lead to drug overuse.

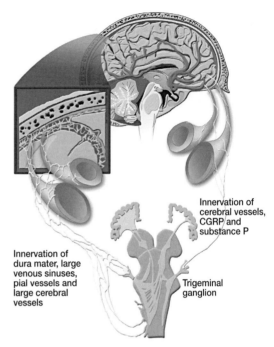

Innervation of cerebral vessels, CGRP and substance P

Innervation of dura mater, large venous sinuses, pial vessels and large cerebral vessels

Trigeminal ganglion

Figure 20.1 Craniovascular innervation. Reproduced with permission from Silberstein, S. D., Lipton, R. B. & Dalessio, D. J. (2001). *Wolff's Headache and Other Head Pain*, 7th edn. New York: Oxford University Press, pp. 6–26; 57–72.

Prescription NSAIDs or combination analgesics may also be used.

Preventive treatments are designed to reduce the frequency, severity, or duration of migraine attacks. These are indicated when acute medications are ineffective or overused, or headaches are very frequent or disabling (Silberstein, 2004). Preventive agents include beta-adrenergic blockers, antidepressants, calcium channel and serotonin antagonists, anticonvulsants, and NSAIDs (Silberstein, 2004).

While daily, oral prophylactic treatments have proven effective, issues such as lack of compliance with daily dosing regimens and adverse effects have limited their usefulness (Blumenfeld *et al.*, 2003; Silberstein, 2004) and resulted in looking for other modalities and agents, including botulinum toxins (botulinum neurotoxins; BoNTs), as potential preventive treatments.

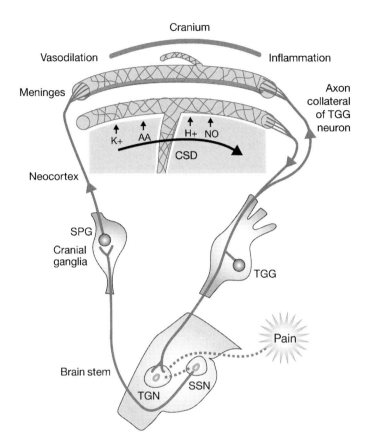

Figure 20.2 Cortical spreading depression. K+ = potassium ions; AA = arachidonic acid; H+ = hydrogen ions; NO = nitric oxide; CSD = cortical spreading depression; TGG = trigeminal ganglion; SPG = sphenopalatine ganglion; TGN = trigeminal nucleus; SSN = superior sagittal sinus. Reproduced with permission from Silberstein, S. D. (2004). Migraine. *The Lancet*, **363**, 381–91.

Mechanism of action of botulinum toxin in headache

The association between botulinum toxin type A (BoNT-A) use and the alleviation of migraine headache symptoms was discovered during initial clinical trials of BoNT-A treatment for hyperfunctional lines of the face (Binder *et al.*, 2000). While the precise mechanisms by which BoNT-A alleviates headache pain are unclear, evidence that it inhibits the release of glutamate and the neuropeptides, substance P and CGRP, from nociceptive neurons suggests that its anti-nociceptive properties are distinct from its neuromuscular activity (Dodick *et al.*, 2005). It is possible that BoNT-A inhibits central sensitization of trigeminovascular neurons, which is believed to be key to the

development and maintenance of migraine (Dodick *et al.*, 2005).

Treatment guidelines

Selecting candidates for BoNT therapy begins with accurately diagnosing and classifying the patient's headache type based on his or her medical history. Botulinum toxin type A therapy may be most appropriate for patients whose disabling headaches interfere with their daily routines despite acute therapy, or for patients who cannot tolerate other preventive strategies. Table 20.1 lists characteristics of headache patients who may be candidates for BoNT-A therapy. Its use is contraindicated for patients with sensitivity to toxins or with neuromuscular

Table 20.1. Candidates for botulinum toxin type A (BoNT-A) therapy for headache

- Patients with disabling primary headaches
- Patients who have failed to respond adequately to conventional treatments
- Patients with unacceptable side effects (from existing treatment)
- Patients in whom standard preventive treatments are contraindicated
- Patients in special populations or situations (the elderly, those at risk of unacceptable side effects from trial drugs or traditional treatments, airplane pilots, students studying and preparing for examinations)
- Patients misusing or abusing or overusing medications
- Patients with coexistent jaw, head, or neck muscle spasm
- Patients who prefer this treatment

Source: Used with permission from Blumenfeld, A. M., Binder, W., Silberstein, S. D. & Blitzer, A. (2003). Procedures for administering botulinum toxin type A for migraine and tension-type headache. *Headache*, **43**, 884–91.

disorders, such as myasthenia gravis (Blumenfeld *et al.*, 2003).

BoNT treatment techniques

Sterile technique should be observed for the entire BoNT injection procedure. Injections do not have to be intramuscular, but we use the muscles as reference sites for injections, which are most commonly administered in the glabellar and frontal regions, the temporalis muscle, the occipitalis muscle, and the cervical paraspinal region (see Figure 20.3).

The injection protocols commonly used are: (1) the fixed-site approach, which uses fixed, symmetrical injection sites and a range of predetermined doses; (2) the follow-the-pain approach, which adjusts the sites and doses depending on where the patient feels pain and where the examiner can elicit pain and tenderness on palpation of the muscle and often employs asymmetrical injections; and (3) a combination approach, using injections at fixed frontal sites, supplemented with follow-the-pain injections (this approach typically

uses higher doses of BoNT-A) (Blumenfeld *et al.*, 2003). Table 20.2 lists recommended anatomical sites of injection for headache and the BoNT (Botox®) dose per site, other formulations may also be used although experience is lacking.

Clinical comparison of efficacy of BoNT in headache disorders

Most studies on the efficacy and safety of BoNT in headache treatment have used Botox. No large, well-controlled studies using other preparations have been published. The following discussion will focus on relevant studies with Botox. Although originally thought to be efficacious, more recent data are not confirmatory. Hence, this therapy cannot be recommended on a routine basis. Selected patients may respond, but the rules for identifying such patients are not yet clear. Clinical trial results discussed below are summarized in Table 20.3.

Some studies support the efficacy of Botox in migraine treatment. A double-blind, vehicle-controlled trial of 123 patients with moderate to severe migraine found that subjects treated with a single injection of 25 mouse units (U) Botox (but not those treated with 75 U) showed significantly fewer migraine attacks per month, as well as reductions in migraine severity, number of days requiring acute medication, and incidence of migraine-induced vomiting (Silberstein *et al.*, 2000). The lack of significant effect in the higher-dose group may be related to baseline group differences, e.g., fewer migraines or a longer time since onset of migraine in the higher-dose group (Silberstein *et al.*, 2000). Another double-blind, placebo-controlled, region-specific study found a significant reduction in migraine pain among patients who received simultaneous injections of Botox in the frontal and temporal regions, as well as an overall trend toward Botox superiority to placebo in reducing migraine frequency and duration (Brin *et al.*, 2000). A randomized, double-blind, placebo-controlled study compared the efficacy of placebo, 16 U Botox, and 100 U Botox as migraine prophylaxis when injected into the frontal and neck muscles (Evers *et al.*,

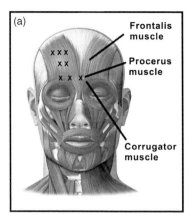

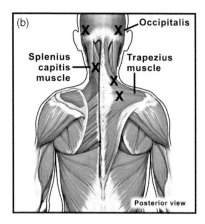

Figure 20.3 Injection site locations for headache treatment. (a) Glabellar and frontal muscles, (b) Occipital and suboccipital muscles, (c) Temporalis muscle. Reproduced with permission from Nucleus Medical Art. Copyright © 2003. All rights reserved. www.nucleusinc.com.

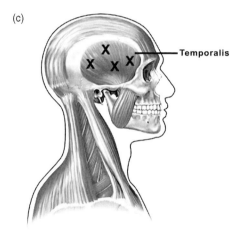

2004). While there were no statistically significant differences in reduction of migraine frequency among the groups, the accompanying symptoms of migraine were reduced in the 16 U Botox group (Evers *et al.*, 2004).

However, more recent studies have failed to demonstrate significant improvements over placebo. One such study of patients (N = 232) with moderate to severe episodic (4–8 episodes/month) migraine compared placebo to regional (frontal, temporal, or glabellar) or combined (frontal/temporal/glabellar) treatment with Botox (Saper *et al.*, 2007). Reductions from baseline in migraine frequency, maximum severity, and duration occurred with Botox and placebo, but there were no significant between-group

differences (Saper *et al.*, 2007). Elkind *et al.* conducted a series of 3 sequential studies of 418 patients with a history of 4–8 moderate to severe migraines per month with re-randomization at each stage and Botox doses ranging from 7.5 to 50 U (Elkind *et al.*, 2006). Botox and placebo produced comparable decreases from baseline in migraine frequency at each time-point examined, with no consistent, statistically significant, between-group differences observed (Elkind *et al.*, 2006).

In the treatment of CDH, several randomized, double-blind, placebo-controlled studies support the efficacy of BoNT. In a large, placebo-controlled study (N = 355), Mathew *et al.* found that while Botox did not differ from placebo in the primary

Table 20.2. Anatomical sites of injection and botulinum toxin type A (BoNT-A; Botox) dose

Muscle	BoNT-A U/Site	Number of injection sites
Procerus*	2.5–5.0	1
Corrugator*	2.5	2 (1 per side)
Medial	2.5	2 (1 per side)
Lateral	2.5	2 (1 per side)
Frontalis*	2.5–5.0	2–4 per side
Temporalis*	2.5–5.0	8–10
		(4–5 per side)
Occipitalis[†]	2.5–5.0	2 (1 per side)
Splenius capitis area*[†]	2.5–5.0	2 per side
Masseter[†]	2.5–5.0	1–2
Trapezius[†]	2.5–5.0	2–8
		(1–4 per side)
Sternocleidomastoid[†]	2.5–5.0	2
Cervical paraspinal muscles[†]	2.5–5.0	1–3 per side

Note:
*For fixed-site or follow-the-trigeminal-nerve protocol; injections should be bilateral.
[†]For follow-the-pain protocol; injections may be unilateral or bilateral, depending on signs and symptoms.
Source: Adapted from Blumenfeld, A. M., Binder, W., Silberstein, S. D. & Blitzer, A. (2003). Procedures for administering botulinum toxin type A for migraine and tension-type headache. *Headache,* **43**, 884–91.

efficacy measure (change from baseline in headache-free days at day 180), there were significant differences in several secondary end points, including a greater percentage of patients with ≥50% decrease in headache frequency and a greater mean change from baseline in headache frequency at day 180 (Mathew *et al.*, 2005). A subgroup analysis of patients not taking concomitant preventive agents (N = 228) found that Botox patients had a greater decrease in headache frequency compared with placebo after two and three injections, and at most time-points from day 180 to 270 (Dodick *et al.*, 2005). In a similar study (N = 702) by Silberstein *et al.*, which utilized several doses of Botox (75, 150, 225 U), the primary efficacy end point (mean

improvement from baseline in headache frequency at day 180) was also not met (Silberstein *et al.*, 2005). However, all groups responded to treatment, and patients taking 150 and 225 U of Botox had a greater decrease in headache frequency than placebo at day 240 (Silberstein *et al.*, 2005).

Studies evaluating the efficacy of Botox in CTTH have been inconsistent. A double-blind, randomized, placebo-controlled study of 300 patients found that while all treatment groups, including placebo, improved at day 60 in mean change from baseline in CTTH-free days per month (primary end point), Botox did not demonstrate improvement compared with placebo at any dose or regimen (50–150 U) (Silberstein *et al.*, 2006). However, a significantly greater percentage of patients in three Botox groups at day 90 and two Botox groups at day 120 had ≥ 50% decrease in CTTH days than the placebo group (Silberstein *et al.*, 2006). Furthermore, a review evaluating clinical studies of TTH supports the benefit of BoNT-A in reducing frequency and severity of headaches, improving quality of life and disability scales, and reducing the need for acute medication (Mathew & Kaup, 2002), while another review, which also included studies with both Botox and Dysport®, concluded that randomized, double-blind, placebo-controlled trials present contradictory results attributable to variable doses, injection sites, and frequency of treatment (Rozen & Sharma, 2006).

Adverse events associated with boNT use

More than two decades of clinical use have established BoNT-A as a safe drug (Mauskop, 2004) with no systemic reactions in clinical trials for headache. Rash and flu-like symptoms can rarely occur as a result of an allergic reaction (Mauskop, 2004). However, serious allergic reactions have never been reported. Injection of anterior neck muscles can cause dysphagia (swallowing difficulties) in some patients (Mauskop, 2004). Dysphagia and dry mouth appear to be more common with injections of BoNT-B (NeuroBloc®/Myobloc®) because of its wider migration pattern (Mauskop, 2004). The most

Table 20.3. Summary of randomized, double-blind, controlled studies of the efficacy of botulinum toxin type A (Botox) in the treatment of headache

Headache type	Study outcome
Migraine	
Silberstein *et al.*, 2000	• Decreased migraine frequency and severity and acute medication use with Botox 25 U but not with Botox 75 U
Brin *et al.*, 2000	• Decreased migraine pain compared with PBO with simultaneous frontal and temporal BoNT-A injections
Evers *et al.*, 2004	• No difference from PBO in decreased frequency of migraine • Greater decrease in migraine-associated symptoms with Botox 16 U
Saper *et al.*, 2007	• Decreased frequency and severity of migraine in Botox and PBO groups with no between-group differences
Elkind *et al.*, 2006	• Comparable decreases in migraine frequency in both Botox and PBO groups with no between-group differences
Chronic daily headache of migraine type	
Mathew *et al.*, 2005	• No difference from PBO on primary efficacy end point – change in headache-free days from baseline at day 180 • A significantly higher percentage of Botox patients had a $\geq 50\%$ decrease in headache days/month at day 180 compared with PBO
Dodick *et al.*, 2005	• Greater decrease in headache frequency after two and three injections compared with PBO
Silberstein *et al.*, 2005	• No difference from PBO on primary efficacy end point – change in headache frequency from baseline at day 180 • Greater decrease in headache frequency for Botox 225 U and 150 U than PBO
Chronic tension-type headache	
Silberstein *et al.*, 2006	• No difference from PBO on primary efficacy end point – mean change from baseline in CTTH headache days • Greater percentage of Botox patients than PBO with $\geq 50\%$ reduction in headache frequency at 90 and 120 days for several doses of Botox

Note:
PBO = placebo.

common side effects when treating facial muscles are cosmetic and include ptosis or asymmetry of the position of the eyebrows (Mauskop, 2004). Another possible, but rare, side effect is difficulty in holding the head erect because of neck muscle weakness (Mauskop, 2004). Headache patients occasionally develop a headache following the injection procedure, although some have immediate relief of an acute attack. The latter is most likely due to trigger point injection effect (Mauskop, 2004). Worsening of headaches and neck pain can occur and last for several days or, rarely, weeks after the injections because of the irritating effect of the

needling and delay in the muscle relaxing effect of BoNT (Mauskop, 2004).

Summary

Headache disorders, including migraine, CDH, and TTH, are common debilitating conditions that profoundly impact quality of life. Existing preventive and acute pharmacotherapies, which may provide some relief to headache sufferers, vary in efficacy and may be associated with adverse events. Overuse and abuse of abortive pharmacotherapies is an important problem in managing these conditions and should be avoided. Clinical studies suggest that, in addition to its therapeutic benefit in disorders characterized by muscle hyperactivity, BoNT-A is a safe treatment and may be efficacious for the prevention of some forms of episodic and chronic headache, including migraine and CDH. Further research is needed to understand the mechanism of action of BoNT-A in headache, further establish its safety and efficacy for these indications, and fully develop its therapeutic potential.

REFERENCES

Bigal, M. E., Rapoport, A. M., Lipton, R. B., Tepper, S. J. & Sheftell, F. D. (2003). Assessment of migraine disability using the migraine disability assessment (MIDAS) questionnaire: a comparison of chronic migraine with episodic migraine. *Headache*, **43**, 336–42.

Binder, W. J., Brin, M. F., Blitzer, A., Schoenrock, L. D. & Pogoda, J. M. (2000). Botulinum toxin type A (BOTOX) for treatment of migraine headaches: an open-label study. *Otolaryngol Head Neck Surg*, **123**, 669–76.

Blumenfeld, A. M., Binder, W., Silberstein, S. D. & Blitzer, A. (2003). Procedures for administering botulinum toxin type A for migraine and tension-type headache. *Headache*, **43**, 884–91.

Brin, M. F., Swope, D. M., O'Brien, C., Abbasi, S. & Pogoda, J. M. (2000). Botox® for migraine: double-blind, placebo-controlled, region-specific evaluation. *Cephalalgia*, **20**, 421–7.

Castillo, J., Munoz, P., Guitera, V. & Pascual, J. (1999). Epidemiology of chronic daily headache in the general population. *Headache*, **39**, 190–6.

Dodick, D. W., Mauskop, A., Elkind, A. H., *et al.* (2005). Botulinum toxin type a for the prophylaxis of chronic daily headache: subgroup analysis of patients not receiving other prophylactic medications: a randomized double-blind, placebo-controlled study. *Headache*, **45**, 315–24.

Elkind, A. H., O'Carroll, P., Blumenfeld, A., Degryse, R. & Dimitrova, R. (2006). A series of three sequential, randomized, controlled studies of repeated treatments with botulinum toxin type A for migraine prophylaxis. *J Pain*, **7**, 688–96.

Evers, S., Vollmer-Haase, J., Schwaag, S., *et al.* (2004). Botulinum toxin A in the prophylactic treatment of migraine–a randomized, double-blind, placebo-controlled study. *Cephalalgia*, **24**, 838–43.

International Headache Society (IHS) Headache Classification Subcommittee. (2004). The international classification of headache disorders: 2nd edition. *Cephalalgia*, **24**(Suppl 1), 1–160.

Lipton, R. B., Stewart, W. F., Diamond, S., Diamond, M. L. & Reed, M. (2001). Prevalence and burden of migraine in the United States: data from the American Migraine Study II. *Headache*, **41**, 646–57.

Mathew, N. T. & Kaup, A. O. (2002). The use of botulinum toxin type A in headache treatment. *Curr Treat Options Neurol*, **4**, 365–73.

Mathew, N. T., Frishberg, B. M., Gawel, M., *et al.* (2005). Botulinum toxin type A (BOTOX) for the prophylactic treatment of chronic daily headache: a randomized, double-blind, placebo-controlled trial. *Headache*, **45**, 293–307.

Mauskop, A. (2004). The use of botulinum toxin in the treatment of headaches. *Pain Physician*, **7**, 377–87.

Meletiche, D. M., Lofland, J. H. & Young, W. B. (2001). Quality-of-life differences between patients with episodic and transformed migraine. *Headache*, **41**, 573–8.

National Institute of Neurological Disorders and Stroke (NINDS) (2002). *Headache: Hope Through Research.* Bethesda, MD: US Department of Health and Human Services, National Institutes of Health; NIH publication 02–158.

Rozen, D. & Sharma, J. (2006). Treatment of tension-type headache with botox: a review of the literature. *Mt Sinai J Med*, **73**, 493–8.

Saper, J. R., Mathew, N. T., Loder, E. W., Degryse, R. & Vandenburgh, A. M. (2007). A double-blind, randomized, placebo-controlled comparison of botulinum toxin type a injection sites and doses in the prevention of episodic migraine. *Pain Med*, **8**, 478–85.

Scher, A. I., Stewart, W. F., Liberman, J. & Lipton, R. B. (1998). Prevalence of frequent headache in a population sample. *Headache*, **38**, 497–506.

Schwartz, B. S., Stewart, W. F., Simon, D. & Lipton, R. B. (1998). Epidemiology of tension-type headache. *JAMA*, **279**, 381–3.

Silberstein, S. D. (2000). Practice parameter: evidence-based guidelines for migraine headache (an evidence-based review): report of the Quality Standards Subcommittee of the American Academy of Neurology. *Neurology*, **55**, 754–62.

Silberstein, S. D. (2004). Migraine. *Lancet*, **363**, 381–91.

Silberstein, S., Mathew, N., Saper, J. & Jenkins, S. (2000). Botulinum toxin type A as a migraine preventive treatment. For the BOTOX Migraine Clinical Research Group. *Headache*, **40**, 445–50.

Silberstein, S. D., Lipton, R. B. & Dalessio, D. J. (2001). *Wolff's Headache and Other Head Pain*. New York: Oxford University Press.

Silberstein, S. D., Stark, S. R., Lucas, S. M., *et al.* (2005). Botulinum toxin type A for the prophylactic treatment of chronic daily headache: a randomized, double-blind, placebo-controlled trial. *Mayo Clin Proc*, **80**, 1126–37.

Silberstein, S. D., Gobel, H., Jensen, R., *et al.* (2006). Botulinum toxin type A in the prophylactic treatment of chronic tension-type headache: a multicentre, double-blind, randomized, placebo-controlled, parallel-group study. *Cephalalgia*, **26**, 790–800.

Wang, S. J., Fuh, J. L., Lu, S. R., *et al.* (2000). Chronic daily headache in Chinese elderly: prevalence, risk factors, and biannual follow-up. *Neurology*, **54**, 314–9.

World Health Organization (WHO) (2004). Headache disorders. Fact sheet No. 277, Available at: www.who.int/mediacentre/factsheets/fs277/en/print.html. Accessed January 8, 2007.

21

Treatment of plantar fasciitis with botulinum toxin

Bahman Jabbari and Mary S. Babcock

Introduction

Plantar fasciitis (PF) is the most common cause of chronic heel pain and is a major health issue in runners and long-distance walkers. Overuse injury may lead to repetitive micro-tears of the plantar fascia near the calcaneus, irritating pain fibers and producing secondary inflammation. Other risk factors include obesity, flat or over arched feet, and improper shoes. The pain usually involves the inferior and medial aspect of the heel (calcaneus), at the medial aspect of the calcaneal tubercle. However, the entire course of the plantar fascia may be involved (Barrett & O'Malley, 1999). Patients describe pain variably as aching, jabbing or burning. In many patients, the application of ice and/or use of heel cup orthosis activity modification and a stretching/strengthening exercise program reduces the pain satisfactorily. Further measures include deep-tissue massage therapy, night splints, and periods of immobilization. Persistent cases may respond to treatment with posterior night splints, ultrasound, iontophoresis, phonophoresis, extracorporeal shock wave therapy (ECSWT), or even local corticosteroid injections (DeMaio et al., 1993). In cases of medical failures, surgery is advocated, with modest results. Approximately 10–12% of the patients fail to achieve pain relief from medical and/or surgical treatment.

Anatomy of the plantar fascia

The plantar fascia is composed of dense collagen fibers that extend longitudinally from the calcaneus to the base of each proximal phalanx (Figure 21.1a). The fascia has medial, central, and lateral parts, underneath which the flexor digitorum brevis (FDB) and the abductor hallucis (AH) muscles reside (Figure 21.1b). The plantar fascia serves to anchor muscles and tendons on the concave surface of the sole and digits, facilitates excursion of the tendons, prevents excessive compression of digital vessels and nerves, and may even aid in venous return (Bannister et al., 1995). The central band of the plantar fascia, AH, and FDB attach to the medial calcaneal tubercle, the site of most pain in PF. Anatomic changes described in PF include marked thickening of the plantar fascia (seen on sonographic studies) (Akfirat et al., 2003), micro-tears related to repeated trauma, and secondary inflammation. The pain may be due to one or more of the following mechanisms: mechanical irritation of pain fibers by plantar fascia thickened from repeated trauma, ischemic pain from chronic pressure of a thickened fascia against digital vessels, and an enhanced reaction to a local pain neurotransmitter/chemical found in the inflammatory response (such as substance P or glutamate). Furthermore, like any other chronic pain condition,

Manual of Botulinum Toxin Therapy, ed. Daniel Truong, Dirk Dressler and Mark Hallett. Published by Cambridge University Press.
© Cambridge University Press 2009.

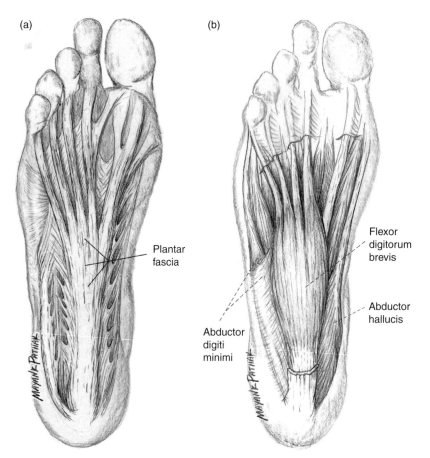

(a)

(b)

Plantar
fascia

Abductor
digiti
minimi

Flexor
digitorum
brevis

Abductor
hallucis

Figure 21.1 (a) Plantar fascia (PF), extending from the heel to the base of all toes. (b) Superficial muscles of the foot after plantar fascia is removed: flexor digitorum brevis (FDB) lies directly beneath PF at the middle of the foot. Abductor hallucis (AH) and abductor digiti minimi (ADM) are seen close to the heel on either side of FDB.

peripheral and central sensitization as well as sympathetic overactivity may play a role in pain persistence.

Rational for using botulinum toxin (BoNT) for treatment of plantar fasciitis

Early observations on the efficacy of BoNT in reducing the pain of spasmodic torticollis suggested investigating the analgesic effect of botulinum toxins in other painful conditions. Emerging literature, for example, suggests efficacy in refractory migraine and myofascial pain syndromes (Silberstein *et al.*, 2000; Foster *et al.*, 2001). Although blockade of acetyl-choline release from presynaptic vesicles plays an

important role in relief of muscle spasms and pain in myofascial syndromes, a number of animal models suggest additional mechanisms. Some of these mechanisms such as the anti-inflammatory action of botulinum toxin type A (BoNT-A) (Cui *et al.*, 2004) and its action against locally accumulated stimulant neurotransmitters (glutamate, substance P) (Sanchez-Prieto *et al.*, 1987) pertain to the pathophysiology of PF.

Randomized, prospective studies of BoNT treatment for plantar fasciitis

We have published the results of the first, prospective, randomized, double-blind, placebo-controlled

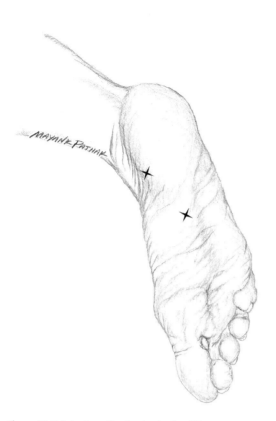

Figure 21.2 Injection sites in plantar fasciitis.

study in PF (Babcock *et al.*, 2005). Patients were adults, mostly walkers or runners with 6 months or more history of heel pain and discomfort, typical of PF. After receiving informed consent, each affected foot was randomized into either the BoNT-A (Botox®, Allergan Inc.) treatment group (A) or the placebo treatment group (B). The Botox solution was prepared by mixing 100 (mouse) units with 1 ml of preservative-free normal saline. Patients in group A were injected with 70 units of BoNT-A (0.7 cc) in two divided doses: 40 units (0.4 cc) in the tender region of the heel medial to the base of the plantar fascia insertion and 30 units (0.3 cc) in the most tender point of the arch of the foot (between the heel and middle of the foot) (Figure 21.2). A 27 gauge, 0.75 inch needle was used for injections. Group B received normal saline at the same locations and of similar volume. Pain

relief was measured by visual analog scale (VAS), pressure algometry (PA), and the Maryland foot score (MFS) at baseline (before treatment) and at 3 and 8 weeks post-injection. Twenty-seven patients participated in the study (11 with unilateral and 16 with bilateral PF). In patients with bilateral PF, one foot received BoNT-A and the other placebo. The pain response to BoNT-A compared to placebo was statistically significant at both 3 and 8 weeks ($P < 0.005$, < 0.001, < 0.0003 for VAS, PA, and MFS, respectively). No patient reported side effects.

In an open-label study, Placzek and colleagues (Placzek *et al.*, 2005) followed nine patients with PF after a single injection of BoNT-A (Dysport®, Ipsen Pharma) for 12 months. They injected 200 units (roughly comparable to 65–70 units of Botox) subfascially in four different directions through one injection puncture into the painful area at the origin of the plantar fascia. Pain response was measured by VAS, Brunner's muscle force assessment, and pain progression stage using Gebershagen score at 2, 6, 10, 14, 26, 29, 39, and 52 weeks. The authors reported significant decrease of VAS scores ($P < 0.05$) for all values obtained after treatment over 52 weeks.

Technique of BoNT treatment for plantar fasciitis: Yale/Walter Reed protocol

We use the technique reported in our 2005 study described previously (Babcock *et al.*, 2005). As noted above, this method includes two injection sites (Figure 21.2) covering both the area of most common pain (medial aspect of the heel) and the central band of plantar fascia with its major underlying muscle (FDB). We encourage physical therapy along with BoNT treatment and no change in a patient's medications during the first month of treatment.

REFERENCES

Akfirat, M., Sen, C. & Gunes, T. (2003). Ultrasonographic appearance of the plantar fasciitis. *Clin Imaging*, **27**, 353–7.

Babcock, M. S., Foster, L., Pasquina, P. & Jabbari, B. (2005). Treatment of pain attributed to plantar fasciitis with botulinum toxin a: a short-term, randomized, placebo-controlled, double-blind study. *Am J Phys Med Rehabil*, **84**, 649–54.

Banister, L. H., Berry, M. M., Collins, P., Dyson, M. & Ferguson, M. (eds.) (1995). Plantar fasciitis and plantar muscles of the foot. In *Gray's Anatomy*, 38th edn. New York: Churchill Livingston, pp. 891–2.

Barrett, S. J. & O'Malley, R. (1999). Plantar fasciitis and other causes of heel pain. *Am Fam Physician*, **59**, 2200–6.

Cui, M., Khanijou, S., Rubino, J. & Aoki, K. R. (2004). Subcutaneous administration of botulinum toxin A reduces formalin-induced pain. *Pain*, **107**, 125–33.

DeMaio, M., Paine, R., Mangine, R. E. & Drez, D., Jr. (1993). Plantar fasciitis. *Orthopedics*, **16**, 1153–63.

Foster, L., Clapp, L., Erickson, M. & Jabbari, B. (2001). Botulinum toxin A and chronic low back pain: a randomized, double-blind study. *Neurology*, **56**, 1290–3.

Placzek, R., Deuretzbacher, G., Buttgereit, F. & Meiss, A. L. (2005). Treatment of chronic plantar fasciitis with botulinum toxin A: an open case series with a 1 year follow up. *Ann Rheum Dis*, **64**, 1659–61.

Sanchez-Prieto, J., Sihra, T. S., Evans, D., *et al.* (1987). Botulinum toxin A blocks glutamate exocytosis from guinea-pig cerebral cortical synaptosomes. *Eur J Biochem*, **165**, 675–81.

Silberstein, S., Mathew, N., Saper, J. & Jenkins, S. (2000). Botulinum toxin type A as a migraine preventive treatment. For the BOTOX Migraine Clinical Research Group. *Headache*, **40**, 445–50.

22

Treatment of stiff-person syndrome with botulinum toxin

Bahman Jabbari and Diana Richardson

Introduction

Stiff-person syndrome (SPS), formerly termed stiff-man syndrome and Moersch–Woltmann syndrome, was first described in 1956 as a condition of muscular rigidity and episodic spasms that principally involved the trunk and lower limbs (Moersch & Woltman, 1956). The idiopathic (typical) form of SPS is now considered an autoimmune disorder, often associated with type I diabetes and increased levels of antibodies against glutamic acid decarboxylase (GAD), the enzyme that catalyzes gamma-amino butyric acid from glutamic acid. Symptoms usually begin during adult life and affect both sexes. Early in the disease course symptoms can be confused with orthopedic conditions, but as the disease progresses, a clear distinction can be made. Increasing symptoms of axial and limb rigidity and painful muscle spasms eventually lead to disability. Electromyography demonstrates continuous and spontaneous firing of motor units in the rigid muscles.

Clinical features

Brown and Marsden (1999) describe a typical form (classic) and several atypical forms (i.e., plus variants) of SPS. The typical form of SPS is characterized by progressive axial rigidity predominantly involving the paraspinal and abdominal muscles along with hyperlordosis of the lumbar spine, and spontaneous or stimulus sensitive disabling muscle spasms of the abdominal wall, lower extremities, and other proximal muscles. Muscle rigidity in typical SPS is attributed to dysfunction of the inhibitory interneurons of the spinal cord. These patients have high incidence of anti-GAD and islet cell antibodies (ICA) (96% GAD-65 antibodies and 89% ICA in Mayo clinic series) (Walikonis & Lennon, 1998). The muscle rigidity partially responds to high doses of diazepam and/or baclofen.

In stiff-person plus syndromes, the rigidity mainly involves the limbs. Patients have other central nervous system symptoms, and their response to diazepam and baclofen is less favorable. Only a minority of these patients demonstrate increased anti-GAD antibody titers in the serum or cerebrospinal fluid (CSF). At least three variants of SPS-plus have been identified:

1. Progressive encephalomyelitis with rigidity (PER). These patients demonstrate additional brain stem and long tract signs, cognitive changes, and CSF pleocytosis. Rigidity and dystonic posturing involves one or more limbs, and some patients have myoclonus. The pathology is an encephalomyelitis which primarily involves the gray matter. The muscle rigidity seems to be related to a release of an inhibitory influence of interneurons on alpha motor neurons (alpha rigidity).
2. Jerky stiff-man syndrome. This variant is characterized by prominent brain stem signs and florid

Manual of Botulinum Toxin Therapy, ed. Daniel Truong, Dirk Dressler and Mark Hallett. Published by Cambridge University Press. © Cambridge University Press 2009.

brain stem myoclonus in addition to symptoms of SPS. Muscle spasms can compromise respiration and prove fatal. Encephalomyelitis or paraneoplastic syndromes are pathological conditions associated with this variant.

3. Stiff-limb syndrome (SLS). Rigidity and painful spasms of the limbs are typical for this variant (Barker *et al.*, 1988). There is a low incidence of increased anti-GAD antibodies, but high incidence of positive rheumatoid factor and auto-antibodies. Patients with carcinoma of the breast or lung (oat cell) may develop SLS with high titers of anti-amphiphysin antibodies (Saiz A *et al.*, 1999). Paraneoplastic associated SPS tends to involve the upper limbs, neck, and cranial nerves (Espay & Chen, 2006). Electromyography usually shows abnormally synchronous discharge of motor units both in low (6–12 Hz) and higher frequencies, a finding which is not seen in typical SPS.

Treatment

In typical SPS, diazepam 5–200 mg, clonazepam 2.5–10 mg, and baclofen 5–60 mg/day (alone or in combination) offer some relief of rigidity and muscle spasms (Gordon *et al.*, 1967; Barker *et al.*, 1988). Patients with high anti-GAD antibodies, rigidity, and muscles spasms may respond to intravenous immunoglobulin treatment (Dalakas *et al.*, 2001). Anecdotal reports claim response to plasmaphoresis or steroid therapy.

Davis and Jabbari (1993) first reported significant improvement of "muscle stiffness" and painful muscle "spasms" with botulinum toxin type A (Botox®, Allergan Inc.) in a 36-year-old-man who developed clinical features of typical SPS over a period of 18 months. The rigidity and painful muscle spasm involved mainly the paraspinal muscles between T12 and L5 levels. His anti-GAD antibody titers (Mayo clinic laboratory) were 1/122 000 in serum (normal < 1/120) and 1/128 (normal < 1/2) in CSF. Treatment with baclofen and high-dose diazepam (100 mg/day) only provided partial relief. Botulinum toxin type A was injected at five levels

(L1–L5) into the paraspinal muscles bilaterally, 40–50 (mouse) units/level for a total of 560 units. Within a week, the patient reported marked reduction in muscle spasms along with improvement of sleep and ambulation. On examination a reduction in the board-like rigidity of paraspinal muscles was noted. Over a follow-up period of three years, four additional treatments of 400 units (200 units per side) maintained relief. In a blinded study by Liguori *et al.* (1997) patients who received Botox showed improvement of muscle rigidity and muscle spasm. Patients were 58 and 59 years old with probable stiff-limb variant of SPS and raised anti-GAD antibodies (titer was not mentioned). In one of the two, a number of lower limb muscles (adductors magnus and longus, biceps femoris, tibialis posterior, gastrocnemius, and soleus muscles) were injected with doses ranging from 50 to 100 units/muscle. The second patient was injected in the trapezius, deltoid, and biceps with doses of 50–300 units per muscle. Both muscle rigidity and muscle spasm showed significant improvement. Authors reported continued responsiveness with smaller doses over a two year follow-up period.

The rationale for treating rigidity of SPS with Botox includes several points:

1. Botulinum toxins block the release of acetylcholine from pre-synaptic vesicles which directly leads to muscle relaxation and reduction of spasms.
2. Botulinum toxins decrease discharge of muscle spindles, the main reporters of muscle stretch to the central nervous system. Reduction of muscle spindle input can reduce central sensitization.
3. Botulinum toxins reduce exocytosis of substance P and glutamate, substances with potential for enhancing muscle spasms.

At the present time no literature exists on treatment of SPS with other types of botulinum toxins.

Anatomy of low back paraspinal muscles

Since typical SPS often involves axial and paraspinal muscles usually in the thoracolumbar area it is essential to understand the anatomy of these muscles for a successful treatment response. In the

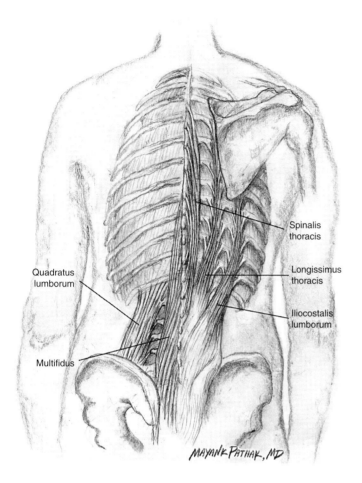

Figure 22.1 Anatomy of low back muscles: as shown in the figure, superficial spinal erecti make a single mass in the lumbar region (right side).

Quadratus lumborum

Multifidus

Spinalis thoracis

Longissimus thoracis

Iliocostalis lumborum

MAYANK PATHAK, MD

low back area the paraspinal muscles are arranged at different levels. The most superficial muscles, erectors of the spine, are long powerful muscles which receive innervation from multiple segments of the spinal cord. These muscles can be felt under the skin and contribute to the board-like appearance of the back area in SPS. The three components of spinal erectors, spinalis thoracis (medial), longissimus thoracis (middle), and iliocostalis lomborum (lateral), with attachments to cervical and thoracic vertebrae fuse and make a large single muscle mass (erector spina; ES) at the level of the upper lumbar region. This single mass of three muscles in the lumbar area ends in a strong tendon which attaches to the sacrum and to the medial

surface of the iliac bone (Figure 22.1). On the lower end, some of the fibers of ES are continuous with that of the multifidus and gluteus maximus muscles (Banister *et al.*, 1995). The multifidus muscle (Figures 22.1 and 22.2) layers deep and medially to erector spinae and is comprised of muscle bands (multifidi) which cross obliquely upward and attach to the whole length of the spine of each vertebrae. The lowest multifidus band is attached to the fourth sacral vertebra. Multifidus bands stabilize and to some degree rotate the spine. Deeper muscles such as rotators (cervicis, thoracis, and lumborum) mainly rotate the spine. Short interspinales and intertransvessali are stabilizers and rotators and play an important role in maintaining posture.

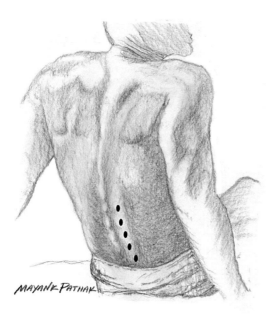

Figure 22.2 In most individuals, spinal erecti are easily visible and palpable in the lumbar area. Figure shows site of injections in one side (40–50 units/site). Patients with SPS usually require bilateral treatment.

Technique of treatment: Yale protocol

Thoracolumbar paraspinal muscles in typical SPS.

In typical SPS with board-like rigidity of back muscles, the superficial paraspinal muscles (erectors of the spine) in the thoracolumbar region are the main focus of treatment. Since some fibers of ES are continuous with the multifidus and glutei in the lumbosacral region, treatment of ES at this level with a sufficient dose theoretically can also affect at least a part of the deeper muscles.

We prepare botulinum toxin type A (Allergan Inc.) with preservative-free saline to the strength 100 units/cc (but other botulinum toxin preparations could also be used). For injection, the solution is drawn into a 1cc syringe, using a 1.5 inch, 27 gauge needle. It is our view that treatment of low back spasms and rigidity in SPS be comprised of multiple site/level injections (at least five) due to the length of the erector muscles (Figure 22.2).

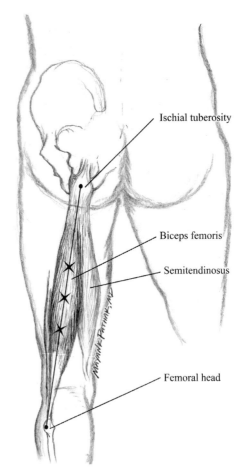

Figure 22.3 For hamstring spasticity injections into biceps femoris may be made in three or more sites with a dose of 30–50 units/site.

Furthermore, an adequate dosage administered in each level is needed in order to ensure sufficient lateral, longitudinal, and depth spread of the solution. After careful inspection and palpation of the back, the silhouette of erector muscles (medial and lateral borders) can be identified in most patients without difficulty (Figure 22.2). Injection into erector muscles is made perpendicular to the surface with the patient either in the sitting position or lying down on the stomach or side. In a thin individual an injection to the depth of 3/4–1 inch is sufficient. In larger individuals the depth of injection varies from 1 to 1.5 inch. We inject five paraspinal levels on each side; 40–50 units/side (total dose per session 400–500 units). In the typical SPS the injected area usually includes L1–L5 or T12–L4 levels.

Treatment of limb muscles in stiff-limb syndrome (stiff-leg, stiff arm) or typical SPS with proximal limb rigidity

Solution preparation, syringe, and needle length are the same as that used for rigid axial/paraspinal muscles. The method of injection is similar to what is currently widely used for treatment of spasticity; i.e., two to four injections in the affected muscles (Figures 22.3 and 22.4). Some physicians use larger volumes of 2 cc (50 units/cc) or 4 cc (25 unit/cc) dilution contemplating better diffusion into the muscle with larger volumes. Comparative studies

are needed to prove the merits of larger volumes. In the case of botulinum toxin type B (Myobloc, Solstice Inc.), we use a ratio of 50:1 (Myobloc to Botox) for treatment of low back or large proximal limb muscles. Electromyography can be used as a guide when injecting paraspinal or limb muscle, but in most instances is not necessary.

Table 22.1 shows doses of botulinum toxin A (Botox, Allergan Inc.) used for the treatment of the proximal rigid muscles often involved in SPS. The recommended doses are slightly higher than that commonly used for spasticity.

Side effects

Potential side effects of botulinum toxin therapy in low back and proximal limbs include transient

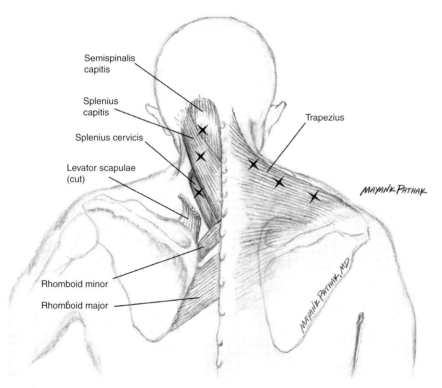

Figure 22.4 Site of injections in the neck and shoulder for rigidity of SPS (20–30 units/site). Injection sites cover trapezius muscle as well as splenius capitis and cervicis. Additional site may be injected around the scapula if necessary to cover levator scapulae and rhomboids.

Table 22.1. Doses of botulinum toxin A (Botox, Allergan Inc.) used for the treatment of the proximal rigid muscles often involved in SPS

	Upper limb	Dose	Lower limb	Dose
Name	Biceps	50–150	Hamstring	100–200
	Triceps	50–150	Rectus femoris	100–200
	Brachioradialis	50–100	Gastrocnemius	100–200
	Deltoid	50–100	Soleus	50–100
	Trapezius	150–200	Tibialis posterior	50–150
	Levator scapulae	50–100	Tibialis anterior	50–150

muscle weakness, pain in the site of injection, focal infection, and transient low-grade flu-like syndrome. These side effects have not been reported from the few patients who received botulinum toxin type A for treatment of SPS. We have not seen spinal instability or problems with ambulation in either these patients or in over 300 patients who were treated with similar doses of Botox into paraspinal muscles in other studies for chronic low back pain. This most likely reflects protection of the spine by a number of powerful deep muscles and ligaments. Furthermore, spinal erectors may not yield to weakness easily due to their exceptional long length and multiplicity of their attachments. Nevertheless, long-term follow-ups are not available and the clinician should inquire about weakness and examine the patient carefully at each visit. Finally, repeated treatments with large doses of botulinum toxins subject the patients to development of antibodies and non-responsiveness. In clinical practice the development non-responsiveness with Botox has become a rare event due to low content of the protein in the new preparation (used since 1997).

REFERENCES

Banister, L., Berry, M., Collins, P., Dyson, M. & Ferguson, M. (eds). (1995). Muscles and Fasciae of the trunk. In *Gray's Anatomy*, 38th edn. New York: Churchill Livingston pp. 809–12.

Barker, R. A., Revesz, T., Thom, M., Marsden, C. D. & Brown, P. (1988). A review of 23 patients with stiff man syndrome: clinical subdivision into stiff trunk (man) syndrome, stiff limb syndrome and progressive encephalomyelitis with rigidity. *J Neurol Neurosurg Psychiatry*, **65**, 633–40.

Brown, P. & Marsden, C. D. (1999). The stiff man and stiff man plus syndromes. *J Neurol*, **246**, 648–52.

Dalakas, M. C., Fujii, M., Li, M., *et al.* (2001). High-dose intravenous immune globulin for stiff-person syndrome. *N Engl J Med*, **345**, 1870–6.

Davis, D. & Jabbari, B. (1993). Significant improvement of stiff-person syndrome after paraspinal injections of Botulinum toxin A. *Mov Disord*, **8**, 371–3.

Espay, A. J. & Chen, R. (2006). Rigidity and spasms from autoimmune encephalomyelopathies: stiff-person. *Muscle Nerve*, **34**, 677–90.

Gordon, E. E., Januszko, D. M. & Kaufman, K. L. (1967). A critical review of stiff-man syndrome. *Am J Med*, **42**, 582–99.

Liguori, R., Cordivari, C., Lugaresi, E. & Montagna, P. (1997). Botulinum toxin A improves muscle spasms and rigidity in stiff-person syndrome. *Mov Disord*, **12**, 1060–3.

Moersch, F. P. & Woltman, H. W. (1956). Progressive fluctuating muscular rigidity and spasm ("stiff-man" syndrome); report of a case and some observations in 13 other cases. *Proc Staff Meet Mayo Clin*, **31**, 421–7.

Saiz, A., Dalmau, J., Butler, M. H., *et al.* (1999). Anti-amphiphysin I antibodies in patient with paraneoplastic neurological disorders associated with small cell lung carcinoma. *J Neurol Neurosurg Psychiatry*, **66**, 214–17.

Walikonis, J. E. & Lennon, V. A. (1998). Radioimmunoassay for glutamic acid decarboxylase (GAD65) autoantibodies as a diagnostic aid for stiff-man syndrome and a correlate of susceptibility to type 1 diabetes mellitus. *Mayo Clin Proc*, **73**, 1161–6.

23

Botulinum toxin in tic disorders and essential hand and head tremor

James K. Sheffield and Joseph Jankovic

Introduction: tics

Tics are brief, sudden movements (motor tics) or sounds (phonic tics) which are intermittent but may be repetitive and stereotypic (Jankovic, 2001; Singer, 2005). Transient tic disorder is the mildest and most common cause of tics. Although these tics usually resolve in childhood, some may persist and become associated with a variety of comorbid disorders such as attention deficit disorder and obsessive compulsive disorder. Tourette's syndrome (TS), considered a genetic and neurodevelopmental disorder, is the most common cause of chronic tics (Jankovic, 2001; Albin and Mink, 2006). There are many other causes of tics which are referred to as "tourettism" or secondary tics. Other causes of tics in particular include insults to the brain and basal ganglia (infection, stroke, head trauma, drugs, and neurodegenerative disorders) (Jankovic & Mejia, 2006). The currently used diagnostic criteria for definite TS formulated initially by The Tourette's Syndrome Classification Study Group (1993) include: (1) multiple motor tics; (2) at least one vocal tic (not necessarily concurrently); (3) a waxing and waning course with increasing severity over time; (4) tic symptoms for at least one year; (5) onset before age 21 years; (6) no precipitating etiologies such as illnesses or drugs; and (7) observation of tics by a medical professional (Jankovic, 2001).

Clinical features

Motor and phonic tics consist of either simple or complex movements that may be seemingly goal directed. Motor tics may be rapid (clonic), or more prolonged (Jankovic, 2001). Many patients exhibit suggestibility and may have a compulsive component, sometimes perceived as an "urge" or a need to perform the movement or sound repetitively until it feels "just right" (Leckman et al., 1994; Jankovic, 2001). Some patients repeat other's gestures (echopraxia) or sounds (echolalia) (Leckman et al., 2001). Many tics are semi-voluntary and are preceded by a premonitory sensation or urge (e.g. crescendo feeling of "tension" before a shoulder shrug, compulsive touching) and may be suppressible (Jankovic, 2005). Such premonitory phenomenon may consist of a generalized urge or sensation in the local area of the tic (Kwak et al., 2003).

Treatment options

The most commonly used effective anti-tic medications, the so-called neuroleptics which act by blocking dopamine receptors or by depleting dopamine, may be associated with troublesome side effects (Silay & Jankovic, 2005; Scahill et al., 2006). These include drowsiness, weight gain, school phobia, parkinsonism, and tardive dyskinesia. While tardive

Manual of Botulinum Toxin Therapy, ed. Daniel Truong, Dirk Dressler and Mark Hallett. Published by Cambridge University Press.

dyskinesia has not been reported with tetrabenazine, a depleter of dopamine, this drug is still not readily available in the United States, even though it has been found to be safe and effective in the treatment of TS (Kenney *et al.*, 2007). There are many other types of drugs used in the treatment of TS, but they all have undesirable systemic adverse effects (Scahill *et al.*, 2006).

Use of botulinum toxin

When oral medications fail to provide relief of tics, local chemodenervation with botulinum toxin (BoNT) offers the possibility of relaxing the muscles involved in focal tics without causing undesirable systemic side effects. Focal tics that are repetitively performed are more effectively treated with BoNT than tics with complex movements that would require injections in multiple muscles. In a pilot study, botulinum toxin type A (BoNT-A; Botox®) (Allergan Inc., Irvine, CA) injections demonstrated marked reduction in the frequency and intensity of dystonic tics in ten patients with TS (Jankovic, 1994). An important observation was that premonitory sensory symptoms were reduced. Kwak *et al.* (2000), in a second open-label study of 35 patients (34 with TS), demonstrated a peak effect of 2.8 on a self-rating scale (range: 0 – no effect, to 4 – marked relief in both severity and function). The effect lasted a mean of 14.4 weeks. The mean dose per session was 57.4 mouse units (U) in the upper face, 79.3 U in the lower face, 149.6 U in the cervical muscles, and 121.7 U in other muscles of the shoulder, forearm, and scalp. Four patients received 17.8 U in the vocal cords. In the 25 patients of the study with premonitory sensory symptoms, 21 (84%) had notable reduction in these symptoms. Complications, which were all mild and transient, included neck weakness (4), dysphagia (2), ptosis (2), nausea (1), hypophonia (1), fatigue (1), and generalized weakness (1).

A randomized, placebo-controlled, double-blind, crossover study of Botox for motor tics was conducted on 18 patients (Marras *et al.*, 2001). There was a 37% reduction in the number of tics per minute within 2 weeks compared to vehicle. The premonitory urge was reduced with an average change in urge scores of −0.46 in the treatment phase and +0.49 in the placebo phase (score range 0–4, which was none to severe). Although 50% of patients noted motor weakness in the injected muscles, the weakness was not functionally disabling. Two patients noted motor restlessness that paralleled the weakness induced by the Botox during the active treatments. Problems with the study included insufficient power to demonstrate significant differences in measured variables such as severity, global impression, and pain. In addition, the patients were only assessed at 2 weeks post-injection and the full effect of the treatment may not have been realized. Finally, the patients did not rate their tics as significantly compromising at baseline indicating that their TS was rather mild.

In an open-label study of 30 patients with phonic tics treated with 2.5 U Botox in both vocal cords (Porta *et al.*, 2004) patient assessments occurred after 15 days and then four times over a 12-month period. Phonic tics improved after treatment in 93% patients, with 50% being tic free. The percent of subjects stating their condition severely impacted their social life reduced from 50% to 13% post-injection and those with tics causing a severe effect on work or school activities reduced from 47% to 10%. In the 16 subjects (53%) experiencing premonitory symptoms, only 6 (20%) continued to have these sensations after injection. Hypophonia, which was mild, was the only side effect of note in 80% of patients (see Table 23.1).

Our experience

Our long-term experience with BoNT in tics provides further evidence that this is a safe and effective treatment modality, particularly in patients with focal tics, such as blinking, facial grimacing, jaw clenching, neck extensions ("whiplash tics"), and shoulder shrugging.

Table 23.1. Selected studies of botulinum toxin injection for tics

Reference	Design	Size	Treatment (technique, dose)	Brand	Follow-up	Outcome	Adverse events	Comments
Kwak et al., 2000	Open-label case series with unblinded assessments	35	57.4 U, 79.3 U in the lower face, 149.6 U in the cervical muscles, and 121.7 U in other muscles of the shoulder, forearm, and scalp. Four patients received 17.8 U in the vocal cords	Botox	Mean duration of follow-up was 21.2 months (range, 1.5–84 months); mean peak effect 115 sessions was 2.8 weeks (range, 0–4); the mean duration of benefit was 14.4 weeks (maximum, 45 weeks); mean latency to onset of benefit was 3.8 days (maximum, 10 days)	Clinical effect on 4 point self-rating scale	Mild and transient, including neck weakness (4), dysphagia (2), ptosis (2), nausea (1), hypophonia (1), fatigue (1), and generalized weakness (1)	Variable protocol based on location of tic involvement Twenty-one (84%) of 25 patients with premonitory sensations derived marked relief of these symptoms (mean benefit, 70.6%)
Marras et al., 2001	Double-blinded, crossover, placebo-controlled	20 randomized 18 completed (2 lost to follow-up)	Variable doses based on clinical judgment	Botox	All outcomes compared week 2 to baseline measurement. Patients reassessed weeks 6, 12, and every 4 weeks until patient and examiners agreed tic disorder had reached baseline and then the patient crossed	Primary measure: number of treated tics per minute on a videotape segment Secondary measures: number of untreated tics per minute, the Shapiro Tourette	50% of patients noted weakness not functionally disabling of the injected muscles. Two patients noted a significant motor restlessness during the active	Observed no pattern to suggest that certain tics respond better than others to botulinum toxin treatment

197

Table 23.1. (cont.)

Reference	Design	Size	Treatment (technique, dose)	Brand	Follow-up	Outcome	Adverse events	Comments
					over to the second phase of the trial	Syndrome Severity Scale score, a numerical assessment of the urge to perform the treated tic (0 to 4), the premonitory sensation associated with the treated tic (0 to 4), and the patient's global impression of change	treatment. Two patients felt the inability to perform the treated tic led to a new tic to replace it	
Porta et al., 2004	Open-label case series with unblinded assessments	30	2.5 IU in both vocal cords; mean number of injections were 1.9 per patient with a mean interval 4.2 months apart	Botox	Assessed after 15 days and then 4 times over a 12-month period	Phenomenology of tics, global impression of changes by physician and patient, number of BoNT-A injections given, interval between injections	Mild hypophonia was the only side effect of note (80% of patients)	Premonitory experiences dropped from 53% to 20%

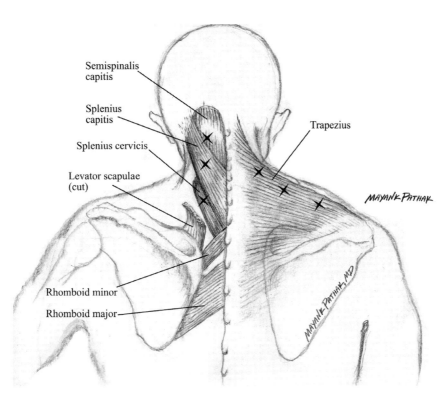

Semispinalis
capitis

Splenius
capitis

Splenius cervicis

Levator scapulae
(cut)

Trapezius

MAYANK PATHAK

Rhomboid minor

Rhomboid major

Figure 23.1 Suggested injection sites for "whiplash tic."

Dosages and muscles injected

The exact muscles and location of injections are determined by considering which movements are of particular concern by the patient, by observing the predominant movement (including severity) of the tic being performed, and by determining whether or not there is a significant localized premonitory sensation or urge associated with the tic. Dosing varies depending on the intensity of the premonitory sensation, force of the contraction, and size of the muscle, but the average starting dose is 25–50 U Botox/Xeomin®, 75–150 U Dysport®, and 1500–2500 U NeuroBloc®/MyoBloc® into the splenius muscle (see Adult Dosing Guidelines and dosage recommendations at www.wemove.org/). On occasion, as patients experience improvement of their BoNT-treated tic, they may have a worsening of tics in other areas.

A common tic seen in TS patients is to have sudden retrocollic jerking of the neck (whiplash tic) which can lead to pain and cervical spine injury (Kwak et al., 2000). This tic can be effectively treated when the splenius capitis muscles are injected as indicated in Figure 23.1. The injection is most efficacious if the patients frequently have a premonitory sensation or urge in the posterior neck just prior to performing the tic.

Introduction: tremors

Tremor is one of the most common movement disorders and essential tremor (ET) is the most common reason for referral to a movement disorders clinic for evaluation and treatment of tremor (Louis et al., 1998; Elble, 2000; Benito-Leon & Louis, 2006).

Clinical features

Essential tremor consists of involuntary, rhythmic, postural movements usually involving the hands, head, and voice, and may be associated with other movement disorders such as dystonia and parkinsonism (Deuschl *et al.*, 1998; Louis, 2001; Jankovic, 2002).

Treatment options

A recent review and practice parameter report by the American Academy of Neurology recommended propranolol, propranolol-LA, and primidone as the only first-line, class A medication therapies for ET (Zesiewicz *et al.*, 2005). Primidone is associated, however, with moderate to high frequency of acute adverse events and a decline in efficacy with long-term treatment in the majority of patients (Koller & Vetere-Overfield, 1989; Sasso *et al.*, 1990; O'Suilleabhain & Dewey, 2002). Propranolol and propranolol-LA are not without side effects and declining long-term efficacy (Cleeves & Findley, 1988). Drugs such as topiramate, pregabalin, and other anticonvulsants are also being evaluated in the treatment of ET (Ondo *et al.*, 2006).

Use of botulinum toxin

When oral medications for tremor have poor efficacy or intolerable side effects, BoNT injections may be used as an adjunctive treatment. There have been more than a dozen studies in which BoNT has been evaluated for efficacy and safety in treating hand tremor. The majority of these have focused on patients with ET, but some have included subjects with Parkinson's disease or parkinsonian rest tremor. There have been two randomized, double-blind, controlled studies to evaluate the efficacy of BoNT-A in treating essential hand tremor. In the first study by Jankovic *et al.*

(1996) 25 patients were injected in both the wrist flexors and extensors with 50 U of Botox and with an additional 100 U four weeks later if they failed to respond. Some of the patients had rest tremors, but all clinically met the criteria for ET. Rest, postural, and kinetic tremors were evaluated at 2–4 week intervals for 16 weeks using tremor severity rating scales, accelerometry, and assessments of tremor improvement and functional disability. A significant ($P < 0.05$) improvement on the tremor severity rating scale 4 weeks after injection was seen in the Botox treatment group compared with placebo. Additionally, at 4 weeks after injection, 75% of Botox-treated patients vs. 27% of placebo-treated patients ($P < 0.05$) demonstrated mild to moderate (peak effect of ≥ 2) subjective improvement in their tremor on a 0–4 rating scale. There were no significant improvements in the functional rating scales. Postural accelerometry measurements showed a $\geq 30\%$ reduction in amplitude in 9 of 12 Botox-treated subjects and in 1 of 9 placebo-treated subjects. All patients treated with Botox reported some mild, transient degree of finger weakness.

In a randomized, multi-center, double-masked clinical trial by Brin *et al.* (2001) 133 patients with ET were randomized to treatment with either low-dose (50 U) or high-dose (100 U) Botox or placebo. Injections were made into the wrist flexors and extensors and patients were followed for 16 weeks. Tremor severity was assessed with the hand at rest and in postural and kinetic positions. The effect of treatment was assessed by clinical rating scales, measures of motor tasks and functional disability, and global assessment of treatment. All assessments were scored on a scale from 0 to 4 measuring severity or disability (0 = none; 1 = mild; 2 = moderate; 3 = marked; 4 = severe). Hand strength was evaluated by clinical rating and a dynamometer. The assessment of tremor severity based on rating scale evaluation indicated a significant difference ($P < 0.05$) from baseline for the low- and high-dose groups for postural tremor at 6, 12, and 16 weeks and for kinetic tremor only at the 6-week evaluation as compared to placebo. Measures of motor tasks and functional disability were not consistently improved, but drawing a spiral and a straight line at 6 and 16 weeks improved. The results of treatment on functional rating scales indicated that low-dose Botox significantly (P < 0.05) improved feeding, dressing, and drinking at 6 weeks and writing at 16 weeks compared with placebo. In the high-dose group, Botox significantly (P < 0.05) improved feeding at 6 weeks, drinking at 6, 12, and 16 weeks, hygiene at 6 weeks, writing at 16 weeks, and fine movements at 6, 12, and 16 weeks. The sickness impact profile (SIP) scores and ratings on speaking, working, embarrassment, and anxiety state were not significantly improved. The subjects had dose-dependent finger or wrist weakness in flexion and extension, with a tendency for greater weakness in wrist and finger extension.

In both placebo-controlled studies, patients had statistically significant finger or wrist weakness in flexion and extension, with a tendency for greater weakness in wrist and finger extensors (see Table 23.2).

Essential head tremor was initially reported to improve with Botox injections into the cervical muscles in 1991 (Jankovic & Schwartz, 1991). This observation was subsequently confirmed by a double-blind, placebo-controlled study (Pahwa et al., 1995). In the first study, both splenius capitis muscles were injected if patients had a lateral oscillation ("no-no" tremor) of the head and one or both sternocleidomastoid muscles if they had and anterior-posterior ("yes-yes" tremor) oscillation. The average dose of Botox was 107 (± 38) U. There was a 3.0 (± 1.1) improvement on a 0–4 scale with 4 indicating complete resolution of tremor. A few patients had mild transient neck weakness (9.5%) or dysphagia (28.6%). In the study by Pahwa et al. (1995) ten patients received 40 and 60 U of Botox injected into the sternocleidomastoid and splenius muscles respectively. Each subject received placebo or Botox on separate injections 3 months apart. Examiner and subject ratings showed 50% vs. 10% and 50% vs. 30% respectively in improvement in tremor between Botox and placebo. Accelerometry

measurements failed to demonstrate a significant difference. Side effects were also mild and transient and included neck weakness and dysphagia.

Our experience

As a result of long-term experience with hundreds of patients treated with BoNT for various tremors, we have modified our protocol and have markedly decreased the dosage in the forearm extensor muscles (to less than 15 U), or completely omit injections into these muscles altogether. With this modification (that is, injecting mainly into the forearm flexor muscles), we now obtain similar benefits in terms of reduction in the amplitude of the tremor without the undesirable extensor weakness. Patients with ET of the head are poorly treated with oral medications and may also benefit from BoNT injections. If the tremor is primarily a "no-no" tremor of the head, injections into the sternocleidomastoid muscles as well as the splenius capitis muscles should be considered, as opposed to the splenius capitis muscles only in a "yes-yes" tremor.

Dosages and muscles injected

We usually inject the forearm flexor muscles predominantly involved, but the flexor carpi radialis and ulnaris muscles are the muscles most frequently injected in ET patients. The average starting dose is 25–50 U Botox/Xeomin, 75–150 U Dysport, and 1500–2500 U NeuroBloc/Myobloc equally divided between the two muscles. Patients with Parkinson's disease resting hand tremor have, and patients with severe essential hand tremor may have, pronation-supination of the forearm. If present, this component of tremor may require an additional injection into the biceps brachii muscle to decrease it by weakening supination. The initial dose injected is based on the severity, but we usually start at the lower end of the range of recommended dosages.

Table 23.2. Class I studies in botulinum toxin injection for treatment of essential hand tremor

Reference	Class	Design	Cohort size	Treatment (technique, dose)	Brand	Follow-up	Outcome (1-primary 2-secondary)	Drop outs	Adverse events	Comments
Jankovic et al., 1996	1	Double-blinded, parallel, placebo-controlled	25–13 12 placebo	50 U If no response, 100 U at 4 weeks	Botox	16 weeks	Tremor rating Investigator/pt subjective rating SIP Accelerometry	1 in placebo due to pregnancy	Finger weakness, mild in 50%, moderate in 42%	Rigid protocol
Brin et al., 2001	1	Double-blinded, parallel, placebo-controlled	133–43 (50 U) 45 (100 U) 45 (placebo)	EMG guided into forearm muscles	Botox	16 weeks	Tremor rating Investigator/pt subjective rating SIP	None	Weakness in 30% of 50 U and 70% of 100 U groups	Rigid protocol

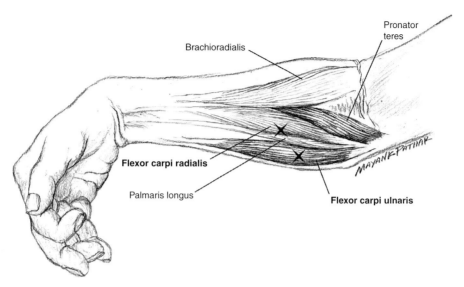

Figure 23.2 Injection sites in the forearm flexors for essential hand tremor.

Figure 23.2 illustrates injection sites into the flexor carpi ulnaris and radialis as would be done for a patient with essential hand tremor.

REFERENCES

Albin, R. L. & Mink, J. W. (2006). Recent advances in Tourette syndrome research. *Trends Neurosci*, **29**, 175–82.

Benito-Leon, J. & Louis, E. D. (2006). Essential tremor: emerging views of a common disorder. *Nat Clin Pract Neurol*, **2**, 666–78.

Brin, M. F., Lyons, K. E., Doucette, J., *et al.* (2001). A randomized, double masked, controlled trial of botulinum toxin type A in essential hand tremor. *Neurology*, **56**, 1523–8.

Cleeves, L. & Findley, L. J. (1988). Propranolol and propranolol-LA in essential tremor: a double bind comparative study. *J Neurol Neurosurg Psychiatry*, **51**, 379–84.

Deuschl, G., Bain, P. G., & Brin, M. (1998). Consensus statement of the Movement Disorder Society on Tremor. Ad hoc scientific committee. *Mov Disord*, **13**(Suppl 3), 2–3.

Elble, R. J. (2000). Diagnostic criteria for essential tremor and differential diagnosis. *Neurology*, **54**, S2–6.

Jankovic, J. (1994). Botulinum toxin in the treatment of dystonic tics. *Mov Disord*, **9**, 347–9.

Jankovic, J. (2001). Tourette's syndrome. *N Engl J Med*, **345**(16), 1184–92.

Jankovic, J. (2002). Essential tremor: a heterogeneous disorder. *Mov Disord*, **17**, 638–44.

Jankovic, J. (2005). Tics and stereotypies. In H.-J. Freund, M. Jeannerod, M. Hallett & R. Leiguarda, eds., *Higher Order Motor Disorders*. New York, NY: Oxford University Press, pp. 383–96.

Jankovic, J. & Mejia, N. I. (2006). Tics associated with other disorders. In J. Walkup, J. Mink & P. Hollenbeck, eds., *Tourette Syndrome. Advances in Neurology.* Philadelphia: Lippincott Williams & Wilkins, pp. 61–8.

Jankovic, J. & Schwartz, K. (1991). Botulinum toxin treatment of tremors. *Neurology*, **41**, 1185–8.

Jankovic, J., Schwartz, K., Clemence, W., Aswad, A. & Mordaunt, J. (1996). A randomized, double-blind, placebo-controlled study to evaluate botulinum toxin type A in essential hand tremor. *Mov Disord*, **3**, 250–6.

Kenney, C., Hunter, C., Mejia, N. & Jankovic, J. (2007). Tetrabenazine in the treatment of Tourette syndrome. *J Pediatr Neurol*, **5**, 9–13.

Koller, W. C. & Vetere-Overfield, B. (1989). Acute and chronic effects of propranolol and primidone in essential tremor. *Neurology*, **39**(12), 1587–8.

Kwak, C. H., Hanna, P. A. & Jankovic, J. (2000). Botulinum toxin in the treatment of tics. *Arch Neurol*, **57**(8), 1190–3.

Kwak, C., Vuong, K. D. & Jankovic, J. (2003). Premonitory sensory phenomenon in Tourette's syndrome. *Mov Disord*, **18**(12), 1530–3.

Leckman, J. F., Walker, D. E., Goodman, W. K., Pauls, D. L. & Cohen, D. J. (1994). "Just right" perceptions associated with compulsive behavior in Tourette's syndrome. *Am J Psychiatry*, **151**, 675–80.

Leckman, J. F., Peterson, B. S., King, R. A., Scahill, L. & Cohen, D. J. (2001). Phenomenology of tics and natural history of tic disorders. *Adv Neurol*, **85**, 1–14.

Louis, E. D. (2001). Essential tremor. *N Engl J Med*, **345**(12), 887–91.

Louis, E. D., Ottman, R. & Hauser, W. A. (1998). How common is the most common adult movement disorder? Estimates of the prevalence of essential tremor throughout the world. *Mov Disord*, **13**, 5–10.

Marras, C., Andrews, D., Sime, E. & Lang, A. E. (2001). Botulinum toxin for simple motor tics: a randomized, double-blind, controlled clinical trial. *Neurology*, **56**(5), 605–10.

Ondo, W. G., Jankovic, J., Connor, G. S., *et al.* Topiramate Essential Tremor Study Investigators. (2006). Topiramate in essential tremor: a double-blind, placebo-controlled trial. *Neurology*, **66**, 672–7.

O'Suilleabhain, P. & Dewey, R. B. (2002). Randomized trial comparing primidone initiation schedules for treating essential tremor. *Mov Disord*, **17**, 383–6.

Pahwa, R., Busenbark, K., Swanson-Hyland, E. F., *et al.* (1995). Botulinum toxin treatment of essential head tremor. *Neurology*, **45**(4), 822–4.

Porta, M., Maggioni, G., Ottaviani, F. & Schindler, A. (2004). Treatment of phonic tics in patients with Tourette's syndrome using botulinum toxin type A. *Neurol Sci*, **24**(6), 420–3.

Sasso, E., Perucca, E., Fave, R. & Calzetti, S. (1990). Primidone in the long term treatment of essential tremor: a perspective study with computerized quantitative analysis. *Clin Neuropharmacol*, **13**(1), 67–76.

Scahill, L., Ehrenberg, G., Berlin, C. M. Jr., *et al.* Tourette Syndrome Association Medical Advisory Board: Practice Committee. (2006). Contemporary assessment and pharmacotherapy of Tourette syndrome. *NeuroRx*, **3**, 192–206.

Silay, Y. & Jankovic, J. (2005). Emerging drugs in Tourette syndrome. *Expert Opin Emerg Drugs*, **10**, 365–80.

Singer, H. S. (2005). Tourette's syndrome: from behaviour to biology. *Lancet Neurol*, **3**, 149–59.

The Tourette Syndrome Classification Study Group (1993). Definitions and classification of tic disorders. *Arch Neurol*, **50**, 1013–16.

Zesiewicz, T. A., Elble, R., Louis, E. D., *et al.* (2005). Practice parameter: therapies for essential tremor. Report of the Quality Standards Subcommittee of the American Academy of Neurology. *Neurology*, **64**, 2008–20.

24

Developing the next generation of botulinum toxin drugs

Dirk Dressler, Daniel Truong and Mark Hallett

Botulinum toxin (BoNT) has now been used for more than 20 years with remarkable success to treat various conditions caused by hyperactivity of muscles or exocrine glands (Scott, 1980; Moore & Naumann, 2003). Its use for treatment of pain syndromes is currently being explored. For most of its indications BoNT therapy is the therapy of choice. For some it has revolutionized therapy altogether. This, together with its exploding use in cosmetics, has generated an industry with annual sales in excess of one billion US dollars. However, 20 years into this therapy, we are still using more or less the original BoNT drugs.

As shown in Figure 24.1 the first BoNT drug was registered in 1989 as Oculinum®. In 1992 its name was changed to Botox®. In 1999 a modified formulation of Botox was marketed without a name change. In 1991 Dysport® was registered as another BoNT type A drug and in 2000 NeuroBloc®/ Myobloc® became available as the first – and so far only – BoNT type B drug. When NeuroBloc/Myobloc was introduced to the neurological community it soon became apparent that it has a much stronger affinity to autonomic synapses than to motor synapses as compared to BoNT type A drugs (Dressler & Benecke, 2003) thus producing frequent autonomic side effects in the treatment of motor disorders. This, together with its high antigenicity (Dressler & Bigalke, 2004), has prevented its large-scale use. In 2005 Xeomin® was marketed in Germany.

Are we satisfied with the existing BoNT drugs? Are there any problems with BoNT therapy where new BoNT drugs could help? Are there any perspectives for future development of BoNT drugs?

Antigenicity

One of the biggest problems of the BoNT drugs is their antigenicity. Antibody-induced therapy failure (ABTF) is rare for certain indications including blepharospasm and cervical dystonia. Frequency of ABTF for the use of BoNT drugs in particularly immunocompetent tissues such as the skin is completely unknown. Largely unknown, too, is the ABTF frequency in high-dose indications such as spasticity or generalized dystonia. Assuming a correlation between ABTF frequency and BoNT doses applied (Dressler & Dirnberger, 2000) the ABTF frequency should be higher than in blepharospasm and in cervical dystonia.

Antibody-induced therapy failure affects the individual patient considerably. Its most profound effect is, however, not seen when it actually occurs, but when strategies to avoid it are considered. Those prevention strategies reduce the real potential of BoNT therapy substantially. This will be demonstrated by some examples: during the dose finding phase the optimal BoNT dose is occasionally not found on the first injection series. Booster

Manual of Botulinum Toxin Therapy, ed. Daniel Truong, Dirk Dressler and Mark Hallett. Published by Cambridge University Press.
© Cambridge University Press 2009.

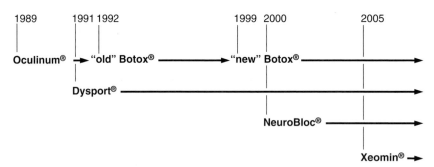

Figure 24.1 Development of botulinum toxin drugs. "Old" Botox® describes the original Botox® preparation, "New" Botox® the formulation optimized with respect to its specific biological activity.

injections, i.e., reinjections administered within less than 3 weeks after the previous injection series, could quickly optimize the treatment result thus avoiding a prolonged waiting time for the patient. However, according to general agreement booster injections should not be used in order to avoid ABTF. When the BoNT effect fades at the end of a treatment cycle reinjections should be applied. Again, according to general agreement those reinjections should not be applied within 3 months after the previous injection series in order to avoid ABTF (premature reinjections). Treating cases of severe dystonia and of severe spasticity often requires use of substantial BoNT doses. Also here, in order to avoid ABTF higher BoNT doses are frequently avoided (adequate BoNT doses). Booster injections, premature reinjections, and adequate BoNT doses could be used if BoNT drugs with reduced antigenicity would be available. This reduction of antigenicity can be achieved using different strategies.

Protein load

One strategy to reduce antigenicity is to limit the protein load of BoNT drugs. All BoNT drugs contain biologically active and biologically inactive botulinum neurotoxin (BNT). The specific biological activity (SBA) describes the relationship between active and inactive BNT (Dressler & Hallett, 2006). Biologically inactive BNT is useless for BoNT

therapy. Nevertheless, it can still act as an antigen. Immunologically improved BoNT drugs should therefore contain as little inactive BNT as possible. With the new formulation of Botox introduced between 1998 and 1999 the SBA could be increased to 60 equivalence mouse units/ng BNT (Jankovic et al., 2003). Subsequently, prospective studies confirmed an improved antigenicity (Jankovic et al., 2003). Comparatively, the SBA is 100 equivalence mouse units/ng BNT for Dysport, 5 for NeuroBloc/Myobloc, and 167 for Xeomin (Dressler & Hallett, 2006). Xeomin, therefore, has the highest SBA of all currently registered BoNT drugs. It should therefore have the lowest antigenicity.

Complexing proteins

Another strategy to reduce the antigenicity of BoNT drugs could be removal of the complexing proteins (Lee et al., 2005). This approach, too, was applied in Xeomin. Whether this strategy is effective in a clinical setting needs to be evaluated.

Other strategies

Shielding of antigenic BNT epitopes could be another strategy. The most effective strategy, however, seems to be the development of high affinity BNT. High affinity BNT could reduce the amount of BoNT applied (and thus the amount of antigen) dramatically. Research into this is currently under way.

Additional development goals

Transdermal BoNT applications

Treatment of hyperhidrosis requires large area intradermal BoNT applications. Given the intradermal diffusion properties of BoNT drugs, three to five injections per $10\,cm^2$ skin area are necessary. These injections are unpleasant but tolerable in the axilla. In the palm and in the sole of the foot, however, they are frequently painful. Skin anesthesia is not practicable in these areas. Currently available BoNT drugs cannot penetrate the skin due to their molecular size and are, therefore, not applicable transdermally. Transdermal BoNT drugs would greatly improve the patient compliance in those indications.

Labeled BoNT drugs

Recently, BoNT application guided by computerized tomography or ultrasound techniques has been suggested. Labeling of BoNT drugs by X-ray, magnetic resonance imaging or ultrasound contrast material could optimize this approach. Optical labeling could improve surface BoNT applications. Radioactive labeling could trace BoNT within the organism. Optical labeling could also improve the handling of BoNT drugs during the reconstitution process.

Ready-made solutions

Of all available BoNT drugs only NeuroBloc/Myobloc comes as a ready-made solution. All other BoNT drugs are powders that have to be reconstituted with $0.9\%NaCl/H_2O$. Avoiding the reconstitution would save considerable time.

Temperature restrictions

In the past all BoNT drugs had to be kept at low temperature to maintain product stability. When Xeomin was introduced, cooling of BoNT drugs became unnecessary for the first time thus improving the handling substantially. Similar product stability should also be possible with other BoNT drugs. Improved product stability could also extend the shelf life of the reconstituted drug thus improving the economics of BoNT therapy.

Shorter duration of action

There are situations where it would be helpful to have a therapeutic effect lasting only a short period of time. This might be the case, for example, when BoNT is used ro allow a fracture to set. Botulinum toxin type F had a shorter duration of action in the few clinical trials in which it was studied (Ludlow *et al.*, 1992). However, it has not been developed commercially.

Longer duration of action

For most of the current indications, BoNT has to be reinjected after approximately 3 months. Once the optimal injection scheme for an individual patient has emerged in the course of the treatment, BoNT drugs with a prolonged duration of action would reduce the number of injection series and thus the costs of the treatment and the discomfort for the patient. It is not clear how this would be accomplished with BoNT, but alternate toxins, like doxorubicin (Wirtschafter & McLoon, 1998) or an immunotoxin (Hott *et al.*, 1998) might be developed further for this purpose.

Rapid onset of action

The therapeutic effect of BoNT typically takes several days to begin and a week or more to reach its maximum. A more immediate onset of action would reduce the time of suboptimal therapeutic effect for the patient and would enable the physician to monitor the BoNT effect more readily thus avoiding repeated office visits of the patient. A rapid onset of action would also be advantageous when post operative paresis is used to improve healing.

BoNT antagonists

Botulinum toxin diffusion may cause adverse effects on muscles adjacent to the target muscle. This might be prevented by protecting neighboring muscles with previous injections of BoNT antagonists. Additionally, antagonists may be used to reverse excessive weakness in target muscles or to correct the effects of misplaced BoNT without the necessity to wait for spontaneous remissions.

Conclusion

Botulinum toxin drugs are not at the end of their development cycle, but rather at their beginning. Currently available BoNT drugs are safe and effective. However, they should be subject to a continuous development process.

REFERENCES

Dressler, D. & Benecke, R. (2003). Autonomic side effects of botulinum toxin type B treatment of cervical dystonia and hyperhidrosis. *Eur Neurol*, **49**, 34–8.

Dressler, D. & Bigalke, H. (2004). Antibody-induced failure of botulinum toxin type B therapy in de novo patients. *Eur Neurol*, **52**, 132–5.

Dressler, D. & Dirnberger, G. (2000). Botulinum toxin therapy: risk factors for therapy failure. *Mov Disord*, **15**(Suppl 2), 51.

Dressler, D. & Hallett, M. (2006). Immunological aspects of Botox, Dysport, and Myobloc/NeuroBloc. *Eur J Neurol*, **13**(Suppl 1), 11–15.

Hott, J. S., Dalakas, M. C., Sung, C., Hallett, M. & Youle, R. J. (1998). Skeletal muscle-specific immunotoxin for the treatment of focal muscle spasm. *Neurology*, **50**, 485–91.

Jankovic, J., Vuong, K. D. & Ahsan, J. (2003). Comparison of efficacy and immunogenicity of original versus current botulinum toxin in cervical dystonia. *Neurology*, **60**, 1186–8.

Lee, J. C., Yokota, K., Arimitsu, H., *et al.* (2005). Production of anti-neurotoxin antibody is enhanced by two subcomponents, HA1 and HA3b, of Clostridium botulinum type B 16S toxin-haemagglutinin. *Microbiology*, **151**, 3739–47.

Ludlow, C. L., Hallett, M., Rhew, K., *et al.* (1992). Therapeutic use of type F botulinum toxin. *N Engl J Med*, **326**, 349–50.

Moore, P. & Naumann, M. (2003). *Handbook of Botulinum Toxin Treatment*, 2nd edn. Malden, MA, USA: Blackwell Science.

Scott, A. B. (1980). Botulinum toxin injection into extraocular muscles as an alternative to strabismus surgery. *J Pediatr Ophthalmol Strabismus*, **17**, 21–5.

Wirtschafter, J. D. & McLoon, L. K. (1998). Long-term efficacy of local doxorubicin chemomyectomy in patients with blepharospasm and hemifacial spasm. *Ophthalmology*, **105**, 342–6.

Index

abductor hallucis (AH) 185, 186
abductor pollicis brevis 105
abductor pollicis longus (APL) 71, 72
abductor spasmodic dysphonia (ABSD) 85, 90
   BoNT doses 89–90
   injection technique 89
acetylcholine 6, 14, 153, 190
achalasia 143–5
adductor pollicis 105
adductor spasmodic dysphonia (ADSD) 85–9
   BoNT doses 89, 90
   injection techniques 86–7, 88
   muscles injected 85–6
adductor (of hip) spasms 110
adverse effects 19–20
aging, facial
   BoNT therapy 135–40
   pathophysiology 133
   see also cosmetic uses
Allergan Inc. 10
aluminum chloride salts, topical 123–4
aminoglycoside antibiotics 19
amputees, phantom limb pain 171
amyotrophic lateral sclerosis 19
anal fissure, chronic (CAF) 149–50
anal sphincter, internal (IAS) 149–50, 151
ankle joint pain 171
antagonists, botulinum toxin (BoNT) 208
anterocollis 29, 37
   muscles involved 33, 36, 38
anti-botulinum toxin antibodies (BoNT-AB) 23
   detection and quantification 23–4
   production 24–5
   see also antigenicity
antibody-induced therapy failure (ABTF) 17, 23, 205–6
   dose injected and 26, 27

   prevention strategies 205–6
anticholinergic drugs 124, 153
antigenicity 17–19, 25–7, 205–6
apraxia of eyelid opening 49, 50
arthritis 171
ataxia 115
athetosis 115
Autenrieth, Johann Heinrich Ferdinand 2
autonomic adverse effects 20
axillary hyperhidrosis (primary) 123
   BoNT injection technique 127–9
   BoNT therapy 125–6, 126–7
   conventional treatments 123–4, 124–5
   treatment algorithm 125

"Bacillus botulinus" 5, 6
back muscles *see* paraspinal muscles
back pain 161, 164
batch 11/79 10
benign prostatic hyperplasia (BPH) 156–7
biceps 107
biological activity 16–17
   specific (SBA) 19, 206
biological weapons 6–7
bladder, overactive 153–5
blepharospasm 49–51, 77
   BoNT treatment techniques 50–1
   clinical features and pathophysiology 49
   differential diagnosis 43
   history of BoNT therapy 10
   muscles involved 49–50
BoNT *see* botulinum neurotoxin; botulinum toxin
booster injections 205
Botox® 16
   conversion factors 16–17
   development 10, 11, 205, 206